Routledge Revivals

Rest, Suggestion

Rest, Suggestion
And other Therapeutic Measures in Nervous and Mental Diseases

Second Edition

by
Francis X. Dercum

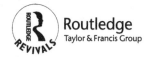

Routledge
Taylor & Francis Group

First published in 1917 by P. Blakiston's Son & Co.

This edition first published in 2019 by Routledge
2 Park Square, Milton Park, Abingdon, Oxon, OX14 4RN
and by Routledge
52 Vanderbilt Avenue, New York, NY 10017

Routledge is an imprint of the Taylor & Francis Group, an informa business

© 1917 by Taylor & Francis

Publisher's Note
The publisher has gone to great lengths to ensure the quality of this reprint but points out that some imperfections in the original copies may be apparent.

Disclaimer
The publisher has made every effort to trace copyright holders and welcomes correspondence from those they have been unable to contact.
A Library of Congress record exists under ISBN:

ISBN 13: 978-0-367-24638-9 (hbk)
ISBN 13: 978-0-367-24642-6 (pbk)
ISBN 13: 978-0-429-28363-5 (ebk)

REST, SUGGESTION

AND OTHER

THERAPEUTIC MEASURES

IN

NERVOUS AND MENTAL DISEASES

DERCUM

REST, SUGGESTION

AND OTHER

THERAPEUTIC MEASURES

IN

NERVOUS AND MENTAL DISEASES

BY

FRANCIS X. DERCUM, A. M., M. D., PH. D.

Professor of Nervous and Mental Diseases in the Jefferson Medical College, Philadelphia; Ex-President of the American Neurological Association, of the Philadelphia Neurological Society and of the Philadelphia Psychiatric Society; Foreign Corresponding Member of the Neurological Society of Paris, Corresponding member of the Psychiatric and Neurological Society of Vienna, Member of the Royal Medical Society of Budapest; Consulting Neurologist to the Philadelphia General Hospital, etc.

SECOND EDITION

PHILADELPHIA
P. BLAKISTON'S SON & CO.
1012 WALNUT STREET

THE MAPLE PRESS YORK PA

PREFACE

The within volume was originally written by the author for the System of Physiologic Therapeutics edited by Dr. S. Solis-Cohen and in which system it appeared as Volume VIII. The present edition has been largely rewritten and revised. Such modifications and additions have been made as the advance in our knowledge has made desirable. As before, emphasis has been laid upon simple physiologic methods of treatment; such as, rest, feeding and psychotherapy. In order that the principles underlying the application of these methods should be clearly appreciated, the author has unfolded, in as systematic a manner as possible, the problems presented by the exercise of function, rest and the various fatigue states. As before he has adopted a purely clinical interpretation of the neuroses, a clear comprehension of which is an indispensable preliminary to intelligent and successful treatment. Attention is particularly called to the interpretation of simple neurasthenia as a fatigue neurosis and to the important distinction existing between the latter and psychasthenia; also, to the lines of differentiation that must be drawn between both of these affections and hysteria and hypochondria; and, finally, to the undeniable claims of both of the latter to independent positions in our nosology.

Throughout, in discussing the treatment of nervous and mental diseases, the author has, to repeat, laid stress upon physiologic measures. He has, however, described in detail and, when necessary, has emphasized, purely medical treatment; as, for example, in the sections on tabes and paresis. In every instance, due consideration has been given to medicines, but, on the whole, these have been assigned a secondary importance.

In the third part of the volume the author has presented the subject of psychotherapy under the general caption of suggestion. Here the object has been to separate the chaff from the wheat. Under "normal suggestion" the great value of psychotherapy has

v

been pointed out and its methods described. In addition a full consideration has been given—and, whenever practicable, a historical résumé—of other and special methods; *e.g.*, of hypnotism, catharsis, psychanalysis, metallotherapy, mind cure, faith cure, Christian Science and mystic and religious methods generally. In each instance, the procedure in question has been submitted to a critical analysis and the inevitable conclusions clearly stated. The aim has been to give the special forms of psychotherapy their true value and to divest the subject of the mysticism in which it has become enshrouded.

In embracing physiologic methods, medicines and psychotherapy in one volume, the author has endeavored to present a comprehensive discussion of the treatment of nervous and mental disorders; especially of those which are functional in character. In how far he has succeeded, must be left to the indulgent consideration of the reader.

F. X. D.

TABLE OF CONTENTS

PART I.—REST

CHAPTER I

FUNCTION AND ITS RESULTS

CHAPTER V

HYPOCHONDRIA

CHAPTER VI

THE APPLICATION OF REST IN CHOREA AND OTHER FUNCTIONAL NERVOUS DISEASES; AND IN ORGANIC NERVOUS DISEASES

PART II.—THERAPEUTICS OF MENTAL DISEASES

CHAPTER I

THE PREVENTION OF INSANITY AND THE GENERAL PRINCIPLES OF THE TREATMENT OF THE INSANE

CHAPTER II

THE TREATMENT OF THE SPECIAL FORMS OF MENTAL DISEASE

PART III.—SUGGESTION

CHAPTER I

NORMAL SUGGESTION

CHAPTER II

SUGGESTION BY MYSTIC AND RELIGIOUS METHODS; SUGGESTION UNDER ARTIFICIALLY INDUCED HYSTERIA—HYPNOTISM; PSYCHANALYSIS

PART I
REST

REST, MENTAL THERAPEUTICS, SUGGESTION

PART I.—REST

CHAPTER I

FUNCTION AND ITS RESULTS

Chemical, Morphologic, and Physical Changes in Functionating Organs and Tissues; Exercise Involves Loss of Substance; Reconstitution by Rest. Physiologic Function of Waste Products; Toxic Action of Waste Products.

In order that we may appreciate fully what is implied by **rest**, it is necessary to consider briefly some of the general facts relating to normal function. Among the various organs of the body, the exercise of function implies varying degrees of activity. There are organs, such as the bones, in which the part played is purely passive, and others, such as the muscles, in which the part played is extremely active. The exercise of function implies a **nutritive change**—a change which is marked in direct proportion to the degree of the activity. Even the bones have been demonstrated to undergo a change, though that change is very gradual and is to be observed only after such lapse of years as marks the transition from one period of life to another. The same is true of cartilage, tendons, ligaments, and other connective-tissue structures. It is, however, in the muscles, the nervous system, the digestive apparatus, the blood, the blood-making organs, and the various glands (both those of internal and those of external secretion) that this fact of change finds its highest expression.

3

Tissue-changes of Function

The change that accompanies the exercise of function may be chemical, morphologic, or physical; as a rule it partakes of all these qualities in varying degree. The most convenient illustration that can be presented, is that offered by the **muscles.** These during functional activity undergo, first, striking **chemical** changes: Thus the chemical reaction, which is neutral or feebly alkaline in a muscle at rest, becomes acid, through the production of phosphoric acid, in a muscle that is active; there is also in the active state a greatly increased elimination of carbon dioxid while the tissue consumes proportionately more oxygen; further, the active muscle contains more water, it yields an augmented quantity of extractives soluble in alcohol, a lessened quantity of extractives soluble in water, a lessened quantity of substances producing carbon dioxid, a lessened quantity of fatty acids and of kreatin and kreatinin, and a lessened quantity of glycogen. Secondly, **morphologic** changes are manifested. The muscle-fiber during activity presents striking alterations under the microscope; the fiber becomes thicker, the transverse striæ approximate each other, and the doubly and singly refractive media of which the fiber is composed exhibit striking differences from the condition observed when at rest. Thirdly, the **muscle as a whole** changes its shape and becomes harder and more resistant. Finally, its **circulatory relations** are modified: its capillaries dilate, it contains more blood, and the blood in its veins differs chemically from that found in its veins when at rest. Certainly no argument is needed to show, at least so far as the muscles are concerned, that the condition of functional activity differs radically from that of rest. Indeed, so great is the contrast in the attending phenomena that function may well be described as the antithesis of rest. This fact, which is so evident as to muscles, is probably equally true as to other tissues, though our knowledge of the details is unfortunately much more meager.

Thus **nerve-substance,** like muscle, when at rest is neutral or feebly alkaline, and when active, is acid. It has not, however, been possible to determine the chemical changes in detail. Not even the exchange of oxygen and carbon dioxid has been demonstrated, though the facts attending vascular supply and temporary obstruction justify the inference that such changes of necessity take place. The effect of temporary compression of the vessels of the brain or of the abdominal aorta in producing arrest of function—of the brain, on the one hand, or of the cord, on the other—is an instance in point. Further, the presence of substances that are the products of retrogressive metamorphosis can have but one meaning. In addition, a number of observers have demonstrated that nerve-cells at rest and in activity present marked differences histologically. Thus, Hodge, Vas, Nissl, Mann, Lugaro, and others have studied the **changes in nerve-cells** that result from function. While the various investigators differ somewhat as to details, they agree as to the essential facts. They have discovered that during rest the chromatic substance in the cells increases in amount, and that during functional activity it is diminished. Activity of the nerve-cell is first accompanied by swelling of the protoplasm of the cell-body, later by a progressive diminution in the size of the cell-body. If functional activity be prolonged, the nucleus undergoes changes similar to those of the cell-body, and this is true of the nucleoli; there is at first an increase in volume, which subsequently gives way to the reducing action of fatigue.

As regards the changes observed in other structures than nerves and muscles, it may be stated as a general fact that **all organs** in which periods of rest alternate with periods of activity, present striking differences, chemical and morphologic, corresponding with these periods. The behavior of the **salivary glands** or of the glands of the **stomach** needs only to be alluded to in this connection. In structures in which function is not periodic, no contrasts of state can of course be found, but the great truth of change, chemical and structural, accompanying functional activity either can be demonstrated or is a matter of logical inference. Again, even in the case of such organs as the **blood-making structures** and the **glands** of **internal secretion,** it is extremely probable that the same degree of activity is neither steadily nor always maintained, and that these organs likewise have periods of maximal and of minimal function.

The changes, chemical and morphologic, taking place in muscles and nerve-cells during the exercise of function indicate a consumption of tissue—a consumption which depends directly upon increased oxidation. In other words, the evolution of energy is the result of increased oxidation. To the physician this physiologic truism becomes of greater significance when restated as follows: **the expenditure of energy means loss of substance.** As opposed to this, **rest,** functional inactivity, is accompanied by the reconstruction of tissue—by the **restitution of substance.** This fact acquires additional force when we reflect that the restitution of substance is really the storing up of energy in a latent form. It is clear, finally, that in order to preserve the physiologic condition known as health, there must be a due proportion between functional activity and rest.

Action of Waste Products

Another factor now presents itself, and that is the rôle played by the products of normal **tissue waste.** It is extremely probable that waste products circulating in the blood in normal amount are not toxic in their action, and in reality exercise an important and beneficial function in the economy. In order to obtain an idea as to the action of such substances, we need but allude to the following experiment: It is well known to physiologists that if a frog muscle which has been completely exhausted by electric stimulation and refuses any longer to respond, is washed out by injecting into its artery ordinary salt solution, the muscle again reacts to the electric current, almost as well as before. Evidently the action of the waste products restrains or inhibits the muscular contraction; and the question arises, May it not be that this is one of nature's methods of preventing undue or excessive fatigue? If it be true that the action of the muscles is inhibited by the waste products resulting from functional activity, this is probably also true of the rôle played by waste products in other organs, more especially in the nerve-centers. Indeed, the probable physiologic action of waste products present in normal amount is to induce rest by retarding activity. Considered in this light the various **fatigue substances** normally thrown into the circulation act as **sedatives** upon the nerve-centers and are among the direct causes of rest and of sleep.   Fatigue is as much an effect of the presence of waste substances as it is of the consumption of tissue.

Excessive exercise of function leads primarily to the excessive consumption of tissue.   Under these circumstances the waste substances thrown into the circulation are present in abnormal amount, and instead of a sedative or retarding influence, exert a toxic action. They no longer act as gentle restrainers of function, as preventives of unphysiologic waste, but as poisons.   In all probability their effect upon the nerve-centers is now that of irritants and excitants, and instead of inducing rest, they disturb or prevent it. Here we have, I believe, the explanation of the nervousness and the irritability of exhausted states and of the insomnia of overfatigue. Moreover, it is extremely probable that excess of function, if persisted in, leads eventually to a perversion of the chemical changes that accompany normal function; and thus arises an additional element of toxicity.   That tissue metabolism is actually deranged in neurasthenia, we shall presently see.

Permanent Structural Changes from Excessive Function

Persistent excess of function leads inevitably to morbid organic changes.   These changes result from two causes: first, the direct effect of the excessive function upon the organ concerned; and, second, the toxic action of waste substances present in abnormal amount or changed in character.   The reaction of nutrition which follows the excessive exercise of function leads at first to hypertrophy; but when certain limits have been passed, hypertrophy is followed by atrophy, by structural weakness, and by degenerative changes.   The ordinary course of hypertrophy and subsequent atrophy in an overused muscle is a case in point: the dilatation, thinning, and weakening of the cardiac walls following a cardiac hypertrophy is another.   The second cause, the toxic action of the waste substances, leads to degenerative changes in the circulatory apparatus, and possibly also in certain glandular structures, especially the kidneys.   In other words, we have here an important factor in the etiology of arterial sclerosis and probably also of some forms of chronic nephritis.   At any rate, the relation which overwork and overstrain bear to degenerative changes in the blood-vessels and kidneys is well known. Finally, instead of being eliminated, waste substances may be deposited in the tissues, and we have here an explanation of some of the vague aches and pains from which neurasthenic patients suffer, and also of the uric acid, alloxuric or gouty diathesis, so commonly met with among them.

CHAPTER II

CHRONIC FATIGUE: THE FATIGUE NEUROSIS

Primary or Essential Symptoms; Secondary or Adventitious Symptoms. Motor, Sensory, Psychic, and Visceral Phenomena.

In order that we may fully appreciate the **principles** upon which **rest** is to be applied as a therapeutic measure, it will be necessary for us to consider in detail the symptoms of **chronic fatigue.** As previously stated, the exercise of function is synonymous with the expenditure of energy and the consumption of tissue; it is evident, therefore, that the means of reconstruction of tissue is to be sought for in rest and in food. Nature determines these factors for herself when the consumption of tissue has been physiologic. It is otherwise when the consumption of tissue has been abnormal. In the demands that modern civilization makes upon the individual, the undue expenditure of energy that results in overfatigue is of frequent occurrence. As a result, a condition is established in which neither physiologic rest nor food suffice any longer to restore the organism to the equilibrium observed in health. Gradually a well-defined neurosis with a definite symptomatology becomes established, and this is widely known among the laity as "nervous prostration" and among physicians as **neurasthenia.** Its symptomatology is essentially the symptomatology of chronic fatigue. So evidently is this the case that the affection well deserves the name of **the fatigue neurosis,** which I have on various occasions applied to it. There is no subject which is of greater practical importance and which at the same time is more neglected. One of the first statements that a patient suffering from this affection makes, is that he becomes tired much more readily than formerly. Often the slightest effort, whether this effort be physical or mental, results in exhaustion. Usually the feeling of exhaustion is general, but frequently it is referred to a certain part of the body, such as the head or back; at other times it is referred to the arms or

9

legs.   The patient also complains of various aches which suggest
closely the achings observed in normal fatigue.   In addition, there
are digestive and circulatory disturbances, all of them characteristic of impaired nervous energy.   Very frequently, too, symptoms
are observed which do not appear at first sight to be indicative of
fatigue; thus, the patient may complain of dizziness, throbbing in
the head or vibratory sensations in the limbs, or of tinnitus or other
strange sensations.

Grouping of Symptoms

As I have elsewhere pointed out, the symptoms of neurasthenia
resolve themselves into two great groups: First, those which belong essentially to the affection and which always present the
phenomena of chronic fatigue; secondly, those which are adventitious or secondary outgrowths of various disturbances of function,
themselves symptomatic of fatigue.   The first, I have termed
primary or **essential** symptoms, and the latter, **secondary** or **adventitious** symptoms.   Viewed in this light, the symptomatology
of neurasthenia becomes clear and readily comprehensible.   The
primary or essential symptoms manifest themselves as weakness
and irritability of various functions, whether these be motor,
sensory, psychic, or visceral.   Thus, the patient almost invariably
complains of **muscular weakness,** which in the majority of cases
can readily be demonstrated to be real.   When tested by the dynamometer, it is usually found that the grip is weak.   Occasionally,
however, the grip at first seems to be normal, but if the patient
be made to repeat the test a number of times in succession, we find
that the grip rapidly grows weaker.   In other words, we can easily
establish the symptom of ready exhaustion.   The various statements which the patient makes are in keeping with this finding.
He will state, for instance, that slight efforts at walking induce
great fatigue, or that slight muscular exercise of any kind rapidly
exhausts him.   Most frequently the weakness is referred to the
legs and back, but occasionally it is referred to the arms.   Decided
local weakness in one arm or one leg is occasionally complained of,
and is then usually due to some peculiarity of occupation.   However, if local weakness be decided, we should at once suspect organic

disease, hysteria, or an occupation neurosis. The weakness of neurasthenia is always more or less general, and this fact cannot be too strongly insisted upon. We should also remember that paralysis never occurs in neurasthenia.

Associated with the symptoms of general muscular weakness we not infrequently find muscular tremor. It is a rather fine intention tremor, and may be elicited by having the patient extend his hands and fingers. While usually limited to the hands, it may be widely diffused over the muscles of the limbs and trunk. At times, too, spasmodic and irregularly recurring contractions of small bundles of fibers, either in the trunk muscles or in those of the face and extremities, are observed. Thus, slight spasms or twitchings are occasionally seen in the orbicularis palpebrarum, in the fibers of the frontalis, and elsewhere about the face. Occasionally twitching may also be noted in the muscles of the extremities, more particularly in those of the calf. Sometimes a spasm or cramp of the calf muscles occurs at night just after the patient has gone to bed, perhaps during the night or just as he awakens in the morning. These symptoms differ widely from those met with in actual organic disease. The muscular twitchings, for instance, are very slight and evanescent and totally unlike the fascicular or fibrillary tremors met with in certain forms of muscular atrophy, e.g., in chronic poliomyelitis.

The muscular weakness observed in neurasthenics is evidently a primary symptom—one that is characteristic of fatigue—while the tremor and muscular twitching now and then observed are to be regarded as adventitious or secondary symptoms; i.e., they are indirect outgrowths of the fatigue.

When we examine the knee-jerks of neurasthenic subjects, we find that in the majority of cases they are decidedly exaggerated. Exaggerated tendon reaction is also noted elsewhere; thus, in the tendons of the triceps and of the biceps and in the various tendons of the wrists. Often, a disappearing ankle clonus may be present. Evidently the exaggerated tendon reactions met with in neurasthenia are to be regarded as primary symptoms. They are the phenomena of motor irritability associated with motor weakness; irritability and weakness always being associated in neurasthenia.

It should be added, however, that in some cases we find that the tendon reactions, though exaggerated, become rapidly less pronounced when the attempt is made to elicit them repeatedly in rapid succession.   In other cases, again, the knee-jerk is found to be normal or even less than normal—this diminution of activity doubtless being due to a decided lowering of the general muscular tone. Even absence of knee-jerk is met with by the ordinary test, but in such case we find that it can readily be elicited by Jendrassik's method of reinforcement.   However, should the knee-jerk after repeated effort at reinforcement remain absent, other symptoms pointing to actual organic disease of the cord or other portions of the central nervous system, should be sought for.   It should also be added that the tendon reaction in nervous prostration varies at different times.   Thus, it is markedly increased by excitement. Increased irritability of the muscles to percussion may also be observed, and in rare instances, light tapping even of the nerve-trunks will produce slight contractions of the muscles which they supply.

In addition to the muscular and tendon phenomena presented, the patient complains of various **abnormal sensations**.   These range from vague generalized feelings, often incapable of description, to others which are definite in character and localized in certain portions of the body.   Usually the complaint will be merely of a general feeling of fatigue or of a sense of more or less marked exhaustion.   Not infrequently this feeling is obscured by special symptoms to which the patient gives prominence.   For instance, he may complain of lightness, of a sense of constriction or of pressure in the head.   At other times he may complain that his head, his arms or legs feel heavy and that he must make a special effort to move them.   Sensations of pressure or constriction may also be referred to certain portions of the trunk or to the limbs, though they are not common in these situations.

By other patients, a feeling of **uncertainty in moving about** is complained of.   Sometimes they complain of being giddy, but actual, *i.e.*, objective, vertigo is rarely, if ever, observed.   The giddiness appears to be due to lessened vasomotor control of the cerebral vessels, so that slight motion or change of posture influence the intracranial circulation. Rarely the sense of uncertainty is so great that the patient grasps at surrounding objects when in reality there is no danger of falling. True staggering and incoördination of movement are rarely observed and being due to weakness they are merely transitory symptoms and not persistent as in organic disease. Dizziness may, however, be very pronounced and continuous and in such case is a very distressing symptom. It may be excited by mental or physical effort, such as reading and writing, by such slight causes as motion in bed or the taking of food.

The generalized sense of fatigue is to be regarded as a primary or essential symptom, while the lightness of the head, the various constricting sensations, and the giddiness, are to be looked upon as secondary or adventitious phenomena—not in themselves essential constituents of neurasthenia, and not always present. It need hardly be added that when true, that is, objective vertigo, is met with in a given case, the latter is not one of neurasthenia and the explanation of the vertigo is to be sought in organic intracranial disease, in disease of the ear, of the ocular apparatus or of some one of the viscera; perhaps in some toxemia.

In addition to these primary and secondary symptoms, the patients complain of various pains which affect the head, the back, or the limbs. They are described generally as dull and diffuse pains or aches which in the severer forms suggest the sensations of simple fatigue; and it is extremely probable that even when they are most pronounced, they are merely exaggerated fatigue sensations. Headache is one of the most common of these symptoms. When present in the milder degree, it is described simply as a dull feeling or dull aching. As a rule, it is not diffused over the entire head, but is referred to the occiput and the upper part of the back of the neck or to the brow, just above the eyes. Occipital headache is, however, by far the most frequent form of headache met with in neurasthenia. Very commonly this occipital headache is associated with a sense of pressure, or even with a feeling of constriction passing around the entire base of the cranium. The headache of neurasthenics, when mild, usually disappears upon the mere cessation of work. When pronounced, however, it may be-

come very persistent and may not be relieved save by prolonged
rest in bed.   Care should, of course, be exercised in regard to persistent forms of headache, to differentiate closely the headaches of
neurasthenia from those due to special causes, such as eye-strain.
Migraine, which not infrequently complicates neurasthenia, is
recognized by the facts that it occurs in paroxysms, that it affects
merely one side of the head, and that it is associated with disturbances of the sympathetic nervous system—such as flushing or
pallor of the affected side, contraction or dilatation of the pupil;
as also by the occurrence of various prodromal symptoms.

Next in frequency to headache, **backache** is complained of.   It
is most commonly referred to the small of the back, though occasionally to the mid-scapular region or to the sacrum.   It is typically
a fatigue sensation, dull and diffuse in character, and varies greatly
in degree.   It is sometimes relieved by lying down and resting.
Frequently it is severe and continuous.   It is brought on or made
worse by exertion.

Instead of or together with backache, there may be aching in
one or more limbs.   Like the headache and backache, this **limbache** is dull and diffuse.   Frequently it bears a direct relation to
the occupation of the patient.   Thus, in a collector, who was in the
habit of walking great distances daily, the fatigue sensations were
most pronounced in the legs.   In a physician who used his right
hand for many hours daily in laryngeal manipulations, the fatigue
sensation was accentuated in the right arm.   In another instance,
a young woman who stood behind a counter for many hours daily
developed an aching in the legs, and for a long time this symptom
was so pronounced as to be the most prominent feature of her case.
I have met with several cases in which aching in the arms, most
painful and persistent in character, developed as a result of excessive piano practice.   Not infrequently the aching is accentuated in,
or limited to, one arm, and in such cases error in diagnosis is not
infrequently made.   Occasionally the distress is referred to a joint
or, more accurately speaking, to the neighborhood of a joint, and
in such instances care should be taken that pain be not mistaken
for rheumatism, organic disease, or hysteria.   I recall the case of a
young man who presented himself with a persistent aching in the

right wrist. Examination failed to elicit increased pain on motion or other evidence of joint affection. Evidences of hysteria were also wanting, but the general examination of the patient elicited various symptoms of neurasthenia. Finally it was learned that his occupation was that of a pocketbook-maker, and that he used his right hand and wrist all day long in folding small pieces of leather. The absence of muscle weakness and muscle spasm, as well as the subsequent history of the case, eliminated a possible occupation neurosis and proved that the pain was a fatigue sensation. Sometimes associated with the backache or limbache there is a feeling of tremor, of fine thrill or vibration which pervades the spine, the back, the trunk, or one or more limbs, as the case may be. Sometimes it seems deep-seated, and at times, when situated in a limb, it may be accompanied by a fine visible tremor. At other times when it is not evident to the eyes, a tremulous sensation may be communicated to the hand of the observer on grasping the limb. It should be added that sometimes the sensation of trembling, thrilling, or purring is present when aching is absent.

In addition to the diffuse aches and other sensations thus far described as characteristic of the fatigue neurosis, **special sensory disturbances,** painful in character, may also be met with. First among these is **spinal tenderness,** so-called spinal hyperesthesia. In many cases of neurasthenia, though by no means in all, we find that the patient flinches when we pass the finger, even though we do so lightly, over the spinous processes. The patient acts as though the spine or the skin above it were tender. Rarely this tenderness extends along the entire spine; more frequently, however, it is limited to small areas. These are found chiefly in certain situations, for example, over the seventh cervical vertebra, over the mid-dorsal region, dorso-lumbar juncture, the sacrum, or the coccyx. The affected area is usually quite small; frequently the painful spot can be covered by the tip of the thumb. Occasionally, however, the tenderness is more widely diffused, and there may also be present spontaneous pain which seems to be deep-seated and burning in character. This spinal hyperesthesia or **spinal tenderness,** as it is termed, is clearly a secondary or adventitious symptom. Less frequently, areas of hyperesthesia are found over the back, the sides of the trunk, the front of the chest, the epigastrium, or the extremities. At times the scalp is exquisitely sensitive; at other times the face, the teeth, the gums, the nipple, or the testicle may be hyperesthetic. Frequently there is also a hypersensitiveness to pain, slight injuries causing a grossly disproportionate amount of suffering.

A subjective sense of **numbness** is also frequently present; as a rule, it is referred to a limb. Its onset is favored by cramped or fixed positions, by garters, tight sleeves, or other local constraint or pressure. Actual anesthesia is, as might be expected, never observed. Sometimes disturbances of sensibility, which are described as prickling, creeping, or velvety sensations, are present. These, together with the numbness and tremor-like sensations, are to be classified with the secondary or adventitious phenomena.

Neurasthenics present, in addition, various disturbances of the **special senses**, which are all of them indicative of fatigue. Thus, patients will complain that they are not able to read for more than a few minutes at a time because of the blurring of the letters that ensues, or because of the headache that is produced. This symptom of fatigue, induced with abnormal readiness, may be due to exhaustion of the accommodative apparatus of the eye, exhaustion of the retina, or exhaustion of the cortical centers; most frequently it is due to all of these factors combined. In addition, symptoms of irritability, such as hyperesthesia of the retina, may be present. The latter frequently leads the patient to protect his eyes against the light by the use of smoked glasses. Various anomalous symptoms may also be present, secondary or adventitious in value. Thus, patients sometimes say that everything appears misty or as though seen through a veil, that objects look dull or excessively bright, that near objects look as though far away or appear excessively small or excessively large. These curious anomalies of sensation are to be referred to the disturbed nutrition of the retina, but more especially to the disordered condition of the nerve-centers. Frequently they unduly alarm the patient.

The sense of hearing presents symptoms comparable to those presented by the sight. Patients frequently complain that they cannot hear properly; that they do not understand what is said to them; though the fatigue in this instance is probably cortical and not peripheral. Auditory hyperesthesia is more frequently met with. Neurasthenic persons are usually very sensitive to sounds; they may suffer exquisitely from noises, even when the latter are insignificant. Tinnitus is also very common and may be very distressing and persistent. The examination of the ears, it need hardly be added, yields a negative result. Both the auditory hyperesthesia and the tinnitus are adventitious symptoms. Disorders of smell and disorders of taste are also present in neurasthenia. Olfactory hyperesthesia, together with paresthesias or perversions of taste, are the more common symptoms. They need not be considered in detail here.

The **psychic disturbances** of chronic fatigue are also exceedingly interesting and significant. At the very outset we have the symptom of ready mental exhaustion—of marked diminution in the capacity for sustained intellectual effort. Just as the patient is incapable of long-continued physical effort so is he incapable of long-continued mental effort. The attempt to do mental work brings on more or less rapidly the symptoms of fatigue. A certain task may be properly begun but soon the patient experiences difficulty in keeping his attention fixed upon it. If the effort be persisted in this difficulty increases until at last, instead of clear and distinct ideas, vague and confused impressions alone are received. At the same time painful sensations are apt to arise, a sense of tension about the head, headache and even giddiness. In a well-established case of neurasthenia, the **difficulty of concentrating the attention** may be so great as to lead to an habitual state of distraction and inattention, associated with a more or less marked dislike for mental effort. It is not uncommon for a patient in this condition to declare that he is "losing his mind" or "losing his memory."

Mental fatigue is also evidenced by a number of other symptoms. For instance, ideas do not present themselves as readily or in the same spontaneous succession as in health. There is a veritable **diminution of the spontaneity** of thought. This the patient himself well recognizes for he often says "I cannot think."

In the man who is chronically overtired there is also a lessening in the strength of the will. The patient does not react as he did while in health to the normal stimuli to effort; he no longer eliminates the energy that effort requires, he lacks confidence and courage and fails of accomplishment. Associated with this state there is also **a lack of decision.** The patient is vacillating and undecided. Often he is incapable of coming to a decision regarding even trivial matters. Indecision and weakness go hand in hand.

Added to the above symptoms, we have those of a **diminished inhibition.** The most trifling causes often excite and anger the neurasthenic patient. He is irritable to a degree. He is also apt to be unusually sensitive and often feels hurt by fancied neglect or oversight on the part of relatives or friends. He experiences changes in the emotions more readily than in health. Totally inadequate causes may provoke marked depression and at other times laughter. A play at a theatre or a newspaper account of a murder may provoke him to tears. In other words, his emotional equilibrium is readily disturbed. This condition differs from the similar state observed in hysteria in that the exciting causes for the emotional changes are always such as would produce the same emotion in health, though to a less degree.

Other symptoms, secondary or adventitious in character, may also be present. Thus, there is a tendency to introspection, noticeable in a large proportion of cases; the patient is apt to dwell upon his symptoms and to be constantly alive to his illness. Quite commonly he becomes depressed and to a certain degree nosophobic. He may think because he has attacks of palpitation of the heart that he has heart disease or because he feels the throbbing of a pulsating aorta that he has some other serious affection.

Again, he may present the symptom of an unusual fear. Fear and weakness are quite closely associated, and it is not surprising that a person in a condition of chronic exhaustion should be morbidly afraid. The symptom may manifest itself in several ways. There may be present a vague generalized sense of being afraid or there may occur, without obvious exciting cause, attacks during which fear becomes, for the time being, greatly accentuated. There is under such circumstances, usually palpitation of the heart and sudden muscular weakness. The patient may sink into a chair or even to the ground. The face becomes pale, the body moist with a cold sweat, the pulse small and rapid, and the respiration hurried, and, if the attack be intense, there may be even relaxation of the sphincters, the bladder and bowels being involuntarily evacuated. Such attacks, though not common, nevertheless recur with sufficient frequency to leave no doubt as to their nature. Quite frequently, unfortunately, they are mistaken by both physicians and lay persons for hysteria. In many cases, the fear assumes a special form and manifests itself only under certain conditions. Especially is this the case if, besides being neurasthenic, the patient be also neuropathic; that is, if there be present also the elements of nervous degeneration, hereditary, congenital, or acquired. A pathologic association may under such circumstances be formed in the patient's mind, so that the emotion of fear becomes definitely linked with certain relations to the environment. Thus, a neurasthenic-neuropathic patient may have an attack of spontaneous fear while he is alone; at subsequent times the mere fact of being alone induces an attack of fear, the attack being accompanied to a greater or less degree by all of the physical signs of the emotion. A patient so afflicted becomes morbidly afraid of being alone. Similarly he may experience fear when in the presence of strangers or of crowds; or he may be attacked by fear when in his own room or when in the street. It is extremely probable also that in some cases of neurasthenia, the faculties are so weakened that the ordinary surroundings no longer give rise to a sense of security. Fear is then a natural consequence. Neurasthenic fears find, as Bouveret long ago pointed out, a fitting analogue in the fear which healthy persons experience when standing at a great height, even though they may be in a perfectly safe position.

To many of the special forms of fear, special names have been given. Thus, some neurasthenics are attacked by fear when they find themselves in open places—**agoraphobia**; in others, the fear comes on when they find themselves in narrow or closed places—**claustrophobia**; the fear of being alone is termed **monophobia**; the fear of crowds, **anthrophobia**, and so on.

Among the secondary or adventitious psychic phenomena of

neurasthenia must likewise be included the **sleep disturbances.** Insomnia is one of the most common of these. It is sometimes one of the earliest symptoms presented. It varies greatly in degree. For instance, a patient may find it difficult to fall asleep; the oncoming of sleep may be delayed many minutes or several hours; or the sleep may be very light or frequently broken, the patient spending the night in alternately falling asleep and awakening. More commonly, however, the picture of the sleep disturbance of neurasthenia is the following, especially in the beginning of the neurasthenic attack. The tired and exhausted patient falls asleep soon after going to bed but awakens at an earlier hour than usual and he finds that his sleep has not been refreshing. If the disturbance of sleep becomes more pronounced, he awakens at a still earlier hour, lies awake for a while and then falls into a heavy second sleep for an hour or two longer and finally awakens greatly depressed, heavy and exhausted. If the trouble becomes more pronounced, the hours of sleep may become progressively shorter and more and more broken until at last a few hours or a few minutes may be the sum total of an entire night of sleep. Sometimes the night becomes entirely sleepless and occasionally the patient may pass several nights and days without any sleep whatever. As a rule such sleep as is obtained is light; occasionally it is heavy and deep. It is always unrefreshing; indeed on awakening the various fatigue sensations are more pronounced than ever.

Not only are neurasthenic patients troubled with insomnia but they are frequently disturbed by **dreams.** Sometimes the dreams deal in a fragmentary way with various experiences of the day. More frequently they are of an unpleasant character. The patient dreams of murders, of terrible accidents, of being pursued by great danger and not infrequently awakens suddenly in a paroxysm of fright. Startling dreams, the nightmare, the incubus, are by no means uncommon.

The psychic phenomena of chronic fatigue form a natural symptom-group; especially is this true of the primary symptoms, ready exhaustion, lessening of spontaneity, lessening of the force of the will, indecision and diminished inhibition. If we add to these the secondary outgrowths of the exhausted state, the general and special forms of fear, the sleep disturbances and dreams, the picture becomes complete.

Just as the various motor, sensory, and psychic phenomena are indicative of chronic fatigue with its outgrowth of secondary symptoms, so also are the various **visceral disturbances**. Thus, the **digestive disturbances** of neurasthenia are primarily those of weakness. The patient having taken a moderate quantity of food feels at first no distress, but after the lapse of a longer or shorter interval of time, sensations of weight, of oppression, and of general discomfort in the epigastrium make their appearance. Quite commonly these are accompanied by distention and eructations of gas, the latter being quite tasteless. The epigastrium may be found slightly sensitive to pressure and, less frequently, pain is complained of, the latter being referred to the epigastrium and to the back between the shoulder-blades. However, if we examine the epigastrium, it is not painful as in ulcer or other organic disease, nor do we find that the stomach is dilated but simply distended. The tongue is clean or at most but slightly coated. If the gastric juice be examined, as a rule, no marked changes in the amount of pepsin or hydrochloric acid are revealed: occasionally, however, a diminution of acid is noted. Thus far the indigestion is merely functional in character. It is an **atonic indigestion,** the result of weakness, of deficient innervation. Digestion may be much delayed and the stomach may not be emptied before it is time to take the next meal. Infrequently some nausea is complained of; vomiting is quite rare.

It is a remarkable fact that the **appetite** of the neurasthenic is almost uniformly good; sometimes indeed it is **increased.** This is in direct contrast with the appetite in melancholia in which it is uniformly diminished and indeed frequently replaced by a disgust for food. This differential point is of great value, as the mental depression which accompanies neurasthenia in some cases, may superficially suggest that of melancholia. **Thirst,** on the other hand, is almost uniformly **diminished,** and neurasthenics habitually consume too little fluid. They rarely drink water between meals and usually very little at meals.

The atonic condition of the stomach is, as might be expected, shared in by the entire intestinal tract. Constipation is the rule. Sometimes there is uncomfortable abdominal distention, meteorism, expulsion of gas.

Not infrequently in atonic indigestion or nervous dyspepsia, as the laity still call it, associated symptoms make their appearance. Sometimes while the indigestion is at its height an attack of palpitation of the heart, often severe, will supervene and thus add greatly to the distress and discomfort of the patient. Again, occasionally during an attack of indigestion the patient may feel heavy and sleepy and more than ever incapable of mental or physical effort. Sometimes giddiness is present.

The digestive disturbances of neurasthenia may gradually become more pronounced and sooner or later a gastric catarrh may make its appearance. The latter must, of course, be looked upon as a secondary outgrowth. The recognition of the relation of a gastric catarrh so arising to a preëxisting and often long-enduring neurasthenic state is of the utmost practical importance.

When we turn our attention to the circulatory apparatus, we are confronted by facts of equal significance and importance. Again we meet with the symptoms of deficient innervation, of weakness and irritability. The disturbances of the circulatory apparatus consist in modifications of the force and rhythm of the heart's action, in the character and the frequency of the pulse and in more or less marked alteration of vasomotor tone. The circulation as a whole is impaired. The patient quite usually presents coldness of the extremities; sometimes lividity is noted. The pulse is commonly soft, rather small and readily compressible, while the blood-pressure is usually quite low. Further, the pulse rate is almost invariably increased and ranges from ninety to a hundred and more. Slight excitement, such as the visit to the physician's office, will sometimes markedly increase its rate. Often the patient will state that he is easily upset and disturbed and that at such times his heart will beat much faster. At other times marked attacks of palpitation of the heart supervene. Indeed such attacks are at times striking features of the affection. As already pointed out it may be associated with digestive disturbances and in such case it usually occurs at that period of digestion when the process seems to have been slowed or arrested and when marked gaseous distention of the stomach has taken place. At other times it occurs spontaneously or as a result of emotional disturbances. During the attack the heart beats violently and with increased rapidity against the chest-wall and there may be marked throbbing of the arteries. Often the patient complains of oppression of breathing, his face is pale, the expression anxious and distressed and very frequently he suffers markedly from fear. If the attack be very severe, he may complain of precordial pain, may be very restless and agitated and may be so frightened as to believe that he is about to die. During the attack the pulse rate rises to 120, 130 or more, but after an interval usually of a few minutes, it falls again, and the patient gradually becomes quieted and relieved.

The average neurasthenic patient presents, as already pointed out, coldness and occasionally lividity of the extremities. At times there are special symptoms present, also indicative of loss of vasomotor tone. Thus, there may be aortic pulsation. The 'patient feels a deep-seated throbbing in the epigastrium and this can readily be verified by the hand of the physician. At times, the throbbing pervades the limbs, the head, or the body generally and may be very persistent and distressing.

When we turn our attention to other organs and functions, we note everywhere symptoms indicative of **deficient innervation.** Thus, the hands of the patient are frequently damp and moist. In addition they are as already stated frequently cold. The amount of moisture may be so great that the patient actually wets or soils objects which he touches. Again, the patient may **sweat** freely upon slight physical exertion, upon slight emotional excitement or mental effort. Thus many neurasthenics on attempting to write and sometimes to read find that the head and neck become moist with perspiration. Again, in some patients sweating occurs only or is especially marked when they lie down or during the relaxation of sleep. Sometimes this is a marked feature at night.

Occasionally, and this is an adventitious symptom, the perspiration is changed in character and becomes unpleasant in odor; this is more especially the case when the sweating occurs in the axillæ or groins.

In other neurasthenics again there is a marked diminution of the perspiration and of the secretions generally. As already pointed out many patients suffer from a deficient thirst and a consequent insufficient ingestion of liquids. In keeping with this fact there is in such cases an unusual dryness of the skin, a deficient secretion of **saliva**, an abnormal dryness of the mouth, together with a diminution of the secretions of the gastro-intestinal tract generally. There is also a diminution in the quantity of **urine**. Further, at times there is an unusual dryness of the joints so that when the fingers or joints are forcibly moved "cracking" sounds are produced. Occasionally such sounds are noted in the back of the neck on suddenly rotating the head and are in such instances to be referred to joints of the articular processes. Another and sometimes very annoying symptom is "cracking" in the maxillary joint occurring during mastication.

Other symptoms both primary and adventitious may be presented by the **sexual apparatus**. Like the other symptoms of nervous exhaustion, they are expressive of weakness and irritability. While more commonly noted in male subjects they are also occasionally noted in women. In the former they relate to loss of power, premature or delayed emission, diminution or absence of the physiological sensations, indifference. In women, lack of response, delayed, diminished or absent orgasm, indifference. Their detailed consideration need not delay us here.

Because of the varied character and large number of the symptoms, it is sometimes declared that in neurasthenia we have not a single affection to deal with but in reality a great variety of diseases. However, it is clear that in their essentials all the symptoms are the same. They are all of them expressive of the two cardinal facts which affect the nervous system, namely, weakness and irritability and they more than justify the term the "fatigue neurosis." It is the application of the principle of rest to this condition that will next occupy our attention.

CHAPTER III

REST IN NEURASTHENIA AND ALLIED STATES

Physiologic Rest. Therapeutic Rest. The General Application of Rest: Degrees of Rest; Exercise and Food. The Special Applications of Rest: Partial Rest Method—Division of Time; Bathing; Massage; Modification of Routine. Absolute Rest Method—Importance of Details; Isolation; Nursing; Adjuvants—Feeding, Bathing, Massage, Electricity, Medicines; Treatment of Special Symptoms; Return to Home. Historical Data—Whyte; Bouchut; Beard; Weir Mitchell. Rest in Neurasthenia Terminalis. Rest in the Neurasthenia of Middle Life. Rest in the Neurasthenia of Old Age. The Neurasthenoid States. Neurasthenia Symptomatica.

We have considered the changes—chemical, morphologic, and physical—that take place in **normal fatigue,** and we have seen how, in the intervals between the periods of activity, **restitution** takes place. In fatigue, for instance, there is, among other things, loss of substance, and during rest this loss is regained. The relation of rest to normal fatigue is quite clear; but this is not the case when the fatigue is pathologic, as we find it to be in neurasthenia. Here physiologic rest no longer suffices to bring about a return to the normal condition, and we are at once confronted with the problem of applying **rest as a therapeutic measure.** How and to what degree shall it be applied? As we shall presently see, rest is a powerful agent, and yet when inappropriately applied, may fail of its object.

REST AS A THERAPEUTIC MEASURE

Elimination of the Causal Factors of Chronic Fatigue

The first practical step toward a successful result in a given case is a careful study to determine the **factors at work** in producing the fatigue symptoms. If the case be one of simple and uncomplicated neurasthenia, it will generally be found that the symptoms owe their origin to some infraction of physiologic living. In the civilization of our day, no cause is more potent than **overwork** and **nervous overstrain.** In many cases, if merely so much of the strain be taken off as is in excess of the patient's strength, nature will gradually reëstablish a normal equilibrium, provided, of course, that the overstrain has not been too long continued. In searching for the cause of a neurasthenia, all of the possible etiologic elements should be inquired into, and in this connection we should remember not only overwork, but also **worry, sexual excess,** and the **abuse of stimulants.** It can readily be comprehended that rest of itself may fail to bring relief, so long as the various unphysiologic strains to which the nervous system has been subjected are not removed.

It is necessary, therefore, in order that rest shall be of benefit, that first of all the patient's **method of living** be carefully regulated and be placed as nearly as possible upon a normal plane. Under such circumstances, merely **physiologic rest**—that is to say, a normal amount of sleep and the slight general rest obtained at the intervals in the work of the waking period that are necessitated by the taking of food, together with rest in the evening—will be followed by a disappearance of the fatigue symptoms. This is true, of course, only of conditions in which the symptoms of overfatigue have not been too long established, and in which they have not become too profound.

Degrees of Rest

The foregoing remarks suggest at once that the term **rest,** in a therapeutic sense, has a very wide range of application. Indeed, the cessation of activity thus implied may be made very slight in degree or it may be made almost absolute. On the one hand, we have that slight degree of rest which is obtained by the elimination of so much of the usual work as is excessive—overwork—or by the elimination of unphysiologic strains; and, on the other hand, the profound degree of rest that is obtained by placing the patient in bed and under such rigid conditions that a minimal amount of activity either mental or physical alone is possible.

Relative Rest.—Under slight rest, it is of importance to mention that relative rest which is obtained by mere change of occupation, or by the introduction of diversity into the occupation. Change and diversity give rest to faculties that are exhausted and stimulation to others that are insufficiently used. The greater the contrast between the kinds of work, the greater is the advantage gained. For example, a man suffering from overwork of the brain is greatly benefited if a portion of his daily labor be converted into out-of-door work of such kind as necessitates physical exertion. When such a change is not possible, advantage may even be gained if the brainwork itself be modified in kind or manner; as, for instance, when dictation is substituted for writing, or when the details and drudgery of business, professional duty, or clerical tasks, are made to vary decidedly at different hours of the day. One reason why physicians maintain so large an average of general health under excessive strain, is the great variety of the labor that is incidental to their calling. Unfortunately, in our present stage of civilization, it is not often possible to institute much change in the character of the work that a given patient has to do, and "relative rest," so-called, has a very limited application.

Exercise and Food

The reader has probably inferred from what has thus far been said, that the principles of rest are closely linked with those of exercise. This is indeed true. Exercise, stimulation of function, in some form or other, even in the most rigid form of rest treatment that can be instituted, is, as we shall see, absolutely necessary. Further, if we recall that overfatigue implies loss of substance—and it should here be interpolated that neurasthenic patients are, as a rule, below weight—we also realize at once that we must attach to the principle of rest, not only the principle of exercise, but also the principle of feeding. We must supply, in addition to rest and exercise, pabulum in some form by which the exhausted tissues can be reconstituted. This principle is all-important; and it cannot be emphasized too strongly that the furnishing of the pabulum can be accomplished only by the administration of food. It is because this fact is not fully recognized that physicians often fail in their treatment of neurasthenic patients. Medicine cannot form tissue, and the various artificial foods and so-called reconstructives that are foisted upon the market have but slight, if any, tissue-building value. It is food, normal food, that is required—food so administered as to be capable of ready digestion and ready assimilation. The much-vaunted specialties of the pharmacist, the so-called nerve-foods, such as the hypophosphites of lime and soda, or the various predigested preparations of the meats and cereals, are but insignificant and feeble adjuvants in the feeding of neurasthenics; under the conditions in which we find the average neurasthenic patient, they are practically valueless. Indeed, I do not hesitate to say that there is rarely a scientific reason for using them It is food that is required—food in bulk, not teaspoonful doses of this or that preparation. The administration of food to neurasthenics often presents problems of difficulty so serious that at first sight they may seem almost insurmountable but the difficulty, no matter how great, does not justify us in losing sight of the fact that food must be administered, and not some makeshift or delusive substitute.

At the very outset, then, of our consideration of the general application of rest, we find that rest is of necessity linked with two other factors—namely, exercise and food.

THE SPECIAL APPLICATION OF REST TO NEURASTHENIA

PARTIAL REST METHODS

It so happens that for a large number of our population an elaborate treatment of neurasthenia by rest in bed for a prolonged period is impracticable, if not impossible. This is true especially of male neurasthenics who are actively engaged in business, as also of many women—mothers and housewives—whose obligations and responsibilities cannot be laid aside or whose circumstances negative the bed method of treatment. In such cases it is obviously necessary to institute a plan of treatment that will embody the general principles of rest, exercise, and food without interfering unduly with the patient's vocation. In other words, the patient is placed on a **partial rest** treatment.   General rules only can be discussed here.   The details will necessarily vary greatly in each case.

Proportion of Rest and Exercise

Let us take, to begin with, an instance in which a patient, a woman, is unable to abandon her home and children and yet is urgently in need of rest.   The physician should first acquaint himself as fully as possible with the various details of the patient's daily life.   By this means he will be able to separate the various duties of the patient into two groups—those which are or seem to be indispensable, and those which she can readily abandon. Among the first are, as a rule, duties intimately connected with housekeeping and the care of children.   Among the others are social duties, not merely participation in social functions, but also in the work of charitable and other organizations, church work, unnecessary correspondence, and the inevitable late hours that social obligations entail.   The necessity of abandoning all but the most imperative cares must be pointed out to the patient. Her consent having been gained, the next step is to increase the number of hours spent in bed.   The patient should go to bed early, say at nine o'clock, and not rise earlier than ten or eleven o'clock the next morning.   In addition, she should again retire immediately after her mid-day meal, remaining in bed for from one to two hours.   In this way from fifteen to sixteen hours, out of twenty-four, are spent in lying down, many of them in actual sleep.   A certain amount of complementary exercise must now be provided, and this exercise should be taken in the open air.   It may consist at first merely of a twenty-minute walk taken between the hours of eleven and one, or between the hours of three and five. Gradually, the amount of exercise should be increased until the patient is walking upward of an hour once, or it may be twice, daily.   In my observation, the error is frequently made of directing the patient to take too much exercise at first.   It cannot be too strongly insisted upon that the amount of exercise should in the beginning be very small.   Very little exercise will suffice, while much inevitably does harm.   Later on in the treatment, the exercise can not only be increased but elaborated at will.   An important guiding principle, however, should be borne in mind. The exercise should always stop well within the limits of the patient's strength. Especially in the early stage of the treatment, should it stop far short of fatigue. If fatigue be induced, the very object of our treatment is defeated. The neglect of this elementary principle leads not only to failure, but frequently to positive harm to the patient.

Details of Feeding

Having carefully prescribed the number and duration of the periods of rest and the extent and character of the exercise to be taken for the time being, we should next turn our attention to the question of food. From what has already been stated, the reader will realize that the amount of the food must, if possible, be large. Secondly, it must be adapted to the peculiarities of nutrition observed in neurasthenics; and, finally, inasmuch as digestion in neurasthenics is enfeebled and delayed, the food should be prepared and administered in such a way as to facilitate digestion and assimilation. Further, in very many cases, a gastric catarrh, usually slight though sometimes pronounced, complicates the neurasthenia and must also be taken into account. The quantity of nourishment that is already being taken can, as a rule, be increased by a very simple expedient. The patient is instructed to add a definite quantity of milk—say from four to six ounces—to each meal and to drink an equal quantity between meals and on going to bed; that is, she should be instructed to take a prescribed quantity of milk six times daily. The amount can gradually be increased until eight, ten, or even more ounces of milk are taken at each feeding. Neurasthenic patients frequently object to milk, asserting that it "disagrees" with them, that it coats the tongue, that it constipates them, or that it makes them flatulent. All of these difficulties can be overcome by various expedients which will be considered in detail in speaking of the treatment of neurasthenia by rest in bed (see p. 40). Suffice it to say here that the generality of patients treated by simple increase of the hours devoted to rest and by exercise in the open air can, as a rule, be brought to digest and assimilate milk readily. Having impressed upon the patient's mind the necessity of taking milk, the next point is to give some general directions with regard to the diet as a whole. Red meats—beef and lamb—are, as a rule, not suitable for neurasthenic patients. In neurasthenia, as has been pointed out, either the output of alloxuric bodies is increased or their elimination interfered with, so that a diet including meat in large quantities is contraindicated. Starchy foods and sweets are also to be avoided: first, because indirectly they favor the formation of alloxuric bodies; secondly, because they give rise to more or less marked digestive disturbances; and, thirdly, because their nutritive value is comparatively low. In regard to meats we should therefore advise the patient to take the red meats, beef and lamb, sparingly. In my experience it is not wise to withdraw them absolutely in the case of patients that are not treated by rest in bed. A certain quantity of red meat is needed, but it should not be taken at more than one meal in a day, and then only in moderation. For a similar reason, the starchy foods and sugars should not be withdrawn absolutely, but their quantity should be regulated. Potatoes and ordinary wheat bread can usually be dispensed with entirely, with advantage. Rice, in moderate quantity, will be found to be a convenient substitute for potatoes, while whole-wheat bread, pulled bread, bran bread, gluten bread, wafers, Zwieback, will be found to be exceedingly serviceable in the place of ordinary wheat bread. Fats should be avoided for a time, and the patient restricted to small quantities of butter. The white meats, fish, chicken, oysters, and the like, should be taken freely, as should also the succulent vegetables. Celery, lettuce, and water-cress, and ripe fruits, except perhaps bananas, should be added. When constipation is a feature, stewed fruits and baked apples, without much sweetening, are of service.

A diet such as that outlined will answer the purpose well in the average case; but some modifications may be necessary to meet individual requirements. We should remember that the physiologic needs of the patient call for a mixed diet, and experience shows that this yields the best result. When difficulties of digestion are marked and decided gastric complications exist, a rigid dietary should, of course, be prescribed in accordance with the indications of the special symptoms. It should not, however, be adhered to too long, lest the ultimate purpose of treatment be defeated. We should remember that liberal feeding, **feeding in excess,** is what is indicated. The diet here outlined is intended for that large number of neurasthenics who cannot resort to a bed treatment or whose condition is not so pronounced as to justify resort to more radical measures. In discussing the full bed treatment, various modifications of its plan and substance will be considered. It is important to add here that the **intervals** between the taking of food should not be too long. The strength of the patient frequently runs down in the long hours between the regular meals, and to give a small amount of food during these hours proves a very valuable expedient. Further, the plan which is now followed so commonly in American families in cities, of converting the mid-day meal into a lunch, reserving the heavy meal or dinner for a late hour of the day, and having the latter take the place of the old-fashioned supper, is decidedly unphysiologic. The mid-day meal should, so far as neurasthenics are concerned, be the most substantial meal of the day. The depression of strength, which is apt to come on in these patients in the latter part of the afternoon, in the neighborhood of four or five o'clock, can frequently be avoided by this means.

The Auxiliary Use of Medicines

The treatment of many cases of neurasthenia can be conducted from beginning to end without the use of any **medicines.** Occasionally, however, because of the atony of digestion, a few drops of the tincture of nux vomica, given before meals—alone or with a little tincture of gentian and of cardamom—will be of service. At other times if gastric catarrh be a factor, a small quantity of bismuth subnitrate can be given before meals; or if the gastric catarrh be pronounced, silver nitrate may be administered in pill form— one-fourth grain of the silver salt with one-fourth or one-half grain of extract of hyoscyamus, twenty or thirty minutes before meals. Should constipation exist, a dose of an effervescent preparation of sodium phosphate, equivalent to about a dram of the active agent, given before breakfast, will prove useful. At other times small doses of fluid extract of cascara may be used—from eight to fifteen drops three times daily after meals. It is not usually of advantage to order this remedy to be taken in one dose at bedtime; its action is most satisfactory when diffused over the twenty-four hours. It is tonic and stimulating to digestion, and after bowel movements have once been regularly established, it may gradually be diminished and finally withdrawn altogether. In regard to other medicines, let me repeat that while some are indicated from time to time, they are never more than adjuvants to the general treatment, and too much reliance should not be placed upon them. A treatment based upon tonics, drugs, and artificial foods will inevitably fail unless the general principles here indicated be applied. As a rule, these remedies do harm not so much of themselves, but because the patient, and I am sorry to say sometimes the physician, deludes himself with the belief that the taking of the medicine constitutes the essential part of the treatment; thus, the really important measures are not carried out, or possibly not even attempted.

The Elimination of Waste Products

We have now considered the application of rest with its concomitant principles of exercise and increased food. Two other points, however, remain, which demand our attention. The elimination of waste products is, as we have already pointed out, generally diminished in cases of neurasthenia. It is, therefore, of the utmost importance that this elimination be stimulated. Many of the vague aches and distressing sensations from which neurasthenic patients suffer, are due to the retention of waste products, notably uric acid and its salts, or perhaps, one should say, more generally, the alloxuric bodies. So far as possible, we should add to the plan of living, simple methods by which the elimination of these substances may be facilitated. Obviously one of the first indications is to increase the amount of liquid which the patient takes. In my personal observation this is a point which physicians too commonly neglect. Its importance becomes especially evident when we remember that neurasthenic patients suffer almost always from defective thirst, and that if left to themselves they habitually drink but little water. It is necessary not only to instruct them to drink water, but also at times to fix the quantity, usually a liberal amount, which they are to consume at stated periods daily. The various table waters may here be prescribed with advantage. The output of urine is by this means decidedly increased. The free addition of milk to the diet, in the manner previously indicated, often accomplishes the same object and renders the addition of water in large quantities less imperative. However, even under these circumstances the patient should be instructed to drink one or more glasses of water between meals.

Stimulation of the Skin.—In accordance also with these general principles, the function of the skin should be stimulated as much as possible, and this can be accomplished very readily in most cases by a liberal use of **baths** and by simple **rubbing.** We should be careful, however, not to use baths so freely as to exaggerate the general weakness and relaxation from which the patient already suffers. As a rule, the use of a simple sponge bath daily, followed by gentle friction, is all that is required. A rapid immersion bath or, if the patient's home facilities afford it, a shower bath of short duration will answer the same purpose. The **temperature** of the bath is a matter of considerable importance. As already pointed out, the circulation of neurasthenics is feeble, the extremities are apt to be cold and livid, and the result is that they do not, as a rule, react well to cold baths. As a matter of actual experience, it is found that the sponge bath taken with water as warm as the patient can bear, the bath not extending over more than eight minutes and followed by gentle but efficient rubbing, is productive of the best results. The bath should be taken in the evening shortly before retiring. At this time it aids in relieving the fatigue of the day and also quiets the patient and prepares him for sleep. In comparatively mild cases of neurasthenia cold water is well borne and followed by a healthy reaction, but in most cases the warm sponge bathing or gentle douching is preferable. The fact that the warm bath favors sleep is of great advantage when we remember that many neurasthenic patients suffer from insomnia in some form or other.

Modifications of Routine

The application of rest is, as we have seen, inseparably connected with the employment of exercise, full feeding, and bathing. I need hardly point out that any one of these adjuvants of rest is capable of very great modification, and that indeed, in special cases, decided modification of the principles here outlined is indicated. In place of the simple exercise of walking, elaborate forms of exercise may be substituted or may be added as the patient improves in strength. Horseback-riding, golf playing, or other out-of-door sports, provided they do not tax the energies of the patient excessively, may be advised from time to time; or the patient may be placed in the hands of a competent physical instructor and a certain amount of time spent in gymnasium work.

The feeding of the patient is likewise capable of great modification, as we shall presently learn in considering the full rest treatment. For instance, in cases in which a marked idiosyncrasy exists with regard to milk, raw-egg feeding may be substituted; raw eggs in a definite and increasing number being added to the daily diet of the patient. Various other modifications both as to the character and the intervals of the feeding may, of course, be employed (see p. 50). In regard to stimulants, alcohol, tobacco, tea and coffee are best withdrawn absolutely, and yet if the patient be placed under such circumstances that he cannot lessen his work, that he is burdened with imperative engagements—carries great responsibilities which must be discharged—the morning cup of coffee may often wisely be allowed, or if marked digestive disturbances exist, a cup of tea may be substituted. As a rule, however, the coffee can be withdrawn and replaced by a cup of cocoa or hot milk. In neurasthenics who are in middle or advanced life and who have been accustomed to a moderate use of stimulants, it will perhaps be wise to permit the use of a small quantity of claret or some generous red wine, such as Burgundy, at dinner. As a rule, however, neurasthenic patients are very susceptible to the ill effects of alcohol. It makes them dull and heavy and renders the discharge of their duties more difficult. On general principles, tobacco should also be withdrawn entirely; in many cases, however, especially in persons who have been smokers for many years, it may be most judicious to cut down decidedly the amount of tobacco that is being consumed but not to interdict its use absolutely.

If our patient be already so neurasthenic that sufficient exercise cannot be taken, it is a good plan to employ **massage**. Massage may in a sense be defined as a form of exercise in which the patient plays a purely passive rôle; it is an expedient which produces effects somewhat similar to exercise without necessitating the expenditure of energy on the part of the patient. It stimulates the circulation, promotes nutrition, without inducing fatigue, and it is, therefore, a most valuable expedient as an adjuvant to rest. However, in the class of neurasthenics that we are at present considering, it may be dispensed with, provided the patient is able to take sufficient exercise. It cannot by any means be regarded as the equivalent of exercise, and, other things being equal, it is distinctly inferior in its beneficial effects. It is sometimes of advantage to employ both exercise and massage in the same case at different periods of the day. At other times, again, associated with the massage, there may be given passive movements of the limbs or occasional movements with resistance. The employment of massage and the details of its application must depend largely upon the judgment of the physician. Both it and exercise may, of course, be modified, elaborated, and varied in numerous ways.

It is hardly necessary to say that the **bathing** of the patient, like the massage and exercise, may be modified in many ways. The primary effect of the application of water is, of course, to cleanse the skin, while the subsequent rubbing with the towel flushes its capillaries. Both of these factors stimulate its excretory power, a function of great importance in neurasthenia, on account of the tendency to defective elimination, already commented on. Other effects are those dependent upon the temperature of the water and the manner of its application. Warm water will dilate the vessels, cold water contract them; powerful effects can be produced by these means. Many neurasthenics are, as already stated, so feeble that a cold bath will depress them, and in such cases simple warm sponge bathing is at first preferable. Gradually, however, the bath may be reduced in temperature, and finally there may be given a rapid bath of 60° to 50°F. (15.5° to 10°C.), which at this time is followed by a prompt and valuable reaction. The arterial tension, which is especially low in neurasthenics in the early hours of the day, is by this means raised; and many of the fatigue symptoms either disappear or are lessened for the time being. Tissue metabolism is also actively promoted, for observation has shown that there results from the stimulus of the cold bath an increased consumption of oxygen and an increased elimination of carbon dioxid. Elaborate hydrotherapeutic apparatus is only infrequently at the command of the physician; but while desirable, it is not indispensable. The patient can usually bring about very satisfactory results by employing simple means at his own home. Thus, he can employ a sponge bath of suitable temperature or a rapid immersion bath may be used. Douching the trunk alternately with warm and cold water while the patient is standing in an ordinary tub is another simple expedient. A small section of garden hose with a nozzle or a sprinkler may be attached to the faucet of the bath tub and may be used as a jet bath or rain bath. Suffice it to indicate here merely the general principles which should guide the physician in the employment of water as an adjuvant to the treatment of neurasthenia by rest. Bathing, as already stated, should always be used in some form; and it may be repeated that we should begin by some simple and gentle application, such as a **warm sponge bath.** Neurasthenics are made worse by measures that irritate and annoy, so that vigorous douching or baths that are too cold may depress and exhaust the patient, especially in the early part of the treatment. Later, **douching** and **cold bathing** may be employed with good result. If there be marked dryness of the skin or persistent fatigue pains, a **dry hot-air bath** (Turkish bath) or a **hot vapor bath** (Russian bath) may be given. When obstinate insomnia exists, a **drip sheet** may prove efficient; the patient stands in a few inches of warm water, while a cold wet sheet is thrown about him; he is then vigorously rubbed with the sheet until a reaction is established. At other times, a **hot wet pack** may be useful; the patient is wrapped in a sheet wrung out of water of a temperature of 110°F.

(43.3°C.), covered with blankets, and allowed to remain in the pack for an hour. Procedures such as these, however, are generally unnecessary. As a rule, simple sponge bathing will answer the purpose from the beginning to the end of the treatment.

Cautions Necessary

We should remember that the cardinal principle in the management of neurasthenia is **rest**, and that exercise, bathing, massage, and electricity are merely adjuvants. Their relative importance is indicated by the order in which they are named. It is important, first, that the patient who is resting should also exercise; next, that elimination and the circulation be stimulated by bathing. If these measures prove insufficient, massage, and later, electricity, may be employed. In the class of cases which we are at present considering—that is, the neurasthenics who are to some extent pursuing their ordinary vocations—electricity can generally be dispensed with. Further, we should bear in mind that the simultaneous employment of every one of the adjuvants to rest, may not merely stimulate nutrition but may also induce fatigue. We must, therefore, be exceedingly careful not to use too many measures at one time, and not to use them too vigorously, especially at first. Exercise, for instance, should in the beginning be exceedingly simple; it should consist at first merely in walking. Secondly, it should always stop far short of fatigue. The last point is the secret of the proper employment of exercise in the treatment of neurasthenia and is too frequently lost sight of. Again, if instead of simple sponge bathing or douching, elaborate hydrotherapeutic measures be employed, we should not forget that even though the patient may react well, he may subsequently feel fatigued, and we can readily understand how the inappropriate or over-vigorous use of bathing may retard increase of weight and strength. Massage also is capable of doing harm if used unadvisedly; rubbing that is unduly severe or unduly prolonged may accentuate the very symptoms that we are endeavoring to remove. I have frequently observed cases of neurasthenia that were being overtreated—by unnecessary medication; or by excessive bathing; or by unnecessary or worrisome applications of electricity; but especially, by excessive exercise; less frequently by injudicious massage. Nature has a wonderful power of recuperation, and if she be wisely assisted and if the patient be placed in simple channels of physiologic living, all that is desired may be gained. Attempts to coerce or hasten the processes of nature lead to disaster. Time is a necessary element, and the patient should be made to realize that his improvement will probably be gradual, though it may be relatively rapid.

Whether progress in a given case is being made will depend upon two facts: first, upon the subsidence of the various fatigue symptoms; and, second, upon increase in the patient's weight. The patient should be weighed, therefore, at intervals, say every fortnight. After a maximum amount of improvement has resulted from the plan of treatment instituted, it may be advisable to send the patient away for a short period. If possible, the patient should be accompanied by a trained nurse, one who is thoroughly familiar with massage and the various forms of physical exercise. The nurse should be fully instructed as to the details of the treatment, especially as to the proportionate time to be spent in rest and in exercise. As a rule, the amount of exercise during the convalescent period should be considerable. In men, the trip away from home, especially if it be during the busy season of the year, may be impracticable; frequently this is the case also with women. In the group of cases we have thus far considered—namely, those in whom the affection is so mild that full rest treatment is unnecessary—this trip away from home may usually be dispensed with.

The management of these relatively simple cases of neurasthenia is of the utmost importance. A very large number of them are not sufficiently ill to demand radical measures, and besides are compelled by the circumstances in which they are placed to meet the obligations of their livelihood. Their successful management is made up of a number of factors, each in itself apparently trivial, but which, when properly grouped, are most efficient in bringing about a restoration to health. The plan of increasing the number of hours spent in bed or in lying down was first instituted by S. Weir Mitchell and termed by him "partial rest," and we have seen how all the other measures—exercise, full feeding, massage, bathing, etc.—group themselves about this central idea. The treatment indeed resolves itself into an application of simple physiologic principles, of which rest is the most important factor.

RADICAL TREATMENT OF NEURASTHENIA BY REST IN BED

In addition to the large class of neurasthenics thus far considered, whose treatment can be successfully conducted without withdrawing them from their ordinary pursuits, there is an equally large number in whom the symptoms are so profound that the general measures described will fail unless supplemented by some more potent restorative influence. The expedient of increasing the hours devoted to rest—prolonging the time spent in bed—is followed by no amelioration of the symptoms, and, moreover, fatigue is so pronounced that it is impossible for the patient to take any exercise no matter how slight. In some cases the neurasthenia has become so grave that even an inconsiderable exertion is followed by pronounced accentuation of the fatigue symptoms. Thus, the patient finds it impossible to walk or stand for even a brief period without inducing backache, or finds it impossible to use the eyes for ever so slight a task without inducing headache. In other cases still, the tired-aches, the nervousness, and the other fatigue symptoms are so pronounced as to be continuous, incessant—and in such cases, rest, involuntary and imperative, is enforced by the very weakness of the patient and yet is not followed by amelioration. In such instances there is no choice but to insist upon the institution of a plan embodying continuous rest in bed, extending over a number of weeks and perhaps months.

Importance of Details
This plan having been determined upon, it must be carried out radically; and the closest possible attention must be given to the execution of the details, lest the whole purpose of the treatment be defeated by some apparently trivial neglect. Every indication presented by the etiology and pathology of neurasthenia

should be followed to the letter. If rest is imperative, it must be made as nearly absolute as possible. The **bed** upon which the patient lies should preferably be furnished with a firmly stuffed horsehair mattress, the latter being supported upon wire springs. As a rule, the patient is merely placed comfortably in the bed with the head resting on a low pillow. He—or she, for frequently it is a woman—is instructed to lie quietly and not to sit up in bed except for the special purpose of taking meals; nor is the patient to leave the bed except for the purpose of emptying the bowels or the bladder. Such a degree of rest maintained for a number of weeks is usually sufficient in ordinary cases. Every now and then, however, cases of neurasthenia are met with, which are so profound that the mere effort of sitting up in bed to eat or of turning from side to side is sufficient to cause great distress. Such patients should, of course, be fed by the nurse, and when there is a desire to change the position in bed, should be gently moved by the attendant. Cases requiring such stringent measures as these are, however, infrequent.

Isolation.—The patient having been placed comfortably in bed, the question arises, Have we now complied with the first indication of the treatment? Not completely. It is necessary for the patient to have not only physical rest but also **mental rest.** The room should be as far as possible a quiet room; which means not only that noises should be excluded, but also that all sources of mental and emotional excitement should be excluded. For this reason it is absolutely necessary that communication with the outside world should be cut off, if not altogether, at least in a very large measure. This necessitates the exclusion of relatives and friends as well as the interruption of all correspondence. In other words, the patient should be **isolated,** and this isolation should be rigid in proportion to the severity of the case. Most patients who present themselves for rest treatment are so worn by the ordinary strains of life, social and otherwise, that they gladly acquiesce in the advice given them in this respect. Occasionally isolation is resisted by the patient, but this is more frequently the case in hysteria than in neurasthenia. Sometimes isolation is violently opposed by some unreasoning relative or friend, and it is against just such friends that isolation is a necessary protection. We have seen in our summary of the symptoms of neurasthenia how the patient is given over to introspection and nosophobia, and it is in this respect that incalculable harm may be done by the injudicious conduct of relatives and friends. The exhibition of anxiety and the constant watching of symptoms serve only to convince the patient that she is seriously ill, perhaps hopelessly so. Sometimes the friend or relative studies and comments on the symptoms more closely than the patient herself, gives to the most trivial occurrences a magnified importance, and, by over-solicitous care and emotional display, serves to bring about a condition of mental invalidism. How much harm such conduct, often mistaken for sympathy, may do, only those know who have come into close contact with it; normal, wholesome sympathy strengthens and encourages, but such false sympathy destroys. It is more especially in hysteria, as we shall see later on, that its influence is pernicious.

Occasionally, the circumstances surrounding a patient are of such a nature that absolute isolation is neither feasible nor wise. A mother, for instance, feels that she cannot consent to an entire separation from an only child for two or three months, and it may be wiser to permit brief visits by the child at stated periods. Other facts of a business nature, especially with male patients, occasionally necessitate modifications of the principle of isolation; but, with due precautions, these modifications are bereft of harm. Isolation, we should remember, is a very powerful expedient. It is true that it insures in the sickroom, other things being equal, an atmosphere of quiet, with freedom from care and from the great nervous drains of life; but occasionally, if carried out unwisely, or too mechanically, isolation may do injury. Especially is this the case when the treatment is attempted without the aid of a special nurse. Upon three separate occasions, I have seen in hospitals cases in which isolation had been attempted without such assistance, and in which for a time decided injury was done by the unrestrained opportunity given the patient for worry and morbid introspection.

In order that a rest treatment should be conducted properly and with advantage to the patient, a special nurse should always be placed in charge. It is her function to devote her entire time exclusively to the one patient. This means that she shall be on duty twenty-two hours out of the twenty-four; *i.e.*, she shall be with the patient during the day, with the exception of two hours for recreation, and shall sleep upon a cot either in the same room with the patient or in a room immediately communicating. The introduction of the nurse into the room constitutes in itself a modification of the principle of isolation, and a very important modification; for the nurse, who, if properly trained and adapted to her work, is of a quiet and restful demeanor, in various ways diverts the patient and leads the mind of the latter gently along pleasant and easy channels. Through the nurse also the unimportant, unexciting, and everyday facts in relation to the outside world gain entrance to the sickroom, and the patient feels her seclusion much less markedly than otherwise she would. The physician likewise, in his visits, acts as a medium through which odinary information is gained. General facts with regard to the patient's relatives—that they are all well, that everything is going on smoothly at home, that the physician is in communication with the family and friends—are conveyed to the patient, and these communications in a large measure contribute to the beneficial effects of isolation by modifying its stringency. The physician and the nurse should be careful, of course, to avoid anything in their demeanor or in their conversation that would in the remotest degree suggest to the patient that there is any unfavorable news from home which is being concealed. The patient is, as a rule, already predisposed to worry and to exaggerate unimportant matters relating to herself or to her family, and this caution cannot be too strongly insisted upon. Under a well-managed isolation, homesickness rarely, if ever, occurs. If it should make its appearance and become a factor in the case, it may easily be relieved by permitting a brief visit from some near relative of the patient's own choosing. If the visitor be trustworthy and has previously been cautioned not to alarm or distress the patient, the incident of the visit will not mar the progress of the treatment. At the very outset of the treatment, the confidence of the patient may be gained and her peace of mind be insured by the promise of the physician that he will at once inform her of any really serious happening at her home; it need not be added that this promise must scrupulously be kept.

General Effects and Necessary Adjuvants of Strict Rest Treatment

Under the correct conditions, the **benefits** to be derived from prolonged rest in bed are both **mental** and **physical.** Nervous tension and anxiety are withdrawn, while the physical strains are likewise reduced to a minimum. Brain-work having ceased, mental expenditure is reduced to slight play of the emotions and an easy drifting of the thoughts; a condition which soon breeds placidity and in most cases contentment. Moreover, the nerve-centers concerned in the function of movement and the muscles themselves are lying fallow; the heart also is resting, for it now drives a stream of blood in a horizontal direction instead of in a vertical column, which means a vast difference in the amount of work imposed. Absolute rest, physiologically speaking, is, of course, impossible; but by continuous rest in bed the expenditure of energy on the part of a patient is reduced to the possible minimum. However, while fully realizing the truth and importance of this general proposition, we cannot but be impressed by the fact that prolonged and profound rest is not without its **dangers.** Prolonged rest in itself is not physiologic. As we have seen, prolonged excess of function is often followed by most serious consequences; on the other hand, the insufficient exercise of function may be followed by results no less disastrous. Just as, on the one hand, excess of function leads to abnormal consumption of tissue, so does the excess of rest, on the other hand, lead to degeneration of tissue. Degeneration of tissue means inevitably a diminution in the capacity for active function, and degeneration and incapacity ensue in direct proportion to the degree and duration of the abnormal inactivity. Diminution of function may be marked and persistent, and may even amount to the total abolition of functional ability. This may be seen typically in a joint placed at rest. The very existence of a joint depends upon its exercise of function as a point of movement. It is well known that in a joint which is placed at rest for a sufficiently long period, limitation of movement ensues, and if rest be persisted in, fixation, absolute loss of function, supervenes. Analogous changes are also observed in muscles that are at rest, and the inference is justified that like changes also take place in the corresponding motor centers. It is hardly necessary to speak of the ill effects of excessive rest upon the heart or blood-vessels, or on the centers which innervate these structures. Like pathologic fatigue, pathologic rest involves its logical dangers. Rest, either local or general, if unmodified and persisted in for too long a period, may inflict serious injury. Rest, therefore, is an instrument as powerful for evil as it is for good, and the problem presents itself as to how this potent agency shall be applied. Evidently it should be applied in such a manner that the patient will receive all its possible benefits without suffering from any of its attendant evils. We are apparently in a dilemma. If we exercise the various faculties of our patient, we expend his energy and still further consume his tissues. If we put him at rest, we may inflict even greater harm. We must, to solve the problem, find a method or methods by means of which the patient's tissues may be exercised in a passive way; and for this purpose we have at our command various expedients.

Massage.—We have already seen that massage may be employed in the treatment of neurasthenia by relative or partial rest; and it has been shown that in the management of the milder forms of neurasthenia, massage is of less value than some forms of active exercise. In the bed treatment of neurasthenia, however, the indication for the employment of massage is imperative. It should always be given, it can never be dispensed with. As pointed out in the previous consideration of the subject, the massage should in the beginning of the treatment be very gentle and superficial in character and should be applied for only a short time. Severe or deep massage, given at first, may greatly increase the general sense of fatigue from which the patient already suffers, while local soreness or rapid action of the heart may add to his distress. Gentle superficial stroking, on the contrary, soothes the patient, and advantage may be taken of this fact by directing the application to be made in the evening. At this time massage strongly favors sleep; it is, indeed, one of the best agents for combating neurasthenic insomnia. Little by little the massage should be increased both in ·epth and vigor, and after the expiration of a variable period, say from a week to ten days, full vigorous massage may be given and its duration increased to about an hour. Some patients, however, are never at any time able to endure a very hard or prolonged rubbing.

Other things being equal, the massage should be given by the nurse. This, of course, makes it necessary that the nurse placed in charge of the case should be thoroughly trained in this measure. If the patient be treated by a masseuse at a given hour of the day, the visit of this third person may act as a disturbing factor; the patient is frequently upset by it, and too often the masseuse is a tactless and garrulous person, capable of working endless harm. In my own experience the masseuse has frequently retarded the progress of the patient. Under exceptional circumstances only is it permissible that the massage should be given by some one other than the constant attendant. For instance, this is the case when the nurse loses sleep at night or when the case proves in other ways to be unusually trying, so that the nurse becomes too fatigued to give the massage properly. The special "method" or "school" followed in giving massage, it may be added, has little influence on the general result.

It is important, however, that this form of passive exercise be applied intelligently, skilfully, regularly, and systematically; and that the special manipulations be judiciously chosen and adapted to the conditions present in the individual case. Here we may note a few facts of salient bearing on our special subject. The nurse should be exceedingly careful not to expose unnecessarily the body of the patient; this is in order that chilling of the surface may not take place. As a rule, the trunk becomes slightly warmer from the rubbing, and this is even more apt to be the case with the limbs; but occasionally the reverse is noted, and in such cases especially, undue exposure is to be avoided.

Toward the latter part of the treatment there should gradually be added to the massage **passive movements** of the limbs, these being flexed, extended, rotated, and abducted from the body in various directions. Finally, the movements should be converted into **movements with resistance.** As a rule, one or two movements, actively resisted, for each limb, are sufficient to begin with. Later their number may be increased and elaborated so as to include, finally, movements of the trunk and neck.

Electricity is distinctly inferior in value to massage. It is merely a useful adjuvant. At the same time its utility cannot be questioned. It also stimulates nutrition and enables us to combat the unfavorable effects of prolonged rest in bed, but, let me repeat, it is vastly inferior to massage and can never be substituted for the latter. Again, it should rarely, if ever, be used in the early stage of the treatment. The patient is, we should remember, exceedingly nervous; electricity is a mysterious agent and the patient is very frequently exceedingly afraid of it. Indeed, in many cases the excitement and irritation which it causes may compel its discontinuance. Its use should not be begun until several weeks after treatment is well under way, and in some cases not until the last weeks of the treatment, preparatory to getting the patient out of bed. At this stage, the exercise that it gives the muscles is undoubtedly beneficial. Earlier it may fatigue and exhaust, besides irritating the patient. Sometimes, indeed, its use is followed by marked general depression and by coldness of the extremities, and if persisted in, may distinctly retard the increase in weight which otherwise takes place. As a rule, it should be applied in the form of a slowly interrupted faradaic current; and the nurse, who has been previously instructed in the more important motor points (points of Ziemssen), makes the application in such a way that each group of muscles undergoes a given number of separate contractions. The applications should at first be limited to the flexors and extensors of the forearms and legs. Later, they may be made to the thighs, arms, and trunk. The duration of the electrization should be not more than from twenty to thirty minutes.

Feeding.—Having considered the modification of rest by massage and by electricity, let us turn our attention to the question of food.

In accordance with what has previously been said, full feeding is indicated. The nutrition of the patient is to be raised to as high a level as possible by furnishing those materials of which he stands in greatest need. As I have pointed out in our consideration of the general application of rest to neurasthenia, the symptoms which the patient presents are complicated either by an excessive formation or a defective elimination of uric acid and allied products. Further, our patient is not exercising, and it can be readily comprehended that she is but little in need of beef or lamb or other stimulating foods. Frequently the red meats can be withdrawn absolutely at first with marked advantage. Starchy foods, potatoes, and wheat bread are also contraindicated for reasons already given. In the class of neurasthenics now under consideration, the atony of the intestinal tract is, as a rule, very marked and is frequently complicated by a more or less pronounced catarrh. It is necessary, therefore, that the food should be as digestible as possible and should at the same time afford the patient abundant nourishment. At first the diet should consist largely, but not exclusively, of milk; later the quantity of other foods may be increased. Milk is admirably adapted as a nutrient to neurasthenics. It represents protein food and yet contains no nuclein and cannot, therefore, take part in the formation of the uric acid group of bodies. Curiously enough, however, many patients object to it and at times strenuously. In the treatment of neurasthenia by rest in bed, however, the use of milk or some of its modifications is almost imperative. In only a few instances may it be dispensed with. It should at first be ordered in small quantities, say from three to four ounces six times daily. When indigestion is very marked, no other food should for the time being be given. Little by little, however, a small quantity of rice, a piece of bread and butter, or some cereal may be added. Soon a soft-boiled egg can be given at breakfast, a small piece of Salisbury steak at dinner, a little boiled rice or some stewed fruit at supper. Chicken, fish, and oysters are next added to the diet and an occasional chop or steak may be permitted. Gradually also one or more of the succulent vegetables, e.g., spinach, squash, stewed celery, are added, and finally peas, string-beans, tomatoes, onions, and the like, until a full diet is reached. Potatoes should for a long time be excluded, as should also wheat bread in any quantity. The neurasthenic is preëminently in need of a mixed diet, one capable of furnishing all that the tissues require: proteids, fats, carbohydrates, vegetable acids, and mineral salts.

The milk is gradually increased in quantity until finally eight, ten, twelve or more ounces are taken six times daily; i.e., with meals, between meals, and at bedtime. In many cases from two to three quarts can be given in addition to a considerable quantity of other food, the patient digesting well the entire amount. Occasionally we find that the patient presents an actual idiosyncrasy with regard to the milk, and is either unable to digest it at all or is able to digest it only with difficulty or in small quantities, even when it is modified in various ways. Under such circumstances it is necessary to resort to egg-feeding. Eggs are best given raw, and should be given in increasing number daily. The procedure is as follows: A raw egg is carefully opened and dropped into a cup in such a way that the yolk is not broken. The patient is then directed to swallow the egg whole with a single effort. As a rule, the trick is readily acquired and the patient experiences no unpleasant taste or other disagreeable sensation. It is best to administer the egg without salt, lemon-juice, or other attempt at flavoring. The white of egg is practically tasteless, and this is all that comes in contact with the tongue so long as the yolk remains unbroken. At first, as a rule, one raw egg between meals is ordered; then the number is increased to two, three, four, five, six or more, as circumstances permit. Afterward raw eggs are added to each meal, the number being cautiously increased to as many as the patient is able to take; the eggs should be swallowed immediately after the food of the meal proper has been taken. In this way six to eighteen or even more eggs a day can be given to neurasthenics, and, strange to say, readily digested by them.

If the feeding be restricted to eggs exclusively the number may be very large indeed. Exceptionally the skin acquires a

4

yellowish tinge.* This may alarm the patient as it suggests an attack of jaundice. However, the discoloration is a brighter yellow than that seen in jaundice and does not involve the conjunctiva. It disappears if the egg-feeding be discontinued or if the yolks be withdrawn and the egg-feeding be restricted to the whites. In a few days the coloring becomes less pronounced and finally fades entirely.

What has been said thus far, indicates in a general way how the feeding of the neurasthenic treated by rest in bed is to be accomplished. Various modifications are, of course, rendered necessary, first by diseases of the digestive tract, and secondly by the idiosyncrasies of the patient. As indicated in the foregoing paragraphs, the digestive disturbance from which neurasthenics most frequently suffer is gastric catarrh—sometimes slight, sometimes pronounced—together with delayed digestion. The indications are generally met by the employment of milk in the manner already outlined, but it may be necessary to modify the milk in various ways; as, for example, by skimming it, or by the addition of a small quantity of sodium bicarbonate or of lime-water. When there is tendency to looseness of the bowels, it is of advantage to boil or "scald" the milk. Hot milk is exceedingly grateful to some persons; taken at night it distinctly favors sleep. Occasionally it is useful to dilute the milk with hot water. At times also malted milk may with advantage be substituted for fresh milk at night or once or twice during the day.

Frequently the addition to cold milk of some alkaline water, still or effervescing, such as Vichy or Selters, makes it very acceptable; this is equally true of the simple carbonated waters, such as Apollinaris or artificial "plain soda water." Sometimes the addition of a little table salt makes the milk palatable; some patients will take and retain salted milk readily when they cannot take simple milk. The milk may also be predigested, or, what is perhaps a better plan, a small quantity of some digestive powder, such as pancreatin and sodium bicarbonate, may be added to cold milk just before the latter is taken. Buttermilk also is of

---

*It appears that in massive egg-feeding some of the protein of the yolk may pass unchanged into the blood.

great advantage, especially in cases in which there is marked constipation. Buttermilk may for a time be given exclusively, or both whole milk and buttermilk may be given separately at various intervals during the day, enough buttermilk being used to keep the bowels open.

In some cases **whey** can be employed with benefit. Although whey does not represent much nutriment, it may prove of service when milk is not tolerated. It is pleasant to taste and can often be given in considerable quantity. It does not answer, however, as a substitute for milk for any lengthy period. Starr's method of preparing whey yields a liquid which is more valuable than when prepared by other methods. He stirs up the curd in the whey and then strains the entire mixture. By this means a certain amount of the curd becomes suspended in the whey and makes it more nutritious. A small quantity of rennet, hock, lemon-juice, or, better still, wine of pepsin, may be used as the coagulant. **Kumyss,** or rather imitation kumyss, is of much greater value than whey, and is frequently retained and well digested when milk, even when modified in various ways, fails. The method of its preparation is exceedingly simple and the nurse should be instructed in the procedure.*

Cream is in my experience of distinctly inferior value to milk; occasionally, however, cream can be given when milk cannot. At times cream may be added to whey, the nutritive value of which it thus increases. It is sometimes better to dilute the cream with hot water.

At times when the difficulty of digestion is very pronounced, it may be necessary to resort for short periods to various meat, oyster or clam broths, or to some of the liquid beef preparations found in the market. It is not necessary to specify any of the latter;

*Dissolve one-sixth of a yeast-cake in a little water; add this to a pint of milk which has been raised to about the body-temperature; add a dessertspoonful of cane-sugar. Pour into a bottle with a mechanical stopper, such as a beer-bottle, filling it as far as the neck. Lay the bottle in a warm place for about twelve hours; then on ice. Kumyss is readily taken by many patients who cannot take milk, and it is of great value in other cases by furnishing a substitute which can be given from time to time when the patient grows tired of milk in other forms.

their number is considerable. They are valuable, of course, in direct proportion to the amount of peptones they contain. Some of the most extensively advertised preparations, however, consist chiefly of alcohol, and the fact of their alcoholic nature must be considered very carefully in prescribing them and in regulating their dosage. The best of them contains but little nutriment. A resort to broths or beef preparations in rest cases can, of course, only be regarded as a temporary expedient necessitated by pronounced indigestion, persistent nervous vomiting, temporary disgust for food, or other complication. How imperfectly these substances answer the purposes of food is proved by the fact that during their exclusive use the weight of the patient inevitably falls. Occasionally one of the peptone preparations can be added to milk in small quantities—a mixture which is occasionally preferred by some patients to whom the ordinary taste of milk is repulsive.

At times we may be forced to resort to **rectal feeding.** Various substances may be used. Peptonized milk, previously brought to the temperature of the body, is very serviceable. The most satisfactory material, however, for rectal injections consists of two parts by weight of finely scraped beef and one part by weight of finely chopped pancreas. The beef is thoroughly mixed with the gland, a little water is added, and the whole mixture gently warmed so as to start digestion. The quantity injected should be rather small; as a rule, about two ounces. The rectum may be made tolerant by the previous injection of a few drops of laudanum or by the use of a half-grain opium suppository. From three to four, occasionally more, rectal feedings can be given in the twenty-four hours without making the rectum sore. Occasionally the bowels should be washed out with a little warm water. Other substances than those here mentioned may, of course, be employed.

A few points of importance in regard to the diet of the neurasthenic remain to be considered. As a rule, the patient continues to take and digest the food well even when the total amount for the twenty-four hours is very large. However, it is wise now and then to diminish the amount for a time. Especially is this the case during the **menstrual period.** During this period the patient can neither be bathed nor rubbed, and it is wise in forced feeding to diminish the quantity of food somewhat until the period is over. In other cases, again, the diet, if too restricted, palls upon the appetite, and in such case small quantities of salted food may be added with advantage. For instance, a few salted wafers may be given with the milk or a small quantity of dried beef or minced ham may be placed on the tray, in addition, of course, to the regular diet; occasionally also a small quantity of grilled bacon at breakfast is very acceptable.

Minor difficulties are sometimes presented by the refusal of the patient to eat certain articles of food. Thus, some patients declare pointblank that the only meat that they will eat is beef; others decline absolutely to eat vegetables, and still others make persistent war upon the milk. The physician should, if possible, educate the patient to partake of a very varied and mixed diet. This object can, as a rule, be accomplished if the physician be not in too great haste to feed the patient large amounts. For instance, if marked peculiarities are noted in the patient, we should proceed somewhat as follows. Milk should, for example, be given whole or in a modified form in very small quantities, say two, three, or four ounces, at intervals of two hours. Other food should during this period be absolutely excluded. Soon the patient becomes quite hungry, and in a day or two takes the milk eagerly. The quantity should then be gradually increased, the patient being kept a little hungry all the time. The victory that is gained is twofold, both physical and moral; as a rule, the patient can later be persuaded to begin taking other foods in small quantities, even when he does not like them. As already stated, however, it is occasionally impossible to give milk no matter how modified, how small the quantity, or what the circumstances. In such cases egg-feeding should be resorted to in the manner already described.

In regard to the use of **stimulants,** what has been said on page 35, when discussing the treatment of neurasthenia by relative rest, applies equally here. The treatment is best conducted from beginning to end without them. Occasionally, however, they may be used by persons who are beyond middle life. White wines or acid wines, for obvious reasons, should be avoided; at most a little claret or Burgundy may be permitted. Occasionally, too, when the period of absolute rest has terminated and the patient has begun to exercise out-of-doors, or when the appetite flags a little, a bottle of light beer may with advantage be substituted for the milk at dinner. This should always, of course, be withdrawn before the patient finally leaves the physician's care.

Bathing.—Just as it is necessary for the neurasthenic who is merely under general rest to bathe freely, so is it necessary to use bathing in the treatment of patients who are resting in bed. As a rule, a sponge bath with warm water, given between blankets, is all that is indicated. Indeed, it is the only bath that is tolerated at first, and as a rule it answers every purpose. Gentle friction with a towel afterward is sufficient to prevent any local depression of temperature. Occasionally, however, it is necessary for the nurse to rub the limbs with her hands moistened with alcohol, friction being vigorously maintained until the limbs feel warm. In this way the coldness and depression which every now and then follow the bath may be avoided. Later in the treatment, tub-bathing may once in a while be substituted, the general principles indicated on page 36 being followed. The caution already expressed as to the feebleness of the circulation in neurasthenics would warn us not to use cold bathing or extensive bathing, especially at first. The cold douche, spray, or shower bath should not be employed until improvement by rest methods has been well established, that is, toward the close of the treatment. In many cases, it need hardly be added, cold or vigorous bathing is never applicable. The method of giving the cold bath is a matter of importance. The patient should stand in six or eight inches of warm water (90°F.) while the trunk, arms, and legs are douched by water of a slightly lower temperature; day by day the temperature of the douche is gradually lowered until about 60°F. (15.5°C.) is reached. In this way the initial shock, so distressing to neurasthenics, is greatly diminished. The nurse may use a basin or a large dipper in giving the douche; if a shower or spray apparatus be at hand, it is to be preferred because of the additional benefit to be gained from the mechanical impact of the water. The expedient of the section of garden hose and sprinkler already mentioned on page

37 may here be substituted. We must, however, repeat the caution that neurasthenics, especially in the early period of their treatment, are made worse by unnecessary handling or fussing, and vigorous bathing should only be resorted to, if at all, after improvement has been well advanced. Finally, it need hardly be added that especial caution should be exercised in the case of patients beyond middle life.

The **degree of progress** that is made in a given case is estimated as in the treatment by relative rest, first, by the subsidence of the fatigue symptoms, and, secondly, by the increase in the patient's weight. The general sense of tiredness and the various local fatigue symptoms as a rule begin to yield from the first. Recurrences, however, are apt to take place from time to time, and not infrequently weeks elapse before these cease altogether. As a rule, the time required for the successful treatment of a case of neurasthenia of such severity as to demand full bed treatment extends over a period varying from eight weeks to three months. It is comparatively infrequent that a really good and durable result can be achieved in six weeks; generally eight, ten, or twelve weeks are required, and sometimes much longer. Usually young neurasthenic individuals require a shorter period of time than those that are older or middle-aged and in whom it is more difficult to stimulate the processes of repair.

In addition to observing the case closely from day to day, the patient should be **weighed** at intervals of every two or three weeks. It is generally of advantage not to begin weighing the patient until at least three weeks have elapsed, as it often happens that the preliminary difficulties presented by indigestion and other disturbances are of such a character as to make pronounced gain in weight at an earlier period improbable. Moreover, unless the gain in weight at the time of the first weighing be marked, the patient is apt to become depressed and to have his confidence in the ultimate result of the treatment diminished. After the first weighing, the patient should be weighed at intervals of two weeks and the progress noted. In the larger number of patients we are able not only to bring the weight up to the normal, taking into consideration the height, age, and sex of the individual, but even greatly in excess of this. Sometimes, indeed, if care be not exercised, the patients become needlessly fat and heavy. A moderate excess of weight is not a disadvantage, however, because it enables us to submit the patient to a thorough system of exercise after the rest treatment is completed.

Conclusion of the Bed-period of Treatment

As the days and weeks pass by, provided the case progresses favorably, various changes are noted. Not only does the patient increase in weight, but there is also a decided improvement in the other physical signs. The muscles become firm, the chilled extremities grow warm, the damp skin becomes dry, and the pallor of the surface gives way to normal flesh tints. At the same time, a change is noted in the mental condition of the patient. After the first week or ten days of the nervousness and restlessness incident to the initial period of the treatment, the patient passes into a condition of placidity, indifference, and contentment. The ever-increasing sense of physical well-being—the luxurious sense of comfort induced by the full feeding, the absolute quiet, and the various physiologic procedures—is such as to induce a state of extreme mental satisfaction. The patient usually remains in this condition until a large degree of improvement has been reached and maintained for some time. Sooner or later, however, a reaction sets in. Mental indifference and placidity now give way to spontaneity of thought and action and to a desire for activity, both mental and physical. The patient begins to be restless and to ask the physician when she may leave her bed or when she may begin to exercise.

As soon as the maximum degree of improvement has in the physician's judgment been attained, the patient should be permitted to sit up for a few minutes daily, say five or ten minutes at first. It is of the utmost importance that the getting up of the patient should be brought about in as gradual a manner as possible. Otherwise she may be distressed by a sensation of weakness and trembling in the extremities, by faintness, or by giddiness. Such symptoms, however, are never observed in cases in which due care is exercised. After a few days the time can be increased by a few minutes, and later the patient can be permitted to be out of bed twice daily. Little by little the time is further increased, the patient also being directed to take limited exercise about the room. In the same gradual manner light calisthenic **exercise,** and finally a full course of Swedish movements, should be instituted. The time out of bed is gradually increased until finally the patient sits up for five or six hours out of the twenty-four. Exercise in the open air by means of walking or an occasional carriage-ride is now added. Finally the patient is up for the greater part of the day, rising late, say at half-past ten or eleven, lying down between two and four, and going to bed again immediately before or after supper. The treatment is best completed by sending the patient away to some nearby point in the **country** or at the **seashore,** where exercise in the open air can be still further carried out. As a rule, two weeks at the seashore or elsewhere are sufficient for this purpose, though sometimes a longer period is desirable. During the stay at the seashore, or shortly before this period, **communication** with relatives and friends can gradually be resumed. The patient is again brought into contact with the outer world and thus prepared for her return to her home. While at the seashore she should, of course, be accompanied by her nurse, who should still carry out general rest methods. However, the nurse should gradually withdraw from the patient assistance in dressing, bathing, and in other matters, so that by the time the patient is ready to leave for home she has become entirely self-dependent. As much as possible, also, the nurse should stimulate the patient to the free exercise of her own judgment and volition, and in this way stimulate self-confidence and self-reliance.

It cannot be too strongly impressed upon the reader that a course of vigorous and persistent **exercise** is necessary in order to bring about a durable result; indeed, the benefits accruing from a rest treatment may be lost if the treatment be not followed by exercise. Happily one of the great advantages of a course of rest treatment away from home is that it frequently and permanently modifies the patient's habits in regard to exercise. The error should not be made, however, of directing the patient to take too much exercise at first. Walking, golf, horseback-

riding, and, occasionally, swimming or surf bathing may be employed according to circumstances. What has been said in this
respect in discussing treatment by partial rest applies equally
here (see p. 29). The exercise should be little at first and
steadily increased, but should always stop well within the limits
of fatigue.

The patient finally **returning to her home,** should be instructed
to live conservatively; a strictly physiologic method of living
should be insisted upon. As a rule, a permanent result follows
a radical treatment, especially if this subsequent course be carried
out. The patient should also seek to fill in her time with some
agreeable and suitable occupation. This point is of the utmost
importance. Sometimes difficulty is experienced in the selection
of the work, but there is no reason why even a well-to-do or wealthy
woman should not take up a course as librarian or private secre-
tary, or should not become proficient in stenography, or, if she
be intellectually inclined, take up a special line of study in history,
art, or literature, or devote herself to some charity. It cannot
be too strongly insisted upon that work is the best guarantee of
mental and physical health—work within physiologic limits and
adapted to the physical and mental constitution of the patient.
An active interest in life insures healthy mental exercise, and this
is as necessary to mental health as is physical exercise to bodily
health. While it is of the utmost importance to prevent the
patient from lapsing into habits of idleness, it is equally important,
on the other hand, to prevent him from again placing himself under
conditions and surroundings similar to those which led to his
illness. The danger of a relapse should be clearly pointed out and
overwork and overstrain, in all its forms, should be carefully
guarded against.

Auxiliary Medication

In the plan of treatment outlined in the foregoing pages, medicines have not been mentioned; in many cases few drugs are
required from the beginning to the end of the treatment—perhaps none at all. Special indications, however, frequently arise
for their temporary use. Some of these have already been con-

sidered in discussing the treatment of neurasthenia by relative rest. Thus, **atony and catarrh of the stomach** and of other portions of the digestive tract are frequently met with. In simple atony small doses of nux vomica, the simple bitters, such as gentian, and carminatives, such as cardamom, may be given. They probably stimulate digestion, but, in addition, like other medicines, they also act by suggestion. Many patients are met with who, if no medicine be prescribed, believe that everything possible is not being done for them, no matter how freely or elaborately the various expedients, such as massage, exercise, electricity, and bathing, may be developed. In cases of this kind, simple remedies, such as are here mentioned, often prove extremely efficient. It is not usually necessary to stimulate the appetite in neurasthenia, for, strange to say, the average neurasthenic has a good appetite; indeed, he sometimes eats excessively. It is only in the graver forms that anorexia is met with. Here, of course, nux vomica, minute doses of strychnin, or the simple bitters, with or without a few drops of dilute hydrochloric acid, may usefully be given. Gastric catarrh, when present, can be successfully combated not only by proper modifications of the diet, but also by the various remedies already considered on page 32; namely, small doses of bismuth subnitrate before meals, or silver nitrate in pill form (say one-fourth grain with one-fourth or one-half grain of extract of hyoscyamus), twenty minutes or half an hour before meals. The silver pill should be swallowed with a small quantity of water, about half an ounce; it is often of decided benefit and may be continued for several weeks. At times when gastric catarrh is marked, and when the stomach is also intolerant to food, small doses of Fowler's solution (from one-half drop to two drops in a teaspoonful of water, ten minutes before taking nourishment) are often of much value. At other times a pill of one-fourth grain of cocain hydrochlorate, ten minutes before meals, is efficacious. Occasionally it is better to give bismuth subnitrate and cocain together in powder. Sometimes a cup of hot water taken before breakfast, or even before each of the meals, is of service. Lavage of the stomach is only exceptionally indicated; it may be employed when the gastric catarrh is very pronounced and very persistent, but even then it should not be resorted to except at somewhat lengthy intervals. If the gastric symptoms do not improve after a reasonable interval, a test-breakfast should be given and the stomach-contents systematically examined. Test-meals, it is true, are rarely necessary in the class of patients under consideration. Every now and then they assist us in differentiating grave organic lesions, as ulcer and carcinoma, from the mere digestive complications of neurasthenia. In this connection it is well to remember that hydrochloric acid may be entirely absent in simple catarrh; and the diagnosis must be made from due consideration of all the facts in the case, including, if necessary, a careful study of the blood.

At times atony and catarrh involve especially the small intestine. In such cases, bismuth beta-naphthol or orphol in ten- or fifteen-grain doses, three times daily, is often of value. This is also true of beta-naphthol, which may be given in capsules of from three to five grains after meals. At other times there is tenderness over the colon and occasionally also a pseudo-fibrinous or mucous exudation which is passed with the bowel movements —so-called mucous colitis or croupous enteritis. In such cases it is often beneficial to use high colonic irrigations; the best solution being simple warm water to which a small quantity of salt (sodium chlorid 0.77 per cent., say a teaspoonful to the pint) may be added. I have never seen any advantage in the use of medicated injections. It is the repeated irrigation and thorough cleansing of the bowel which are of value. Mucous and catarrhal conditions of the large intestine are not of themselves serious complications of neurasthenia, but the presence of mucus in the movements is often noted by the patient, who may become unduly alarmed. Many patients, already nosophobic, begin to watch their stools closely from day to day. The condition, it need hardly be added, improves hand in hand with the general health, and eventually disappears altogether.

In a large number of cases of neurasthenia, **constipation** is present. At times this is successfully combated by the diet and by massage. Frequently it is necessary to employ some simple laxative. If catarrh of the stomach and intestines be present, it is of advantage to use sodium phosphate, preferably the effervescent preparation, in dessert or tablespoonful doses, freely dissolved in water, about thirty to sixty minutes before breakfast. Other mild laxatives, such as Hathorn or Friedrichschall water, may also be employed. There is, however, a decided disadvantage in the long-continued use of salines, no matter how mild, in patients whose weight we are trying to increase. It is wiser, therefore, when we are obliged to use a laxative for some time, to give some simple vegetable preparation, such as a pill containing small doses of compound extract of colocynth, aloes, and belladonna, or the well-known pill of aloes, belladonna, and strychnin; in cases in which a more decided laxative is required a pill containing podophyllin may be administered. As a rule, the laxative pill should be given at night. In the majority of cases of neurasthenia, however, simple atony of the bowel is the difficulty which confronts us, and this is best met by some preparation of cascara. At times the aromatic fluid extract, which is pleasant to take, answers every purpose. More frequently, however, the simple fluid extract, because of its greater efficiency, is to be employed. It should, as already mentioned on page 33, be given in small doses after meals rather than in a single decided dose at bedtime. As a rule, eight to fifteen drops after each meal is sufficient. By giving the remedy after meals, its action, which is tonic and stimulating to the intestine, is diffused over the entire twenty-four hours. The fluid extract is greatly to be preferred over cascara in pill form because of the nicety with which the doses can be regulated. As a rule, the constipation in neurasthenics rapidly improves, and the dose of cascara can be diminished drop by drop until it is finally withdrawn altogether.

In all cases in which constipation is present, thorough **massage of the bowel** should, of course, be employed. This should be given not only with the patient lying in bed upon the back, but, especially in obstinate cases, also with the patient upon all fours or with the shoulders and arms resting upon the back of a chair; by these postures, the abdomen is made more or less pendulous and can be manipulated very vigorously. Occasionally **electricity** is also of service; one pole of the faradaic battery should be placed over the lumbar region and the other over various points on the abdominal wall—especially in the neighborhood of the navel.   A rapidly interrupted faradaic current is most serviceable.   Instead of placing one electrode over the small of the back, a properly protected metallic electrode (a rectal electrode) may be inserted as far as possible into the bowel.   This procedure, however, is rarely necessary and is attended with considerable discomfort to the patient.

It need hardly be pointed out here how in various digestive disturbances the alkalies, the mineral acids, the digestive ferments, or the antispasmodics, camphor and asafetida, are to be employed. These subjects are dealt with in works upon materia medica and upon diseases of the digestive tract.

Occasionally in spite of the rest, the bathing, and the massage, the various fatigue sensations, pains, and aches of which the patient complains persist for an unduly long period.   Pains thus persisting are probably due to the **retention of waste products**, especially of the uric acid or alloxuric group.   This point I regard as of great importance and of special significance because of the close relation existing between neurasthenia and the so-called uric acid diathesis.   Indeed, it has become my rule to regard aching pains in neurasthenia, when persistent, as of diathetic origin and demanding diathetic treatment.   Usually they yield more or less readily to such measures.   Some salicylate which is well borne by the stomach should be given, such as aspirin, salophen, or salol.   Aspirin in five- to fifteen-grain doses three or four times a day is usually very efficient.   When the stomach is in good condition, sodium salicylate, ten or fifteen grains, with an equal or slightly larger quantity of sodium bromid may be given in a large quantity of water after meals.   The salicylates are efficacious not only in the backache and limbache of neurasthenia, but also in many of the persistent headaches.   An alkaline treatment by means of lithia waters may also be instituted, or, what is better, piperazin, lycetol, or atophan may be given along with large quantities of water.

Occasionally a **headache** is so severe that it is necessary to use some analgesic; in such case it is better to avoid the use of the coal-tar products if possible.   Trial should first be made of small or

increasing doses of a trustworthy fluid extract of cannabis indica—
say from one to five drops repeated every two hours until the pain
is relieved. This drug possesses the great advantage of not producing any depression in the patient. Sometimes, however, its
physiologic effects become manifest, and these may cause the patient considerable distress and alarm. The initial dose should,
therefore, be small, one drop or less, and it should only gradually
be increased and not repeated at too short intervals. When the
cannabis indica fails, or when it cannot be tolerated, fluid extract
of gelsemium should be given in its place. From five to ten drops
of this drug, repeated in two hours if no impression has been made
on the pain, are very frequently efficacious. In large doses gelsemium is a motor depressant, and it should not be used too freely in
neurasthenia. It is also a less valuable remedy than cannabis indica. In many cases of headache we are forced to make use of one
of the coal-tar products—preferably phenacetin. These are also
of benefit in relieving backache and limbache. They are best
given alone; at times, however, they may be advantageously combined with a bromid—ammonium or strontium; thus ten grains
of antipyrin with twenty grains of ammonium bromid. If there
be much depression produced by the pain or the drug, a grain of
caffein may be added; camphor monobromate (one to three grains)
is also a useful adjuvant. These remedies should, however, for
obvious reasons be avoided if possible, and if employed be discontinued promptly.

Occasionally electricity is of service, together with massage, in
relieving aching in the back or in the limbs. The constant galvanic
current should be used, the positive electrode, which should consist of a large flat disc, being applied over the painful area. Sometimes, as over the spine, the pain is complicated by hyperesthesia;
here the galvanic current used in the manner described is often of
decided value. If the pain be diffused in character and evidently
involving the muscles, a mild, rapidly interrupted faradaic current
is useful. Local hot wet packs over the painful area are also at
times followed by good results.

In cases in which pain persists in spite of diathetic or other
treatment, local or special causes should be sought for. It is hardly

necessary to point out, for instance, how often persistent headache is due to some affection of the **eyes**—an anomaly of refraction
or of the ocular muscles. An examination of the eyes should, therefore, be made in all such cases, though correction and other interference is generally best deferred until the close or the latter part of
the rest treatment. In other cases the **nasal cavities,** the **teeth,**
or it may be the **pelvic organs,** will demand our attention. Neurasthenics, because of the extreme irritability of the nervous system, react excessively to slight causes of peripheral irritation, and
comparatively trifling local disturbances may be instrumental in
keeping up a headache. Frequently, however, the true neurasthenic character of the pain is shown by the fact that it persists
after the local trouble has been corrected. The relation of local
affections to neurasthenia is fully considered in the discussion of
neurasthenia symptomatica and the neurasthenoid states (pp. 81
to 84).

When special pains or aches fail to respond to diathetic and
other treatment, and when they are not related to local or visceral
disease, **hysteria** should be suspected and the stigmata of this
affection carefully sought for. In such case, of course, the patient
would not be suffering from a neurasthenia simplex but from one
complicated by hysteria, or possibly from hysteria alone (see
chapter on Hysteria).

An annoying complication of neurasthenia is every now and
then presented by **insomnia.** In many cases the mere taking of
food has a soporific or sedative influence; occasionally a glass of hot
milk or of hot malted milk has an extremely soothing effect.
Massage given at night also favors sleep in most cases. Sometimes a hot tub-bath or the hot wet pack (see p. 37) is successful in
bringing about the desired result. In other cases the "drip sheet"
entirely overcomes the insomnia. The patient stands in a few
inches of tepid water in a tub. A linen sheet, dripping with water
at a temperature of 60° or 50°F. (15.5° or 10°C.), is wrapped loosely
about the patient, and the nurse now makes vigorous friction
through and with the sheet. As a rule, the surface and limbs of
the patient soon become warm, and on drying the patient and
placing him in bed, a quite refreshing sleep is apt to ensue. Again,

neurasthenic patients are commonly, and sometimes keenly, susceptible to suggestion; and placebos are, therefore, often followed by the most gratifying results. There are few hypnotics, for instance, more potent than a ten-grain capsule of starch given under proper conditions and with an *indirect* but *strong* suggestion. Striking and almost incredible results are sometimes achieved by this means in cases in which insomnia has previously been a very marked feature. Frequently, however, this and other means fail, and the insomnia then persists as a most distressing symptom. Under these circumstances it is wise to use one of the milder hypnotics for a short time. By this means the sleep habit is reëstablished and the drug can, as a rule, be readily discontinued. The victory over the patient is often greatest if the remedy can be given without his knowledge; he is then apt to believe that sleep has been produced by the other measures adopted and he continues the habit of sleep subsequently when these measures alone are used. A drug frequently efficacious under these circumstances is hyoscin; it may be given in doses of from one two-hundredth of a grain to one seventy-fifth of a grain. It may be dissolved in the bedtime milk or in the last drink of water which the patient takes at night. It is not usually followed by any unpleasant reaction, though in exceptional cases it produces a slight dryness of the mouth and throat. Scopolamin (Merck), which closely resembles hyoscin, has in my hands proved somewhat more efficacious than the latter. The dose necessary appears to be somewhat smaller, while the sleep is somewhat longer. Unfortunately, neither hyoscin nor scopolamin is a very certain hypnotic, and when they fail, we are obliged to fall back upon other remedies. Physicians recognize that sedatives should not, save exceptionally, be used over long periods of time. Their obvious application is to secure the immediate relief of a distressing insomnia. Frequently after such relief has been secured, the patient, as just indicated, continues sleeping without the medicine or sleeps under the influence of a placebo. In given cases, should this not be the result, the remedy should still be suspended and if later a sedative is necessary an entirely different one should be given.

The choice of the sedative is important and here general prin-

5

ciples should guide us. An ideal remedy would be one which would induce sleep approximating the normal sleep and which would not be followed by depression or other unpleasant symptoms. As a matter of fact we are to-day in possession of quite a number of remedies more or less closely fulfilling these conditions. For example, adalin gives rise to a sleep which is light and gentle and is unattended by any other concomitant or subsequent effects. It has further the advantage of usually being efficacious in relatively small doses, *e.g.*, five grains, although not infrequently fifteen grains are required. Another such remedy is medinal (veronal sodium). This is more decided in its action but the sleep again approximates the normal sleep and there is no depression or other unpleasant after-effect, for it is very rapidly eliminated. Veronal itself, especially in too free a dose, may give rise to a sleep that is too prolonged and is in some instances followed by heaviness and hebetude. Of late years a new and very valuable remedy belonging to the same group has been added to our list, namely, luminal. In three-grain doses the latter is very gently sedative and induces a most satisfactory sleep. In larger doses, five or ten grains, it acts very decidedly and marked physical relaxation may follow the sleep. Large doses are not necessary and are not adapted to neurasthenic cases.

The sulphonal group likewise presents several valuable sedatives, each of which has special advantages. Trional acts kindly and without unpleasant after-effects. Sulphonal acts slowly and is of especial advantage when it is desired to procure a prolonged sleep. It is slowly absorbed and slowly eliminated and after full doses some hebetude may persist for a time after awakening. Tetronal closely resembles trional in its action. Porphyruria, said to follow the too free administration of the sulphonal group, I have not met with.

The alcohol group of sedatives—as they are termed by Eager— alcohol, paraldehyd, amylene hydrate, chloral hydrate and butyl chloral hydrate, may all be dismissed as not adapted to neurasthenics. In any event they are greatly inferior to the veronal or sulphonal group.

The bromid group also can be readily dismissed. As hypnotics the bromids are obviously not suitable and not as useful as other remedies in our possession. Finally, opium and its alkaloids have no place in the armamentarium of neurasthenia.

In practice when simple physiological expedients, massage, bathing, hot milk-feeding and the like fail to relieve a distressing insomnia, recourse may be had with advantage to trional, to veronal sodium or to sulphonal. Both trional and veronal sodium (medinal) are suitable to cases in which the patient has difficulty in falling asleep and lies awake for a long time before sleep finally comes on. Again, many neurasthenics fall asleep readily, but awaken in the early morning hours or at various intervals throughout the night. In such cases sulphonal in small doses—five or ten grains—often acts admirably. Again, not infrequently it is of advantage to use trional and sulphonal together or veronal sodium and sulphonal, adjusting the proportions of the remedies to suit the individual case. Sleep once having been established the medicine may be discontinued and capsules of starch substituted or the replacement of the remedy by starch may be made more gradual.

Occasionally, the **nervousness** of the patient persists for an unusually long period after the institution of rest methods, and in such cases it is justifiable to make use of moderate doses of one of the bromids. Strontium bromid or, better still, ammonium bromid, because it is the least depressant of all the bromids, may be given in fifteen- or twenty-grain doses, in a large quantity of water after meals. In bad cases the bromid may be associated for a short time with five- or ten-grain doses of antipyrin. Such a combination exerts a decidedly steadying effect upon the nervous system. It should, of course, be gradually but rapidly withdrawn so soon as the nervousness has been controlled. Many persons are very susceptible to the bromids and in such cases bromid acne or other annoying skin manifestations may make their appearance. For this reason and also because of the undoubted depressant action of the bromids when long continued, their administration should be very guarded. An excellent remedy for the lessening of the nervousness of the patient is presented by luminal in small doses; three-quarters to one and a half grains given once, twice or three times daily. Such small doses exert a wonderfully soothing and quieting effect upon the nervous system without the slightest depression or any other untoward symptom. Sometimes other remedies may be employed; for instance, a three-grain pill of asafetida may be given three or four times a day, especially when the nervousness is associated with intestinal disturbance. When complaint is made of sinking sensations referred to the epigastrium, a capsule containing two or three grains of camphor given after meals may have a most beneficial effect.

It is largely the custom to employ tonics in neurasthenia. I believe them to be of comparatively little value in this affection provided that rest measures are efficiently carried out. They are rarely indicated. The appetite of the patient is already good and the wants of his tissues are best met by food. It is a common custom to prescribe iron, and yet in neurasthenia there is no affection of the blood; its specific gravity, the percentage of hemoglobin, and the blood-count are normal, or present but trifling variations from the normal.* The surface pallor noted in so many neurasthenics is not indicative of anemia but is merely due to the feebleness of the surface circulation. A drug very frequently prescribed is strychnin. The philosophy of its employment is difficult to understand; it can only help the patient temporarily; it is not a food and cannot build up tissue; and it has the disadvantage of occasionally increasing the nervous tension from which the patient suffers. Many patients come to the physician making the statement that they cannot bear strychnin and requesting that it be not prescribed. Under certain conditions, however, it should be employed; for example, when there is unusual feebleness of the heart. It should then be prescribed in large doses, i.e., from one-thirtieth to one-twentieth of a grain, three or four times daily. Cod-liver oil also is unnecessary. The fatty matters contained in the food and in the milk, or, if fatty elements be especially indicated, in the cream added to the milk, are in most cases sufficient. Similar remarks apply to the various malt preparations; at best they are merely adjuvants to feeding and are only infrequently indicated.

---

*Occasionally the blood-count reveals an unusually large proportion of lymphocytes, a fact the significance of which it is difficult to interpret.

Management of Obese Patients

A difficult problem is now and then presented by patients who, instead of being thin, are overfat, and who notwithstanding are so profoundly neurasthenic as to demand treatment by rest in bed. As a rule, these patients present not only excessive muscular weakness but also great feebleness of the circulation. They are soft and flabby, with pallor of the surface and coldness of the extremities, and have but feeble powers of resistance. By a careful application of the methods already discussed, a very remarkable change can be brought about in them. The carbohydrates and hydrocarbons, the starches and fatty foods, should, of course, be excluded from the diet, or permitted only in minimal amount. The diet should consist at first of the white meats and of the succulent vegetables. The patient should be instructed to drink little or no water or other liquids with his meals. Water, whey, or milk that has been thoroughly skimmed may be permitted between meals. At the same time massage should be instituted, directed especially to the fatty deposit; the fat rather than the muscles should be kneaded, squeezed, and rubbed. By these means much of the soft subcutaneous fatty tissue is gotten rid of, and if, later on, when the general progress of the case justifies it, exercise, first slight and later vigorous, be instituted, striking changes are observed. The patient becomes smaller, the tissues grow hard and firm, and in addition the neurasthenic symptoms gradually disappear. Usually the patient loses weight while the general reduction in bulk is taking place, but in other instances an actual increase in weight accompanies the diminution in size. As a rule, dietetic measures with properly applied massage and exercise are all that is required, and thyroid extract can usually be dispensed with. Now and then, however, it may with advantage be employed, but it should be given in moderate doses; we ought not to lose sight of the fact that in decided doses it is both a cardiac and cerebral excitant, with toxic and depressing powers not yet well understood. It sometimes produces an actual, morbid denutrition.

Historical Résumé

The picture of neurasthenia presented in the foregoing pages, as well as the discussion of the principles of its treatment, render it necessary to speak at this point of the part taken by American physicians, especially by George M. B. Beard and by S. Weir Mitchell, in the recognition of the disease and in the development of its treatment. Although medical men had vaguely recognized the existence of the affection so early as the sixteenth century, definite knowledge in regard to it is quite recent. According to Arndt, the first writing in which neurasthenic symptoms are mentioned is that of Fernel. It bears the title "De Abditis Rerum Causis," was published in 1540, and ascribed the symptoms to vapors arising from altered sperm or menstrual blood. Later writers were equally obscure and no less fanciful in their pathology. This is implied by the titles of their works; for instance, Lange, "Treatise on Vapors, their Effects and their Remedies," Paris, 1687; Joly, "Discourse on a Strange Malady, Hypochondriac and Gaseous," Paris, 1689; Hunauld, "Dissertation on the Vapors and Gases of the Blood," Paris, 1716; Blackmoore, "Treatise on the Spleen and Vapours," London, 1725; and by the titles of other works, too numerous to mention, up to the latter part of the eighteenth century. These writings reveal a knowledge of quite a number of neurasthenic symptoms, such as giddiness, cardiac palpitation, constriction of the head, and states of fear; but these are associated with signs which to-day would lead to the diagnosis of other functional or even organic nervous diseases. The subject remained in a condition of gross confusion until 1765, when Robert Whyte, of Edinburgh, differentiated between neurasthenia, hysteria, and hypochondria. In his work on these nervous disorders he says clearly: "The complaints of the first of the above classes may be called simply nervous; those of the second, in compliance with custom, may be said to be hysteric, and those of the third hypochondriac." Notwithstanding this lucid statement, and despite the great number of subsequent publications, little further progress was made until the beginning of the second half of the nineteenth century, when there appeared the writings of Bouchut. This author in 1857 published a paper "On the Nervous State in its Acute and Chronic Form," in the "Bulletin de L'Académie de Médecine," and subsequently other writings upon the same subject, in "L'Union Médicale" and the "Gazette des Hôpitaux," the last appearing so late as 1869. Bouchut maintained that an affection, which he designated as *nervosisme*, and which had heretofore been confounded with hysteria, hypochondria, the psychoses, and with various forms of organic disease, was really an independent affection and was just as much a disease as hysteria or epilepsy. He maintained that it did not depend upon organic changes in the nervous system but was purely a functional disease. He distinguished between an acute and a chronic form, and it is here that he fell into error. He recognized under the acute form various active febrile states occurring in weakened and in debilitated individuals after slight and often inconsequential causes. Under the chronic form, however, he grouped the manifold symptoms which are observed as persistent phenomena in nervous individuals; the special symptoms noted in a given case depend upon the form which the nervousness takes, and there are to be distinguished not only a *nervosisme cérébral, spinal, cardiaque, laryngé, gastrigue, utérin, séminal, cutané, spasmodique, paralytique, douloureux*, but also a *nervosisme simple, hystérique, hypochondriaque*, etc. Bouchut's recognition of an acute or a febrile form is unfortunate; it embraces diverse febrile or inflammatory affections occurring in nervous individuals. In the recognition of the chronic form, however, he approaches remarkably near, as Mueller points out, to the modern conception of neurasthenia. His division into the forms above enumerated closely calls to mind some of the well-known clinical forms recognized at the present day, such as the spinal and gastro-intestinal forms. Others of his forms, however, such as the *nervosisme paralytique, spasmodique*, and *douloureux*, prove that he still confounded other affections with neurasthenia. Great as had been the step forward, much was still left to be desired; Bouchut's writings were simply rough indications along pathways still undefined.

It remained for an American physician, George M. B. Beard, to give to the affection under consideration a true individuality and a name by which it subsequently became known to the entire civilized world—namely, neurasthenia. The introduction of this word at once gave definiteness to the conception of the disease, while the descriptions given by Beard added much to our knowledge of its symptoms. Although Beard, like his predecessors, made many statements which increasing experience proved to be erroneous, he notwithstanding had clear conceptions as to the nature of the affection. He believed it to be a chronic functional disease, the cause of which lies in a diminution of nervous strength, this in turn being dependent upon an impaired or defective nutrition of nervous tissues. He also recognized clearly that it was not caused by anemia. He ascribed the various symptoms observed by him to reflex phenomena in which the sympathetic and the vasomotor nerves played important rôles. Beard's writings attracted great attention, especially abroad, and numerous papers by Continental writers tended, some to further elucidate our knowledge of the disease, and others, to increase confusion. The conception of neurasthenia, however, became firmly engrafted upon medical literature.

The first use of the word neurasthenia in this connection, it should here be added, was not made by Beard, but, as C. H. Hughes of St. Louis has pointed out, by E. H. Van Deusen, of Kalamazoo, Michigan, who first used the word in the supplement to the Biennial Report of the Michigan Asylum for the Insane for 1867. He says, among other things: "Our observations have led us to think that there is a disorder of the nervous system, the essential character of which is well expressed by the term given above, and so uniform in development and progress that it may with propriety be regarded as a distinct form of disease." Van Deusen, however, did not follow up his suggestion, and it is also quite certain that Beard, although his first publication did not appear until 1869, in the "Boston Medical and Surgical Journal," had no knowledge of Van Deusen's views. The word neurasthenia, though perhaps invented independently by both Beard and Van Deusen, is apparently much older. Thus, it is found in the first edition of "Dunglison's Medical Dictionary," published in 1833; contemporaneous English, French, and German dictionaries, however, do not contain it.

Beard's publications were very numerous and extended from 1869 to 1881. He was the first writer to present a separate treatise on nervous exhaustion. While he advanced many views which to-day are untenable—for instance, that neurasthenia is a modern disease, that it is an American disease, that neurasthenic persons suffer less from febrile and inflammatory affections than others or that they are especially predisposed to disease of the teeth, that they are mostly persons of fine physical development, that they are persons who are capable of an unusual amount of work, mental and physical, that neurasthenics are more youthful in appearance than other persons, and similar partial observations—he nevertheless was the first writer to entertain clear conceptions of the disease; and when we reflect upon the great importance of the subject, we can justly claim for Beard that he initiated a new epoch in practical medicine.

The contributions of Beard to our clinical knowledge of neurasthenia were destined to be supplemented by a still greater achievement in the field of therapeutics. Time had waited for the genius of another American physician, S. Weir Mitchell, to apply in the treatment of this disease, and a kindred affection, hysteria, the principle of rest. Dr. Mitchell's first publication on this important subject appeared in 1875 in Seguin's Séries of American Clinical Lectures, volume I, No. IV, on "Rest in the Treatment of Nervous Diseases." Subsequently, in a treatise entitled "Fat and Blood, an Essay on the Treatment of certain Forms of Neurasthenia and Hysteria," and in his "Lectures on Diseases of the Nervous System, especially in Women," he published his views and methods in greater detail. It is difficult at this day, more than forty years after Weir Mitchell's first utterance upon the subject, to appreciate the importance and the radical character of this innovation in therapeutics. In the treatment of chronic affections, as in that of acute diseases, physicians had been in the habit of relying almost exclusively upon medicines; and when other remedies, such as massage or electricity, were employed, they were used in an independent and isolated manner. They were not incorporated as parts of any one method or plan of treatment, and, as regards rest, it is safe to say that up to the time of Mitchell no one had had any adequate conception of its importance or of its great therapeutic power. No one had ventured to employ it in so radical a manner nor in a way involving weeks and months of continuous stay in bed. The ill effects of excessive rest—of insufficient exercise—had been vaguely recognized, but no one had attempted to combat the disadvantages of rest—to rob it of its harm by the application of corrective procedures; no one had attempted to formulate a plan of treatment in which rest should be the main therapeutic measure—rest so guarded and corrected that none of its evils, only its benefits, should accrue to the patient. It is this achievement which belongs to Weir Mitchell, an achievement which is distinctly and solely his. The rest cure is essentially a cure by physiologic methods, and this alone is sufficient to give it the stamp of originality.

We have seen, in considering the general application of rest to neurasthenia, that the treatment must be based upon broad physiologic principles. Rest must be supplemented by exercise, either active or passive; the starved tissues must be supplied with food; waste products must be eliminated. In the application of these principles, no one method can be followed. Each case demands a special application in accordance with its individual needs. Some cases demand relative rest with active exercise; others, again, rigid seclusion with passive exercise. Further, the rest cure, as well as the treatment by relative rest, must be expanded so as to include all of the physiologic methods at our disposal. Especially should the treatment include some method of facilitating the elimination of the waste products. How the latter tend to accumulate in neurasthenia, and how injuriously they affect the organism by their retention, we have seen. Evidently there should be added to the treatment, the free ingestion of liquids, and some form of hydrotherapy. How efficacious the methods of hydrotherapy are in assisting the elimination of waste products has more than once been stated in these pages, and the importance of this point cannot be too strongly accentuated. Rest methods not infrequently fail if means are not taken to stimulate the elimination of uric acid and its metabolic congeners. The rôle which the diet plays in the attainment of this end we have already dwelt upon. Finally, we should bear in mind that into every plan of rest treatment, even the most rigid, exercise must sooner or later enter, and that exercise in some form or other must be persisted in subsequently.

REST IN NEURASTHENIA TERMINALIS

When neurasthenia persists for a long time, and especially if it be profound, it no longer remains a purely functional disease. Prolonged and persistent derangement of function is inevitably followed by tissue changes. A heart that is constantly overacting, that is subjected to repeated and violent attacks of palpitation or perhaps more or less persistent tachycardia, may undergo hypertrophy; subsequently degeneration of the cardiac walls and dilatation may ensue. Similarly, changes, degenerative in nature, take place in the blood-vessels. Actual organic changes also occur in the digestive tract. How readily gastric catarrh becomes superimposed upon a pure gastric atony, we have already seen, and if gastric catarrh persist sufficiently long, the function of the stomach may become permanently deranged. That alterations also occur in other structures, such as the muscles, there can be no doubt; indeed, not even the bones are exempt. The changes in the muscles and bones are analogous to those seen in the blood-vessels; they are those of premature senescence. The muscles of the limbs become flat and flabby, while the changes in the cranium and face suggest the shrinkage of old age. Like the lesions of senescence, the changes here described are permanent in character, and this fact is of the utmost importance as regards prognosis and treatment. The clinical picture presented is that of a profound and chronic neurasthenia, to which I have given the name of neurasthenia terminalis. It is probable that the lesions are the result not only of persistent nervous and physical overstrain, but also of the various toxic substances present in the blood, themselves the result of excessive or perverted tissue metabolism. The presence of waste products in excess easily explains the existence of degenerative changes in the vessel-walls and in the organs, such as general arteriosclerosis, sclerotic changes in the kidneys, and perhaps changes in other organs, including the nervous structures. Of course, if undoubted degeneration of the substance of the heart is present the case must be classified as one of myocarditis; if true and evident arteriosclerosis exists, the case must be classified as one of arteriosclerosis; if undoubted interstitial changes are present in the kidneys the case must be classified as one of contracted kidney. If there are present merely the general changes of early and premature aging together with the history and symptoms of chronic nervous exhaustion extending over a long period of time, the case deserves to be classified under the caption of neurasthenia terminalis.

Terminal neurasthenia is established, as a rule, only after a simple neurasthenia, profound in character, has existed for a number of years. Occasionally, however, it comes on in a relatively short period. An important factor in its development is the age of the individual, the disease being more readily induced in persons at or beyond middle age. It is, however, occasionally seen in young persons; thus it is met with not infrequently in the breakdown of athletes who have persistently overtrained. The neurasthenia in such cases is usually very persistent, and very difficult of treatment.

The **prognosis** in neurasthenia terminalis is, of course, never so favorable as in neurasthenia simplex. There are forms so grave that the degree of improvement possible is very limited. Nevertheless, profound as are the symptoms, some improvement, and at times very marked improvement, follows a properly adapted and elaborate plan of treatment.

The **treatment** by **rest** must be **modified** in several important particulars. First, it must be pointed out that absolute rest, in neurasthenia terminalis, is not devoid of danger. Great and persistent weakness may ensue if a patient with terminal neurasthenia remain persistently in bed for a long time; indeed, through the injudicious application of rest, an individual still able to be about and otherwise capable of considerable improvement may be converted into a bedridden invalid. The mere employment of massage and electricity may not suffice to prevent this result. Rest in such cases should never be absolute, save for a very short time. The patient should be permitted to get out of bed and to exercise gently about the room once or twice daily soon after beginning treatment—sometimes within a few days. In other words, in addition to massage, exercise, though small in amount, must be added to the treatment. It is important also to bear in mind that these patients frequently do not bear massage well; even when not vigorous, massage may excite rather than soothe, or may increase the fatigue sensations. For this additional reason exercise should be employed early. Indeed, in pronounced terminal neurasthenia, exercise, gentle in character, should be instituted in the beginning; partial rest methods only should be employed at first, and as the treatment progresses the amount of rest may be cautiously increased; but let me repeat that it should never be made absolute for a prolonged period.

It is further important to bear in mind that the other physiologic methods at our disposal cannot be used so vigorously as in the case of simple neurasthenia. This is especially true of the bathing. As a rule, the latter must be limited to a warm sponge bath daily. It is but rarely possible to use cold douching or spraying. The patients react badly and are easily depressed.

Finally, rest methods should be pursued in terminal neurasthenia for a very long time, and, after the greatest possible improvement has been attained, a careful hygienic plan of living should be adopted, which the patient should follow subsequently.

Persons with terminal neurasthenia often take spontaneously to their beds and in the course of time become confirmed bedridden invalids. Such cases, especially if they have been bedridden for a number of years are, of course, those which present the greatest difficulty in treatment, and yet remarkable victories may be gained, even under these circumstances, provided that all of the conditions necessary to a successful rest treatment be complied with by the patient and the patient's friends; among these conditions, it should be added, isolation is of the utmost consequence.

In cases in which the patient has been lying in bed for so long a period that exercise has become next to impossible, gentle bathing and gentle massage should, of course, be instituted, but most important of all is the stimulation of the excretion of waste products.

In terminal neurasthenia the deficient thirst, already observed as a prominent symptom of simple neurasthenia, is most pronounced. The patient consumes but small quantities of liquids as well as grossly insufficient amounts of solid food. The first indication therefore is the **free ingestion of liquids**—milk and especially water. Gentle saline laxatives and at times irrigation of the bowel should be employed. At the same time the general **dietetic** principles already considered in discussing the treatment of simple neurasthenia should be applied. Piperazin, the lithia waters, or the milder salicylates, salophen, or aspirin, may be administered. By these means, especially by the thorough washing out of the system produced by the free and continued ingestion of liquids, it may be possible to start the patient on the road to improvement. A slight gain is made especially in the lessening of fatigue sensations, and, this being carefully followed up by the feeding and massage, it is frequently possible after a considerable time to get the patient out of bed. **Exercise,** very gentle, of course, can then be instituted and a marked degree of improvement—a relative cure —be brought about.

REST IN THE NEURASTHENIA OF MIDDLE LIFE

The neurasthenia of middle life differs in several particulars from the neurasthenia of youth and early adult life. In middle life, nutrition is no longer so active as in earlier years. Metabolic and tissue-forming processes are on the eve of involution. Strains are less well borne, reaction is less prompt, repair is less complete. If, therefore, at this period the organism be subjected to unphysiologic conditions, to overwork, to insufficient sleep, to social dissipation, to sexual excess, or to other exhausting factors, a condition of more or less profound nervous exhaustion is induced. Further, this exhaustion is, as a rule, very persistent; it always lasts a number of months and not infrequently several years. In women its symptoms are commonly confounded with the **menopause.** The relation between the neurasthenia of middle life and the menopause is, however, merely one of concomitance. Sexual involution is a perfectly physiologic procedure and does not of itself induce neurasthenia. Further, the neurasthenia of middle life is not by any means limited to women, but occurs quite frequently in men. The symptoms are those of ordinary simple neurasthenia, to which in women the signs of the menopause may be added. The symptoms may, it is true, be accentuated at the times of the menstrual epoch, or may be influenced by metrorrhagia or other complications, but in a large number of neurasthenic women in middle life, the menopause plays no rôle whatever.

Applying **rest principles** to the treatment of this condition, we should bear in mind, first, the diminished activity of the nutritive processes; secondly, the tendency of the symptoms to persist for a long time; and, thirdly, the tendency of women at middle life to accumulate fat. In response to the first indication, we should whenever possible institute **full rest treatment**; that is, continuous rest in bed. For patients whose circumstances, pecuniary or otherwise, make a full rest treatment impossible, **partial rest methods** may be instituted, but, as might be supposed, these are far less efficacious; as a rule, they yield a very imperfect result. In many cases, indeed, no impression whatever can be made upon the symptoms. Strict rest methods, elaborate and detailed, are required in the larger number of patients. Secondly, the rest treatment must be **prolonged**. We soon notice that our patient reacts less readily and gains more slowly than does the younger neurasthenic. The various symptoms are not only persistent but often tenacious and obstinate. Absolute rest, careful massage, the thorough washing out of the tissues by the free ingestion of liquids, the use of electricity, and, especially, the carrying out of rigid isolation are the means which must be employed. They must, as a rule, be extended over a long period—three or four months or more. In some cases the treatment should be followed by partial rest methods with persistent exercise for many months longer.

Many women who are neurasthenic at middle life, like younger patients, are very thin and much below weight; others, however, tend to accumulate fat, and in these cases the general principles already indicated for the management of obese cases should be followed (see p. 69). It is well to bear in mind also that the adiposity may be in direct relation with deficient ovarian and thy-

roid activity. Here, a careful and judicious use of thyroid extract
or of lutein may prove of advantage.

REST IN THE NEURASTHENIA OF OLD AGE

As we approach the latter period of life, that ebb in the tide of
nutrition, which begins in middle life, becomes gradually more and
more pronounced. Little by little the ability to expend energy in
large amount is diminished. It is hardly necessary to state that
the man of sixty or seventy is no longer able to do the mass of work
of the man of thirty or forty. Changes inevitable, physiologic and
consequent upon life itself, gradually diminish the power for sustained work. We are hardly called upon here to enumerate the
changes that take place in the tissues as the last decades of life are
reached, to dwell upon the alterations in the blood-vessels, the
wasting of the muscles, the brittleness of the bones, the atrophy of
glandular structures, in short, the degenerations, atrophic, sclerotic,
and fatty, met with in old age; nor should it be necessary to point
out that in old age nervous exhaustion can very readily be induced.

The problem of treatment in the neurasthenia of old age is
essentially a problem of physiologic living. As a matter of course,
rest must be employed, and yet, for obvious reasons, rest should not
be absolute or unduly prolonged. The treatment is essentially
that of neurasthenia terminalis (see pp. 75 *et seq.*). As in the
latter affection, continuous rest for long periods is not devoid of
danger. The weakness of senile neurasthenia may be increased if
rest be too rigidly instituted. Here again we are confronted by
the question of rest and **gentle exercise** properly proportioned.
As a rule, a very large amount of rest—rest but little short of continuous rest—is well borne, provided it be broken by short periods
of sitting up out of bed or walking about the room once or twice
daily. As soon as practicable, exercise in the open air, either
walking or carriage-riding, is to be undertaken, and later on this
exercise is very gradually to be increased.

Massage, so useful in other forms of neurasthenia, should in
old age be used with much discretion. It must indeed be begun
in a tentative way; it should at first be very light and not too deep.

Should unpleasant sensations, faintness, dizziness, or restlessness follow, it must, of course, be discontinued. By many old people, however, massage is well borne, and in such cases continuous rest in bed may for a time be instituted. Bathing should be limited, as a rule, to the daily warm sponge bath between blankets. The general principles indicated in the diet of simple neurasthenia, modified by special indications, should also be followed. Full feeding should be practised, but great care is necessary not to over-feed. The quantity of food should at first be relatively small and should only be increased very gradually. Milk, as in other forms of neurasthenia, is of great value. Errors of digestion, constipation, the gouty diathesis, must be borne in mind. In the way of medicines, the simplest and most necessary only should be employed. These have already been fully considered. Hypnotics, it should especially be remembered, should be used very cautiously, and in the beginning in tentative doses only.

Little by little the amount of rest should be diminished and the hours of outdoor living increased, but in many cases a more or less permanent adherence to measures embodying early going to bed, late rising, and rest during the middle of the day will be found necessary. While senile neurasthenia offers, on the whole, a much less promising field than other forms, it is remarkable how great a degree of improvement can frequently be attained, and this improvement is often synonymous with an actual prolongation of life.

THE NEURASTHENOID STATES

Thus far we have discussed rest methods in relation to neurasthenia alone. It will be necessary to say a word as to the exact position which neurasthenia occupies toward related states. At the present day there still exist, not only in the mind of the general practitioner, but often in the minds of specialists, the most vague and ill-defined notions concerning neurasthenia. Not only do we hear from clinicians of the highest standing allusions made and views expressed in regard to neurasthenia which disclose that this all-important affection has never received serious study at their hands, but this is true even of some neurologists and alienists.

Neurasthenia, as we have seen, presents itself as a well-defined symptom-complex. While the picture is somewhat varied in different cases and often complicated by the appearance of secondary symptoms, its essential and underlying features are always those of a chronic exhaustion, a persistent fatigue. Further, the picture that has been outlined in the preceding pages is that of an exhaustion affecting an organism otherwise normal, and to this affection the term neurasthenia simplex should be applied. That the clinical picture must be more or less modified when the organism has been previously neuropathic, would seem probable on *a priori* grounds and this the facts prove to be actually the case. An individual who is not neuropathic may from overwork or other nervous overstrain develop nervous exhaustion, but, if he happen to be neuropathic, special symptoms are developed which by their prominence dominate the clinical picture, indeed, often to such an extent that the factor of the nervous exhaustion is lost sight of. Neuropathy, we should remember, is expressive of basic morphologic and functional deviations and weaknesses, of deficiencies and aberrations inherent in the nervous system. When such a nervous system is subjected to exhaustion, the symptoms of the resulting neurasthenia are much modified; indeed, this goes without saying. Thus, fear may now present itself as a phobia, an obsession, an anxiety; hesitation and lack of decision as a veritable insanity of indecision; weakness of will as a pronounced aboulia, while deficient inhibition may lead to the picture of a compulsion neurosis. I have given to this group of cases the appellation "neurasthenic-neuropathic" or "neurasthenoid." Janet has applied to it the term psychasthenia. We will return to their detailed consideration in the second part of this book.

Another group of cases to which the term neurasthenoid may be applied is made up of individuals who are likewise neuropathic by heredity but who never develop well-defined clinical pictures. They betray by their weaknesses and deficiencies their lack of inhibition, excessive irritability and other vagaries, the abnormality from which they suffer and which has perhaps in ancestral or collateral lines expressed itself in definite mental disease. The condition may be described as a congenital psychopathic state.

It is a true organic, constitutional inferiority. It may manifest itself as an innate, **constitutional nervousness**, or it may be especially featured by an habitual morbid depression, or perhaps by an habitual, constitutional excitability. The organism as a whole is weak and its resistance to depressing influences of all kinds deficient. Frequently a history of excessive illness in childhood is present and is significant, other things equal, of feebleness of resistance to infection. Frequently, too, there is a history of delayed and defective dentition, of a tendency to delirium or convulsions, of disturbed sleep, of night terrors, of excessive dreaming or of somnambulism. Puberty is at times much delayed and in females is established with difficulty and often with much general disturbance. At other times puberty makes its appearance too early and the patient manifests unusual sexual precocity. The patient is frequently of slight and delicate physique and sometimes bears upon his person the stigmata of arrest and deviation. School is attended with indifferent success, at times with retardation and study is frequently interrupted by illness. On the other hand, the patient may present a history of unusual precocity, and yet as adult life is approached his capacity is found to be limited, perhaps below mediocrity. Occasionally the intelligence appears to be normal or the patient may even be gifted, but too often fate relegates him to the rank of the incapables. Aimlessness, lack of persistence, change of plans, incompleted undertakings, spasmodic efforts, are common in the personal history. As a rule the patient is thin and below weight; less frequently he is obese and anemic.

It is evident, of course, that the states above described have no relation with true neurasthenia, although medical writers—especially the Freudians—habitually confound the two conditions. Inasmuch as the psychopathic organization is attended by a more ready exhaustion than that of the normal individual, the two states present certain resemblances; namely, rapid appearance of fatigue phenomena and increased irritability. Further, inasmuch as neuropathic subjects are quite prone to develop states of exhaustion, the resulting clinical picture may—as I have already pointed out on page 82—be a compound of neuropathy and neurasthenia. Notwithstanding, as Kraepelin also maintains, we cannot ignore the fundamental difference between congenital neuropathy and acquired neurasthenia. In the latter there are present merely the simple facts of exhaustion, while in the former there are present in greater or lesser degree those changes in thinking, acting and feeling which are expressive of degeneracy and insanity.

Physicians must also be careful to distinguish from neurasthenia the vague nervous symptoms which are present in the long prodromal periods of various psychoses; such symptoms are **neurasthenoid**, never truly neurasthenic; it is a mistake, for instance, to say that a patient who passes into melancholia after a long prodromal period of nervous and hypochondriacal symptoms has had a neurasthenia which has deepened into melancholia. The patient has merely passed through a prodromal period. As a matter of clinical fact, neurasthenia simplex never eventuates in mental disease. The above considerations are of the greatest practical importance. Especially is this the case from the standpoint of prognosis. Acquired neurasthenia in the previously normal subject offers under given conditions a uniformly favorable prognosis. In neuropathic subjects, on the other hand, the prognosis must be guarded in proportion to the existence and prominence of symptoms indicative of the preëxisting neuropathy. In the second part of this book the treatment of neuropathic-neurasthenic states is considered in detail. Suffice it to say here that it is based upon general rest and psychotherapeutic principles.

NEURASTHENIA SYMPTOMATICA

It goes without saying that visceral or general somatic disease may be—and frequently is—attended by weakness or exhaustion. It is conceivable that serious local disease—for example, organic disease of the stomach or pelvic disease—should weaken the entire organism, and with it the nervous system; and that various signs of nervous weakness should be present is but natural; but these signs do not make up that disease which we know as neurasthenia simplex. They are symptoms of nervous weakness such as accompany other diseases, either local or general. They are seen, for instance, in tuberculosis, in chlorosis, in the various anemias, in the toxemias due to infection or metallic poisoning, and in other grave disturbances of nutrition; but they form in such cases a very subsidiary and very unimportant group of the symptom-complex. At most, they constitute merely a **neurasthenia symptomatica.** Here, again, the diagnosis is to be made, first, by the absence of, or departure from, the typical fatigue syndrome; and, secondly, by a careful and systematic internal examination. Physicians are not wanting who fall into the gross error of regarding all neurasthenia as directly due to some local condition; *e.g.*, a movable kidney or a displacement of the uterus. Thus, the view was formerly entertained that various nervous disorders, and among them neurasthenia, were the direct result of **pelvic lesions.** However, an increasing knowledge has not borne out this belief. It is found, for instance, that the nervous symptoms caused by pelvic disease are not at all those of neurasthenia and are quite limited. There is present pelvic pain, pain referred to the back, hips, and thighs, together with more or less marked impairment of the general health, but the symptoms do not constitute a nervous disease, and least of all, neurasthenia. They are part of the pelvic disease itself and are directly symptomatic of it.

On the other hand, the physician must be warned against making the opposite error of mistaking a symptomatic neurasthenia for a simple neurasthenia. Here the failure to recognize the true nature of the case may lead to irreparable loss of time; *e.g.*, in the ill health attending a chronic appendicitis or a disease of the gall-bladder.

If a serious operation is to be performed concerning which there is no urgency, a preliminary course of rest in bed may be of value, especially when the condition of the patient is unsatisfactory. More frequently, however, it is of value after the operation, and if carried out radically may add greatly to the improvement of the patient's health.

CHAPTER IV

HYSTERIA

Hysteria, a Hereditary and Innate Neuropathy. Mental Character of the Symptoms. Sensory, Motor, Visceral and Mental Phenomena. Etiologic and Pathologic Factors. Treatment by Rest and Physiologic Methods. Psychotherapy. Attitude of Physician to Patient. The Nurse. Auxiliary Measures—Feeding, Bathing, Massage, Electricity. Treatment of Special Symptoms. Hysteria and Accident Compensation.

THE NATURE OF HYSTERIA

In order to discuss intelligently the treatment of hysteria, it will be necessary as in the case of neurasthenia first to acquire a clear conception as to the nature of the affection. Our knowledge of hysteria has been of very slow and gradual evolution. The story of the early views, their gradual modification and the final recognition in recent times of the actual truth forms one of the most interesting chapters in the history of medicine. The early Greeks believed that the explanation of the phenomena which they witnessed was to be sought in the behavior of the uterus. They believed, for instance, that during a hysteric attack the uterus becomes detached from its moorings and goes wandering about the body seeking sexual satisfaction. Plato informs us that the uterus is an organism which ardently desires to engender offspring and that when it remains sterile for a long time, it can bear the fact with difficulty, becomes exasperated, runs about the body, obstructs the air passages, arrests the respiration, throws the body into extreme dangers and causes various diseases, until desire and love, uniting man and woman, bring about the birth of fruit.*

* See Gilles de la Tourette, "Traité Clinique et Therapeutique de l'hysterie," 1891, p. 2.

Hippocrates tells us that if the uterus goes to the liver the woman at once loses her voice, clenches her teeth and her color becomes dark; further, that these attacks come on suddenly in full health and that they occur especially in the unmarried and widows. The theory of the uterine origin of hysteria finds expression also in the writings of Celsus, Galen and others. Galen, however, treated as absurd the view attributed to Plato of the ascension of the uterus during a hysteric attack. His anatomical knowledge apprised him that the uterus could not travel from the vulva to the xyphoid cartilage. Galen appears also to have been the first to recognize that hysteria is not confined to women.

For us the chief interest in the **uterine theory** of hysteria lies in the fact that it has served to fasten the name hysteria derived from hystera (ὐστέρα, the Greek word for womb) upon the affection. It is interesting to note that while the crude theory of the wandering uterus has long been abandoned, ideas as to the sexual origin of hysteria have persisted, in modified forms, up to our own day. Unsatisfied passion, unrequited love, genital irritation and, lastly, repressed memories of sexual peccadilloes in childhood—advocated by the Freudian school—have in turn served to befog the subject, to surround it with a veil of mystery and to lend it a prurient interest. However, from the days of Sydenham to those of Charcot, it became increasingly evident that the symptoms of hysteria are nervous or mental in origin, and, further, that they bear no relation to the sexual organs. Operations upon the sexual organs of women, such as the removal of the ovaries or uterus, leave the hysteria uninfluenced; and it has been known for a long time also that hysteria occurs in men as well as in women.

Interesting, also, though of less importance for our purpose, are the accounts of the **epidemics** of hysteria occurring in Europe during the sixteenth and seventeenth centuries. Hecker describes an epidemic which occurred at Aix-la-Chapelle in 1574. Troops of men and women coming from Germany offered in the streets and in the churches a very strange spectacle. Holding hands and no longer in control of their senses, they danced entire hours and continued this behavior unrestrained by the presence of bystanders until they fell exhausted to the earth. Then they complained of great pain and groaned as if they felt the approach of death. This was kept up until their abdomens were tightly constricted by sheets after which they came to themselves, being at once relieved of their trouble. This procedure seems to have been suggested by the tympany which made its appearance after the fit. Sometimes a more simple method was resorted to, the patients being given severe blows with the fist or the foot upon the belly. During the dance, they had apparitions, they neither saw nor heard what was going on about them, and their imaginations made them see spirits the names of which they spoke or rather hurled forth. When the attack was completely developed, it began by a convulsion. The patient fell to the ground, panting, unconscious and frothing at the mouth. Soon he got up by bounds and commenced his dance accompanied by hideous contortions. In the course of some months, the epidemic spread to the low countries. Analogous epidemics occurred in the tarantism of Italy and in the demoniac possession which invaded the convents of Germany from 1550 to 1660. France, too, suffered from similar outbreaks. The salient feature which these epidemics illustrate is that hysteria under given circumstances may become contagious.

Little progress at first was made in the knowledge of hysteria. Ambroise Paré writing in the sixteenth century still describes the uterus as the seat of the affection, and Fernal reproaches Galen for having said that the uterus did not move about and thus produce the hysteric attack. However, in 1618 a French physician, Charles Lepois (Carolus Piso), made a definite break with the past and described hysteria as a nervous disease. Sydenham in England took the same stand, as also did Willis. Louyer-Villermay writing in 1816 again adopted the theory of the wandering uterus and attributed the symptoms to a spermatic plethora! The occurrence of hysteria in man was denied as late as 1833 by Dubois and again in 1846 by Landouzy, while Hufeland maintained that hypochondria was the corresponding affection in man. Romberg explained the symptoms of hysteria as reflex from an irritation of the uterine system. He declared that women must be sexually ripe to have hysteria and, further, naturally restricted hysteria to the female sex.

Ollivier, Todd and Isaac Porter recognizing the nervous character of the symptoms maintained that hysteria had its origin in the spinal cord. Georget, writing in 1821, declared that inasmuch as it could be produced by psychic causes, it must have its origin in the brain. Briquet, however, in 1859 was the first to make a clear presentation of hysteria in the modern sense, basing his account on a close systematic study of the affection. He regarded hysteria as a dynamic affection of those portions of the brain that have to do with the affects and perceptions. He declared that the excitability of these portions is increased so that affective reactions no longer pursue a normal course but are excessive, disordered, and perverted; that the uterus and stomach are never the seat of hysteria, and that these organs never reveal anything except when the brain directs toward them its manifestations.

Briquet's views are remarkable for the emphasis which he lays on the morbid action of the emotions and his denial of any rôle to the spinal cord, the peripheral nerves or the viscera.

The pathway leading in the direction of the truth clearly lay, henceforth, in the clinical study of the symptoms. Charcot, it will be remembered, studied not only the hysteric convulsion, but also studied his patients in the intervals between the attacks and thus arose quite naturally a division of the symptoms into those of the paroxysms and those of the interparoxysmal period. Now began a most elaborate study in which not only the name of Charcot but that of his pupils, Paul Richer and Gilles de la Tourette, became historic. In the interparoxysmal period disturbances of sensation, of motion, of the special senses, of the viscera were elaborately recorded, mapped out and charted. Very soon the world was presented with a detailed symptomatology. Accurate descriptions were given of the various "stigmata," the painful spots and hyperesthesias, the anesthesias, palsies, spasms, the contraction of the visual fields—in short a remarkable presentation of the most varied symptoms. In their ensemble they formed a structure of fascinating interest and which led logically and inevitably to the discovery of the final truth, a truth as revolutionary as it was unexpected and astonishing. Charcot clearly divined something of the nature of hysteria when he drew an analogy between hys-

teria and hypnosis, and, also, when he emphasized the hysteric
nature of the "traumatic neurosis." Moebius, however, appears
to have been the first to maintain that all of the symptoms of hysteria were of **psychic origin.** He pointed out that the hysteric
person reacts, without being hypnotized, like one under hypnosis.
It remained, however, for the genius of Babinski to make the next
great advance.

A symptom frequently elicited in persons presenting hysteria
is a loss of sensation, an anesthesia in a limb or in some portion
of the body. Quite commonly the loss of sensation embraces an
area covering a hand and part of an arm like a glove, or a foot and
a leg like a sock or a stocking. Such a sensory loss is, of course,
totally at variance with the anatomical facts of nerve distribution
and supply. We need but recall the distribution of the ulnar and
median nerves to realize how radically different would be the result
of lesion of the median or ulnar nerve in producing an anesthesia.
A lesion of the ulnar nerve, for instance, would give rise to a loss
of sensation involving the little finger, the outer half of the ring
finger and of corresponding areas of the hand and forearm. Similar definite facts obtain in regard to lesions of the other nerves of
the arm, and, in addition, there are associated facts of palsy and
wasting of special muscles and gross disturbances of nutrition which
make each picture of actual organic nerve lesion characteristic;
not by any possibility could a glove-like or stocking-like anesthesia
be brought about. Further, the same is true of lesions of the spinal
cord. Losses of sensation in a limb, due to a lesion of the spinal
cord, assume the direction of stripes running up and down, in the
direction of the length of the limb, each stripe, so to speak, being
definitely related to certain segments of the cord. It is obvious,
therefore, that a glove-like sensory loss of the hand or arm, for instance, cannot be due to a lesion or disturbance of the spinal cord.
If we attempt to correlate a glove-like anesthesia with a lesion of
the brain we find ourselves equally at fault. Lesions of the sensory
pathway conveying sensory impressions to the cortex of the brain
give rise to a loss of sensation involving one-half of the body and
the arm and leg on the same side; never to a glove-like loss. The
same is true when the lesion involves portions of the surface of the

brain. Depending upon the area involved, the patient may, for instance, be unable to recognize by touch familiar objects, although sensation may in many respects be well preserved; that is, there may be present an astereognosis; under no circumstances is there present a glove-like sensory loss. Only one inference is possible; namely, that a glove-like sensory loss is mental, not physical. The same fact, it may be now stated, is equally true of all the other phenomena presented by hysteria; all are of mental origin.

The next step in the interpretation of the symptoms was the recognition of the fact that they owe their origin to **suggestion**. It is here that Babinski made his great advance. As is, of course, well known a symptom frequently noted in hysteria is hemianesthesia. Babinski in testing 100 consecutive cases of hysteria *not previously examined by physicians*, for hemianesthesia, and being careful to avoid the making of any suggestion, failed to elicit the symptom in a single case. Again, the hemianesthesia is usually found upon the left half of the body. Babinski pointed out that the physician being usually right-handed, has the camel's hair brush, pin or other instrument, in his right hand and, facing his patient, naturally tests the left side of the patient first, thus suggesting the very hemianesthesia he is trying to discover. Quite commonly the examination is accompanied by the question "Do you feel this?" a question which naturally suggests to the patient that the doctor has a doubt upon the subject and is expecting the patient not to feel the pin-point, and soon the answer comes, "No, I do not feel it;" or "I hardly feel it at all."

In other words the supposed hemianesthesia is an artefact. It has no previous existence in the patient. It is directly produced by the physician. What is true of hemianesthesia is true, as we shall see, of all of the other phenomena of hysteria. All are the result either of **medical** or of other **suggestion**.

Another point becomes evident upon further investigation. If the physician test a healthy or normal individual for hemianesthesia making at the same time free use of suggestion both direct and indirect, he invariably fails to develop the symptom. In other words, the normal individual repels, the hysteric individual accepts the suggestion. It is this vulnerability to suggestion which is the most striking feature of hysteria. To the consideration of the neuropathy of hysteria we will presently return. Suffice it to say here that it always preëxists, is always innate in the individual.

Further, the anesthesia of hysteria presents a number of remarkable peculiarities. Thus, the patient previously unexamined never comes to the physician complaining of his anesthesia. Before the examination he has no knowledge of its existence. Again, even after it has been elicited during the medical examination, the patient does not conduct himself either during the examination or subsequently as though the part in question were really anesthetic. Thus, immediately after an examination, a patient who has been partially disrobed will not infrequently use an anesthetic hand in dressing herself in a most natural manner and apparently without the slightest impediment. Buttons, hooks, pins are adjusted without hesitation as though the patient had full knowledge of the position and physical qualities of these objects through touch. Spontaneously, too, the patient may without thinking perform various acts which would be incompatible with true sensory loss. Thus, a patient in whom an anesthesia has been well established may, when her case is not under discussion, pick up a kitten and stroke its fur or may possibly resume an interrupted piece of sewing, knitting or fancywork. Further, the hysteric anesthesia never becomes the seat of injury as is the case in organic anesthesia. The patient never burns or bruises the anesthetic part as is so frequently the case, for instance, in syringomyelia.

Again, when we study the symptoms of a given sensory loss closely, e.g., a hemianesthesia, we usually find that the patient does really feel, but says that he does not feel as well upon the anesthetic as upon the opposite side of the body; in other words, the symptom developed is that merely of a diminished sensation, a condition which has received the name of hypoesthesia or hypesthesia. When the test is being made, the question of itself—for the test is a question even when the physician does not ask it in words—arouses first a doubt in the patient's mind, followed immediately by a realization that the physician expects to find no feeling in the part and finally that there is no feeling. The mental phases are in rapid succession; "Do I feel it?" "I don't feel it as well as on the other side." "No, I don't feel it." In keeping with this fact, a sensory loss mild at first—a hypesthesia—frequently passes into one that is pronounced—an **anesthesia**. Especially is this apt to ensue in a much-examined case.

Further, areas of hysteric anesthesia are not fixed. Their distribution, boundaries, location, change and shift about with great frequency. It is not unusual, for instance, to see a complete transference of the hemianesthesia from one side to the other. It is not surprising, therefore, that examinations of the same case by different physicians yield different results. This is indeed just what our previous consideration of the subject would lead us to expect. In this connection it is interesting, also, to learn that cases of hysteria in a ward often change decidedly when the medical service changes; in other words, the cases vary with the examinations made by the changing chiefs and internes.

Finally, that the sensory loss of hysteria does not really exist is further proven by the following facts. Quite frequently during an examination, as we shall see, **painful superficial areas** are developed over various portions of the body; for instance, beneath the breast, over the groin and elsewhere over the trunk and limbs. It is an astonishing fact that commonly after a hemianesthesia has made its appearance, such painful areas can be developed on the very side in which loss of sensation has just supposedly been demonstrated.

That which is true of the development of the symptoms of sensory loss by suggestion is equally true of all of the other symptoms of hysteria, whether these consist of palsies, of symptoms referable to the various organs or to the general conduct or attitude of the patient. The origin and mechanism of a suggestion is not always so easy to trace as in the development of an anesthesia. Frequently, too, the suggestion is indirect in action and unexpected by those about the patient. This is well illustrated by the following case. Some years ago, Professor Raymond of Paris presented at the Neurologic Society of that city, a young woman suffering from a hysterical hemiplegia with contractures. The history of the case was that the patient and her husband, recently married, had spent their honeymoon at the seashore, and it so happened that in their daily walks they met an old man suffering from hemiplegia. No comment was made by the young woman, but some time after returning to her home, she began to walk as did the old man, while her limbs also assumed the positions of fixation and contracture. Obviously, such a result could only have occurred in a person in whom hysteria had preëxisted.

The facts justify no other conclusion than that hysteria is an affection which is **innate** in the individual; the hysteric woman or hysteric man is born, not made. It is a neuropathy which is characterized among other things by a pathological susceptibility to suggestion. This is a fact which has long been recognized. Moebius expresses it by saying that the hysterical person without being hypnotized reacts like a hypnotized person. The comparison gathers in force when we recall that Charcot and Gilles de la Tourette declared that the state of hypnosis is but a state of hysteria artificially induced.

Just as the reaction of the hysteric subject is so excessive as to be pathological, so is his reaction to emotional stimuli excessive and pathological. That the hysteric patient laughs and cries more readily than do normal persons is a fact of common experience. Emotional instability and exaggerated emotional expression are symptoms of every-day observation. The hysteric person is more readily frightened than is the normal person. The fright is commonly out of all proportion to its cause. Very frequently the latter is trivial; so much so, at times, as to be practically non-existent. Among the many causes other than fright which may induce excessive emotional reaction, are joy, annoyance, anger, disappointment, mortification, fancied slights, wrongs or insults, grief, shame, the shock of sexual experiences, the worry over sexual peccadilloes, and kindred matters.

Given a reaction to suggestion and to emotional stimuli that is excessive, it follows as a physical corollary, that the mental state should express itself outwardly in an excessive physical reaction. Thus, the outward manifestations of fright are commonly very great; sometimes so much so as to appear to be in excess of any possible emotion. What is true of fright is, of course, true of all the other mental states. It is for this reason that an idea communicated by suggestion expresses itself with such extraordinary ease and rapidity in some corresponding outward reaction.

Another fact remains to be pointed out, namely that the duration of the outward reactions is very variable. This may be so brief as to be transient or even evanescent or it may persist a long time. When the matter is investigated we find that the symptoms persist so long as the suggestion which called them forth persists or remains uncorrected. This is seen typically in the hysteria developed in persons claiming compensation for alleged injuries. Here the symptoms persist until the claim is tried out in court, settled or otherwise disposed of. The hysterical plaintiff neither gets well nor improves, no matter what treatment is adopted, so long as his claim remains unsettled or so long as there is any hope of settlement.

A final word as to the neuropathy of hysteria remains to be said. First, hysteria is a neuropathy of degeneracy. Hysterical persons are relegated with few exceptions to the ranks of the incapables. It is characterized by lack of endurance, lack of persistence, lack of fixity of purpose, lack of those staying qualities which are necessary to bear the strain of life—necessary to success in the struggle for existence. The hysterical woman makes an inefficient servant, an inefficient wife and housekeeper, an inefficient mother; the hysterical man an inefficient workman, an inefficient provider for his family, an unsuccessful member of the community. The various faculties of the mind may reveal no special peculiarities; frequently, however, there is present a distinct mental subnormality.

In keeping with the above facts, it is not surprising that heredity is a marked factor. The hysterical strain can very commonly be traced from a hysterical mother through her various children. Again, the family histories may reveal other neuropathic disorders, mental disease and alcoholism. Charcot and his pupils regarded hysteria as an affection always inherited; all other factors have merely the value of "agents provocateurs;" they are merely incidental factors which may arouse the slumbering hysteria; they can never produce it.

A fact of great significance remains to be stated. Cases of hysteria presenting crass hemiplegia, hemianesthesia, contractures, blindness, deafness and like symptoms are found almost exclusively in the out-patient departments of hospitals and hospital wards. The private rooms rarely contain them. Neither are they found among the better middle or higher classes. The hysterical claimants in the courts, too, are, with rare exceptions, at the level of the out-patient class. Surely, we have here a fact of profound biological significance and one in keeping with the view that hysteria is a neuropathy of degeneracy. Hysteria when met with in the upper classes usually expresses itself by a more recondite and more purely psychic group of symptoms. When it expresses itself physically, if it does so at all, it commonly assumes the form of some visceral disturbance.

Résumé of the Symptomatology.

The above considerations of hysteria have made it clear that the detailed symptoms are always the result of suggestion, medical or other; they are always the outward expression of suggestion received. It becomes important that when once developed we should be able to recognize their spurious character, should be able to differentiate between them and the symptoms due to actual organic disease.

It is obvious that they may express themselves as sensory, motor, psychic and visceral disturbances. The **disturbances of sensation** may consist of anesthesia, hyperesthesia and less frequently of paresthesia. As already pointed out they bear no relation to the facts of anatomy. Thus, as we have seen, an anesthesia may involve the hand or hand and arm like a glove or the foot and leg like a stocking; or it may involve merely a segment of a limb; e.g., it may extend from the wrist to the elbow, being absent in the parts below and the parts above. Such an instance is spoken of as a segmental anesthesia. It may, on the other hand, be limited to a patch upon the trunk, limbs, or face; such an instance is spoken of as an islet-like anesthesia and if it have a regular shape like a circle, triangle or square, it is spoken of as a geometric anesthesia. Such vagaries, however, are very rare at the present day, doubtless due to a difference in the methods of medical examination.

Quite frequently, as we have seen, the anesthesia involves one-half of the body, constituting a hemianesthesia; very rarely it involves the entire body or almost the entire body. Some years ago a young woman appeared at my clinic with the statement that she had "universal anesthesia," that it involved every part of her body except her nipples, that she knew this was the case because she had been carefully examined by Dr. Blank while in the wards of ———— hospital. She recited in great detail the time the doctor had spent upon her case and the various instruments he had used in making his tests.

A hysteric hemianesthesia is distinguished from one of organic origin by two features: first, it is very sharply defined in the middle line of the body; secondly, it is of even intensity throughout its distribution. The sensory loss is just as great near the middle line of the body as it is over the distal portions of the extremities. In an organic hemianesthesia, for instance, one due to a lesion of the internal capsule and adjacent structures, the anesthesia is most pronounced over the foot and hand and grows progressively less as the trunk is approached upon which it may finally disappear long before the middle line is reached.

It should be added that the sensory losses of hysteria usually include all forms of sensation, but sometimes, though rarely, syringomyelia is simulated; that is, the patient, while admitting that he feels tactile impressions, may deny that he feels heat, cold or pain. Finally, it should be emphasized that the patient most frequently does not state that he does not feel at all in the part examined, but merely that he does not feel as well as elsewhere; in other words, merely a hypesthesia is present (see p. 92).

What has been said of the sensory losses of hysteria applies equally to the exaggerations and perversions of sensation. Most frequently the hyperesthesias of hysteria are developed in certain situations as isolated patches. These may be developed upon various portions of the trunk or limbs. Certain situations, however, are especially favored; especially a small oval area over the

7

ribs just beneath the mammary gland and another immediately over the groin. It is suggestive, too, that these painful areas are developed more frequently upon the left side of the body than upon the right and possibly for the same reason that, as Babinski points out, hemianesthesia is also found so frequently upon this half of the body. When found below the breast, the area is often spoken of as "**inframammary tenderness**" and when found over the groin, as "**inguinal tenderness.**" This so-called inguinal tenderness at one time gave rise to much confusion. It was early termed "ovarian tenderness," being supposedly due to a painful ovary, but experience soon showed that it had nothing whatever to do with the ovary. Years ago the French called the women presenting this symptom "ovariennes." Time and again, in this country and elsewhere, the ovary was removed by the surgeons, and notwithstanding, as a matter of course, the tenderness persisted.

Painful areas are developed with great frequency over the spine, e.g., in the neck, over the seventh cervical vertebra, between the scapulæ, in the lumbar region, over the sacrum or at the very end of the spine over the coccyx. Quite commonly, too, they are elicited to one side or other of the spine below the inferior angle of the scapula; at other times in small patches upon the scalp. In the latter situation they are usually quite small and at one time received the name "clavus hystericus," a term now no longer employed. Occasionally, if the vagina or rectum be included in the medical examination, patches of painful tenderness are developed in the mucous membranes of these structures. If in the vagina, the patient may state that she cannot have intercourse; i.e., may claim the symptoms of what has been termed vaginismus. That the mucous membranes reveal no change in appearance to the naked eye nor to any other examination need hardly be stated. In the case of vaginismus, the tenderness may be limited to small areas or it may involve the entire vagina and also the vulva. The purely psychic origin of vaginismus is well illustrated in an instance observed by the writer in which a young woman suffering from hysteria developed this symptom during the continuance of which she refused to receive her husband. She was visited by a sister, also a young married woman. The patient's recital of her symptoms was followed in the sister almost immediately afterward by an attack of the same symptoms, and she for a time likewise refused to receive her husband. Strangely enough in the hysteria of accident litigation similar conditions are claimed to exist. Time and again it is alleged that the marital act has become painful and that the plaintiff can no longer be a wife to her husband, and yet in more than one instance in the writer's experience, the plaintiff has become pregnant and been delivered of a child in the long delay pending trial.

Painful areas are sometimes developed in other situations, both upon the general body surface or the mucous membranes, but wherever occurring they are always the result either of the medical examination or of suggestions received previously from other sources.

The painful sensory areas are interesting historically because when occurring in the epidemics of the sixteenth and seventeenth centuries, they received the name "devil's spots," stigmata diaboli, and up to modern times the word **stigmata** (from στίγμα, spot or brand) has unfortunately been retained in speaking not only of the sensory phenomena but also of the symptoms of hysteria generally.

The unreal character of the tenderness, *i.e.*, the absence of tenderness, becomes apparent as soon as we begin to investigate it. If the finger of the examiner comes lightly in contact with the supposedly painful area, the patient reacts excessively—acts as though she were suffering acutely; but, the patient's attention having been directed to some other part of the examination and the finger or hand be now allowed to rest upon the supposedly painful area, no response is elicited, and this is equally the case if deep pressure be gradually made; the patient pays no attention to the area which a moment before appeared to be so painful. For instance, if painful areas or points of tenderness are elicited over the back or spine, and if the hand or fingers of the examiner be allowed to rest on these areas at the same time that the patient's attention is drawn to the front of the chest, to the abdomen or elsewhere—as when the physician, his hand still resting upon the tender area over the spine, proceeds to auscult the heart and in his conversation directs the attention of the patient to the heart's action—no response is made by the patient whether the supposedly painful area be pressed upon or not.

Because of the frequency and ease with which painful areas are developed over the back and spine in accident cases, three years ago gave rise to the term "railway spine." Among other terms that were formerly employed are "spinal tenderness," "spinal irritation," "spinal concussion," and vague theories of spinal anemia, spinal congestion, inflammation of the membranes of the spinal cord or of its substance, were made to do duty to explain the symptoms.

Another and very important sensory symptom remains to be considered. At times a patient will hold a limb in a fixed position and will complain of pain whenever an attempt is made to move it, the pain being referred to a joint; for instance, the ankle or the knee. The examination soon reveals that there is no tenderness in the joint at all. The patient who has her eyes upon every movement of the doctor, flinches whenever the skin covering the joint is touched, though ever so lightly, while a jar through the limb given stealthily and at a moment when the patient's attention is actively directly elsewhere is not followed by any reaction. Frequently also "hysteric joints" are associated with fixation and contracture of muscles. To this we will presently return. Naturally hysteric joints are more frequently observed in the lower extremities due to the more frequent incidence here of suggestion from trauma. They are also met with elsewhere.

The **motor phenomena** may manifest themselves as palsies, contractures, tremor, incoördination. Like the sensory phenomena they bear the impress of their mental character. Thus, the palsies bear no relation to the facts of anatomy and never conform to the symptom-groups observed in the organic palsies. A paralysis, like a hysteric anesthesia, may involve one limb—a monoplegia—or only a segment of a limb, e.g., the hand. It is never limited to individual muscles or a group of muscles. Palsies referable to a single nerve, e.g., the musculospiral or the ulnar nerve, are never witnessed. Again, the paralysis may involve homonymous portions of the body, for example both legs, and thus give rise to a paraplegia; or it may involve one-half of the body and give rise to a hemiplegia.

The palsy of hysteria may vary from a mere weakness to an apparent total loss of power. Most commonly it is attended by relaxation or flaccidity, though at times, the paralyzed part is rigid or spastic. When rigidity is pronounced, it may give rise to a marked fixation or contracture of the limbs. Usually, the nutrition of the muscles remains unaffected, but in cases of long duration, some diminution in volume, such as results from want of use, may be observed; a true degeneration of muscles, however, never occurs. A reaction of degeneration is, therefore, never present.

Very frequently the patient associates in his mind loss of power with loss of feeling and in such cases, the part involved may present both palsy and anesthesia. Not infrequently, if there be rigidity, fixation or contracture, the patient reacts as though the part were painful. The sensitiveness, tenderness or pain—however it may be described—is typical in that it is superficial and presents the other characteristics of painful hyperesthesia which have already been described. It is frequently associated with the so-called "hysteric joints" (see p. 100).

Hysteric paralysis is very variable in duration. Sometimes it is very persistent. This is seen typically in cases involving a claim for damages for supposed injuries. Here the palsy persists until the claim is disposed of, no matter what form of treatment may be adopted. A paralyzed arm, for instance, remains paralyzed until the case is settled; that is, the money actually paid over.

Very remarkable facts are also observed in connection with hysteric palsies. Not infrequently after an examination in which the palsy of a limb, say an arm, has been determined, the patient may, the case being no longer under discussion or apparently under observation, use the supposedly paralyzed member in resuming his clothing. The story of the plaintiff who was suffering from a paralyzed arm and who being asked to indicate how far he could raise the arm, moved it a very little and then being asked how far he had been able to move it before the accident raised the arm above his head, is corroborated by an instance in my own experience. Here the plaintiff, a woman, allowed the arm to remain hanging helplessly at her side, but being asked as to her control of the paralyzed member previous to her injury, unconsciously or forgetfully, showed me by moving the paralyzed arm instead of the sound one. Dejerine and Gauckler relate the following interesting instance.

A patient who was able to stand erect only a few minutes at a time, and who could not extend her arm longer than three seconds without the latter falling helplessly to her side, daily dressed her hair with great skill, this procedure consuming one hour. She did not, of course, realize the contradiction in her conduct. Lewandowsky speaks of patients who are able to exercise actively in the open air for hours at a time without fatigue, and who cannot perform the same exercises in their rooms longer than a few minutes before becoming completely exhausted.

It is hardly necessary to point out the special features which distinguish hysteric hemiplegia and paraplegia from the organic conditions which they grossly simulate. For instance, in a **hysteric hemiplegia** the arm is most frequently flaccid or nearly so and does not assume the position of secondary contracture usually met with in organic hemiplegia; the leg is usually more involved than the arm, is held somewhat stiffly or is dragged in walking as though it were dead and helpless; or curiously enough it is shoved in advance of the patient as he walks. The gait only superficially resembles that of organic hemiplegia.

Further, the muscles of the face are never paralyzed. There is never any involvement of the lower half of the face as in organic hemiplegia, and a total palsy of one-half of the face, such as is met with in Bell's palsy, likewise never occurs. The tongue when protruded sometimes deviates from the middle line, but in such case, it always deviates not to the paralyzed but to the sound side, exactly the reverse of that which occurs in a true hemiplegia, *i.e.*, in an organic hemiplegia in which the face is paralyzed on the same side as the arm and leg. Again, the palsy in hysteric hemiplegia is equally marked in all of the segments of the limbs. In true hemiplegia we know that the palsy, like the sensory loss, is most pronounced in the distal portions of the extremities and less marked in the portions proximal to the trunk. Thus, the hand and forearm are more affected than the arm and shoulder; the foot and leg, more than the thigh and hip.

Hysteric **paraplegia** is likewise as a rule readily differentiated from organic paraplegia. If the patient with a hysteric paraplegia walks, he usually makes use of canes or crutches. Quite commonly he handles the latter in such a way that they cannot be of any possible assistance either in bearing the weight or in locomotion. Frequently, he calls for his canes or crutches and when they are handed to him, rises from his chair before he has adjusted them. Quite commonly, too, he subconsciously withdraws his attention from his crutches, releases them and resumes his chair without their assistance. The gait, also, is very variable. Sometimes the legs are held stiffly and a spastic gait is simulated; at other times, though less frequently, the legs are handled as though merely weak; in either case the patient drags or shoves them along the floor. In other instances still, he throws them wildly about or moves them in some very irregular and grotesque manner.

Quite often the patient will declare that he is utterly unable to walk or even to sit up and, in such case, will remain continuously in bed. Under these circumstances he moves his legs about more or less spontaneously, especially when not under observation. Being urged by the physician to raise one of his legs off the bed, he may with much show of effort move it very slightly. If, while this test is being made, the physician slips his hand under the opposite limb, it is found that this limb although supposedly paralyzed is depressed into the bed, often with force. The procedure should then be repeated with the opposite limb. The test is especially valuable in hysteric monoplegia. If, in such instance, the physician having placed his hand under the paralyzed leg, directs the patient to raise the sound leg from the bed, the paralyzed leg is depressed into the bed in proportion to the degree and force with which the sound leg is elevated.

Again, in a true paraplegia the involuntary muscles are involved as well as those which move the limbs; namely, the sphincters. In hysteria the sphincters are never involved save in so far as they are under the control of the will. A true paralysis of the sphincters, such as occurs in a destructive lesion of the cord, never occurs in hysteria. An organic incontinence of the bladder with its constant overflow of urine, excoriation of the genitals and infection of the bladder, is never met with in hysteria. This is also true of the bowel, with its leakage and spontaneous and helpless evacuations into the bed. When examining a case of hysteric paraplegia, the absence of urinary or fecal odor or of stains of urine or fecal matter upon the clothing or bedding of the patient is a noteworthy fact. Physicians cannot, however, be too careful in making their examinations; especially reprehensible is conversation upon the question of the sphincters during the examination. The hysteric individual is remarkable for the readiness with which new symptoms are assumed and added to those already present. In several instances, I have known a patient presenting hysteric paraplegia, and in whom the sphincters were obviously intact, but who had been asked the question whether he could hold his water, subsequently to allow the urine to escape into his clothing or bedding, or even during the examination, upon his person. Similarly, though less frequently, we may meet with hysteric retention of urine. Both conditions are, of course, spurious and bear the earmarks of their mental character. Hysteric simulation of paralysis of the bowel I have not met with, but I have little doubt that under given conditions it could be produced. There is one condition, however, which hysteria does not simulate, and for obvious reasons, and that is the bed-sore. The back, the sacrum, the coccyx may become reddened and sensitive from continuous lying in bed, but the trophic sore with its sloughing base, its ragged edges and infected surfaces does not occur.

Finally, the motor phenomena of hysteric paraplegia have as their accompaniments, sensory phenomena which belong to the type of the stocking-like and segmental losses already described.

The **tendon reactions** in hysteria do not present constant phenomena. They may differ from the normal; they may be somewhat exaggerated though never, unless the patient has been trained by suggestion, to the degree seen in organic disease. On the other hand, they may be less than normal. They are never really lost, though here a caution is necessary. There are some persons, rare to be sure, who, though in apparent health, never have a knee-jerk. There are others, equally infrequent, in whom the knee-jerk is feeble and it is perfectly conceivable that under mental influences it may disappear altogether. Finally, the knee-jerk is normally absent in many children.

Similar remarks apply to the Achilles-jerk and to the ankle clonus. An ankle clonus is not infrequently elicited in hysteria, but it is usually of short duration. Occasionally, however, it is persistent, and this is not surprising when we realize how readily a persistent ankle clonus may be simulated by persons in perfect health. Finally, in studying the tendon reactions in hysteria, we must remember that the muscles called into play are under the influence of the will and that the reactions are, therefore, keenly sensitive to medical and other suggestion.

The **cutaneous reflexes** are almost uniformly preserved; they may, however, be lessened and in a few instances disappear. The latter, however, is never the case in those reflexes which are beyond the influence of the will. For example, in an anesthesia no matter how profound, the nipple will react, when touched, by contraction or erection, and this is also said to be true of the clitoris. Finally, the cremaster reflex is never influenced by hysteria; it likewise is a reflex independent of the will. Loss of the abdominal reflex, which has been described, but which I have never seen, may probably be due to the fact that the patient holds the abdominal wall tense and that he also closely observes the words and procedures of the doctor. It may be here stated that in performing many of the tests the patient should be so placed that he cannot see what is being done.

Not infrequently the plantar reflex is slight or lost. This reaction, however, loses much of its significance when we realize that in many adult persons it is normally absent. When, in a hemianesthesia, the plantar reflex is diminished or lost on the anesthetic side, and not on the sound side, we must bear in mind that the patient is very much alive to the reflexes on the normal side and that these may be, by contrast with the affected side, unusually pronounced, and finally the ever-present element of suggestion must be borne in mind. If the patient believes that his side is "dead," that he has lost power in it, which to his mind means both loss of motion and sensation, it stands to reason that the examiner will have great difficulty in eliciting any sensory or motor reactions into which psychic influences enter.

An invaluable sign is the absence of the Babinski reflex. This consists, as is well known, in the fact that when in an organic case of hemiplegia or other lesion of the pyramidal tract the sole of the foot be gently stimulated or irritated, the toes, especially the great toe, become extended. If the same test be made in a normal individual, the toes either do not move at all or they are flexed, i.e., are turned downwards. In hysteria, as just stated, this sign is necessarily absent. Caution, however, as in making other tests, must here be exercised. If the physicians indulge in conversation or discussion concerning the sign, the patient may promptly respond by extending the great toe and perhaps the others. In other words, the patient may be indirectly trained to produce the symptom. This I proved conclusively in a case in which obvious hysteria existed, but in which the toes responded by a prompt and full extension. The fact that the extension of the toes usually takes place rather slowly, is indeed often a little delayed, suggested to me that the reaction observed was not genuine. However, apparently accepting the symptom and concerning the presence and importance of which the attending physician was very voluble, I stroked the sole of the foot rapidly in succession with the tip of a wooden toothpick. Each stroke was followed by a prompt extension of the toes. I then repeated the test, again stroking the foot in rapid succession, but now while still making the gesture with my hand, I suddenly omitted to touch the sole of the foot. The patient promptly responded by an extension of the toes just as though the sole had been stroked, thus clearly demonstrating the spurious nature of the reaction.

As already stated, a paralyzed limb may instead of being flaccid present spasticity and contracture. The position assumed may be exceedingly bizarre or there may be flexion of the forearm upon the arm, with or without flexion of the hand, wrist and fingers upon the forearm. Similar phenomena may be observed in the lower extremity, though here the tendency is usually to rigidity with extension. The contractures only infrequently simulate those of organic disease. Particularly is this true of the positions assumed by the legs and feet. Here not infrequently grotesque and apparently impossible positions are assumed such as suggest gross deformity. In organic paralysis, *e.g.*, hemiplegia, the contractures are most marked in the distal portions of the extremities, *i.e.*, the forearms, hands and fingers, the legs, feet and toes, while the muscles proximal to the trunk are less involved. In hysteria such a distinction may not obtain, a limb being equally involved as a whole.

Tremor may also be noted in hysteria; it may be fugitive and transient or quite persistent. It is of variable rapidity, ranging roughly speaking from four to twelve in a second. Quite commonly the tremor ceases when the plaintiff is not under observation, and reappears when the patient finds himself under observation; the extent of the movement also increases at such times. This is likewise true when the plaintiff is asked to make a voluntary effort.

Now and then **incoördination** is noted. This may involve all of the extremities. Much more frequently it involves both legs and then we have present the picture of a hysteric ataxia, an astasia-abasia. Usually the incoördination becomes evident only when the patient makes an effort; for instance, when he attempts to stand or to walk. When the patient is lying down or sitting in a chair, there is power to move the legs normally in all directions, but when he attempts to rise, ataxia at once becomes manifest, and, if he tries to walk, it commonly becomes very pronounced. The gait does not resemble that of tabes in the slightest degree. There is great irregularity of gait; wide, oscillatory, coarse or grossly bizarre movements of the legs, arms and trunk commonly supervene. Usually these phenomena are associated with a demeanor and conduct on the part of the patient as though he were afraid of falling. Quite frequently, too, he becomes emotional during the effort.

The phenomena presented by the **special senses** are kindred to those already considered. Their history is most interesting. Formerly, one of the most common clinical findings was a contraction—a concentric diminution—of the visual field, as though the peripheral portion of the retina were the seat of anesthesia. Every now and then a patient claims that he cannot see at all with one of his eyes, a **blindness** hysteric in nature being present. Such losses of vision are, of course, unreal as is easily demonstrated by simple ophthalmological tests; such as covering the affected eye with a plain glass and the sound eye with a glass of such refractive power that the patient cannot possibly see distinctly through it. He is then asked to read and proceeds to comply with the test entirely unconscious of the fact that he is reading with his supposedly blind eye. **Contractions** of the visual field, it should be pointed out, are suggested to a hysteric patient with the greatest ease, just as is a hemianesthesia. Everything depends upon the manner in which the examination is made. The test object should invariably be carried from the center outward and the fact of failure to see determined by indirect questions. Never should the test object be held in the periphery of the field and the question asked, "Do you see this?" For reasons pointed out in discussing hemianesthesia, the answer will naturally be "No." In other words, contraction of the visual fields is another of the numerous artefacts which increasing knowledge has laid at the door of physicians. However, the story does not end here; a remarkable finding termed "reversal of the color fields" for many years claimed engrossing attention and to-day must be grouped with the artefact "contraction" of which, in reality, it is but an elaboration.

Quite commonly, and for similar reasons, a contracted field is developed upon the same side on which a hemianesthesia has already been elicited. At times, too, the limitation of the field assumes a character which at once demonstrates its mental character; *i.e.*, the area of the contracted field remains of the same size whether the perimeter is held near or far from the patient; *i.e.*, a so-called "tubular vision" is observed.

Hysteric losses may also be developed in the function of

hearing. Hysteric **deafness** may follow suggestion and may be an accompaniment of hemianesthesia. Quite frequently its unreal character can be demonstrated by means of a binaural stethoscope. The ends of the tubes are introduced closely into the ears of the patient; the operator stands back of the patient and converses with the latter by speaking into the stethoscope in a low and, later, barely audible voice. The sounds are, of course, conveyed to both ears of the patient and the latter replies to questions or complies with various instructions. If, now, the physician compresses the tube leading to the sound ear and the patient continues to hear, he must, of course, hear with the hysterically deaf ear. Usually hysterical deafness is, like the loss of vision, incomplete. Bone conduction is, of course, well preserved, though its existence may be denied and may not be demonstrated save by stealth. It is a suggestive fact also that hysteric deafness is quite commonly, if not indeed always, accompanied by hysteric anesthesia of the external ear.

Loss of the senses of **smell and taste** may likewise be elicited in hysteria. A patient, especially one in whom anesthesia has been developed, may stoutly maintain that he is unable to smell or taste upon the hemianesthetic side; sometimes loss of smell and taste are complained of by patients who do not present anesthesia. In a given instance, a patient when tested with various sapid substances will maintain that he does not taste them upon one or, perhaps, both sides of the tongue. If irritating substances be now applied or if physical irritation, such as pricks with a pin be employed, the patient likewise denies that he perceives them. In other words, he makes no distinction between gustatory and tactile loss. Quite commonly, too, such a patient not only fails to respond when tested for tactile impressions upon the tongue, but also when the gums, the mucous membrane of the cheeks and inside of the lips are tested. Similar remarks apply to the loss of the sense of smell. Here the loss is associated in the patient's mind with tactile loss, and no distinctions are made by him between loss of smell and loss of those sensations which are only aroused by purely physical or mechanical impressions.

The picture presented by hysteria every now and then is

such as to direct attention forcibly to the viscera. Here again
the symptoms are such as to be clearly mental in character.
Among them are vomiting, belching, regurgitation, globus hystericus, loss of appetite, anorexia nervosa, tachycardia, various
vasomotor phenomena, rapid breathing, coughing, yawning, sneezing, retention of urine, anuria, phantom tumor, aphonia, spurious
aphasia and the like. Space forbids any but a brief consideration
of these phenomena.

Hysteric **vomiting** may be so severe as to simulate vomiting,
the result of organic disease. Pain may be complained of and
may lead to the erroneous diagnosis of gastralgia or of gastric
ulcer. Occasionally, the vomited matter is tinged with a few
drops of blood usually readily traceable to the gums. When a
history of hematemesis is given it should, of course, be regarded
with suspicion; investigation proves it to be fraudulent. It need
hardly be added that test-breakfasts and microscopic examinations of the stomach-contents reveal no evidence of real disease,
and this is, of course, true of all the gastric disturbances of
hysteria.

Loss of appetite may be present and when very pronounced is
known as **anorexia nervosa.** The patient declines to take food,
declares that it nauseates her and rejects it if administered, but
strangely enough, she reveals little change or impairment of
nutrition. Indeed, in many instances in which the protests of
the patient are loudest and her conduct most dramatic, her
nutrition continues of the best. In other instances, however, in
which secret access to food is not possible, there may be a loss of
weight, sometimes very pronounced; especially, if the insufficient
taking of food be long continued.

Tachycardia may occur as simple attacks of palpitation or
may be quite persistent. The palpitation may be, and frequently is, associated with flushing of the face. Sometimes pallor
and coldness of the surface of the body and the extremities may
be noted. Hysteric rapid breathing is also occasionally observed. The increase in the rate may be very great; as many as
ninety respiratory acts to the minute have been counted. It may
or may not be accompanied by tachycardia. Indeed, most

frequently there is no disturbance of the pulse rate, nor is there any dyspnea nor any evidence of cyanosis.

Hysterical **cough** is a not infrequent symptom. As a rule this cough is dry. It is not accompanied by any physical signs. Sometimes instead of cough, curious cries or sounds are emitted, which suggest the barking of a dog, crowing of a cock, or other bizarre sounds. In other cases, again, frequent and excessive yawning may be observed. As a rule, the act of yawning is very greatly exaggerated and prolonged. Hysterical sneezing which is often very persistent should be added to this category.

At times the patient loses his voice; at other times he is mute and utterly unable to speak. In both of these conditions, hysterical **aphonia** and hysterical mutism or aphasia, the signs themselves are of such a character and the other phenomena present usually so pronounced and unmistakable, as to leave no doubt as to the nature of the symptoms.

Among other symptoms, fever has been ascribed as occurring in hysteria. However, after an experience of thirty odd years spent in the hospitals, I am compelled to deny its existence. Fraudulent tricks with the clinical thermometer are met with, true fever never. Trophic disturbances have also been claimed. These, likewise, I have never observed. So-called hysterical ulcers and other skin lesions disappear as soon as the patient's access to them is prevented by a plaster of Paris bandage or other mechanical device. Now and then the muscles of a limb which has been disused for a long time, show some diminution in size. This diminution is, however, never very marked and cannot in any sense be termed trophic.

Dermatographia, local flushing, and kindred phenomena are but part and parcel of the other circulatory disturbances admittedly the result of mental and emotional influences. Blushing, pallor and other vasomotor perturbations can hardly be termed trophic. This is also true of the slight swellings or edemas which are at times noted as occurring in a disused extremity.

Very often the patient presents the symptom of increased frequency of micturition. Less often he asserts that he cannot hold his water; however, as has already been pointed out, if the clothing and bedding of such a patient be examined, it presents no evidence of having been soiled or stained, nor is there any odor of urine. Wilful deception may, of course, be practised. Now and then retention of urine is complained of, but it is a retention which is usually not real and which when ignored leads to no evil results. True paralysis of the bladder or sphincter, as we have already seen, is never observed.

Many hysteric patients present the symptom of **polyuria;** occasionally large amounts of urine are passed, especially after a hysteric paroxysm or emotional disturbance. The urine in such cases is light-colored and of low specific gravity. Less frequently, the amount of urine is greatly diminished and in given instances the claim of absolute suppression of urine is made. That such statements are fraudulent goes without saying. Patients with hysteric anuria never present the symptoms associated with actual suppression of urine; unconsciousness, coma, convulsions, death, are conspicuous by their absence. Further, when such persons are observed by stealth, it is found, that although the night vessel is not used, it may be that a soap dish or pitcher or other article about the room has been utilized and the urine subsequently surreptitiously disposed of when the patient believed herself free from observation.

Now and then distention of the abdomen is noted. At times this distention is very marked so that the patient may present a superficial appearance of pregnancy. Sometimes the distention is so great that if its character were not recognized, it would constitute a really alarming symptom. At times, also, due to an irregular contraction of the abdominal muscles, the distention is irregular in outline and in this way a so-called **"phantom tumor"** may be produced. Occasionally spurious tumors are produced by a limited contraction of a single muscle; for instance, a contraction of a belly of the rectus.

Patients, at times, call attention to their genital functions. Particularly is this the case in hysteric litigants claiming compensation for alleged injuries. Men, for instance, not infrequently claim that they have become impotent. Women, as we have already seen, may complain of their inability to receive their husbands, alleging that coition is attended by suffering. That there is a great field here for gross misstatement and wilful deception, need not be pointed out. It is usually impossible either to verify or to disprove the assertions of the patient However, it has occurred on more than one occasion in the writer's experience, that during the long delays pending trial, a woman making such a claim has become pregnant and given birth to a child. Similarly in the case of men claiming to be impotent, their wives have borne children; for example, in the case of a man presenting hysteric hemiplegia, there were two trials. In the first the claim of entire loss of sexual power was made. For some technical reason, a second trial was granted; the second trial was not reached for another year. In the meantime the wife gave birth to a child the paternity of which, at the second trial, the plaintiff admitted. Many such instances could be adduced.

All of the symptoms of hysteria are, as has been pointed out, mental in character. The essential features of the mental condition itself have also been discussed. It still remains to consider various special mental or psychic phenomena that present themselves. These, like the sensory, motor and visceral symptoms, at once impress us with their unreality and unessential character. In fact, there is something about them which even to the lay mind suggests their true nature. The simulation of abnormal mental phenomena is grossly imperfect. States of emotional excitement are very common, but the shrieks, screams, wild cries and weeping deceive no one. At most, a delirium or mental confusion may be simulated, but here as in the case of the physical signs, the symptoms have the appearance of something that is not genuine, something assumed, something voluntarily and artificially produced. This is usually quite obvious in the ordinary **hysteric paroxysm.** Hysteric attacks may vary greatly in intensity, as well as in the symptoms which they present. They may be limited to comparatively slight emotional disturbances attended by weeping and laughter, or by transient changes in speech and conduct in which the emotional factors are so evident that even the laity recognize the attacks as hysteric.

8

In the description of the hysteric attack Charcot and Gilles de la Tourette, as in other matters, led the way. There can be little doubt at this day that the elaborate picture which they drew was largely based on artefact. Certain it is that just what they saw has never been seen in any other clinic; and in Paris itself, I am credibly informed, it no longer exists. However, a definite residuum has remained. Thus, the entire attack may be limited to the slight or transient phenomena above detailed. Instead, however, it may be more pronounced and perhaps also prolonged. Thus, the patient may betray that her emotional equilibrium has been much disturbed. For a few hours, or it may be for a day or two, the patient acts as though she were out of sorts, is nervous, depressed and irritable, is uncommunicative and avoids the members of her family; perhaps she becomes angry or weeps upon slight provocation; or she may become excited, restless, perhaps a little exuberant or boisterous, or she may laugh and weep by turns. Not infrequently she complains of choking sensations, clutches at her throat, says that she cannot breathe, complains of headache or other distressing feelings. These symptoms after persisting for a time may constitute the entire attack and may gradually subside.

On the other hand, a convulsion may set in, or the latter may make its appearance without prodromata having been observed. The **convulsion** begins by the patient slipping from a chair or falling to the ground. It is characteristic that she never hurts herself, as for instance, does the epileptic. The convulsion begins by the patient stiffening all of her muscles. The limbs and trunk may become rigidly extended; this may be so great that an opisthotonos may be simulated. The latter may become so extreme that the patient may rest upon her heels and shoulders or occiput (?) forming what the French have called the "arc de cercle." This tonic contraction persists for a variable period, usually for a few minutes only. Soon it is followed by clonic movements, which are much greater in extent than those seen in epilepsy and of themselves suggest a voluntary character. Hysteric attacks are of very variable duration; some are brief, others more prolonged, and, in the latter, the patient may contort the body into various bizarre positions, or may make gestures and movements clearly expressive of volition and purpose. Sometimes the patient tears her clothing, dishevels her person, assumes dramatic and passionate attitudes, shrieks and weeps. Little by little she becomes quiet, welcomes the sympathy and ministrations of her friends, and conducts herself normally, or, perhaps, goes to sleep.

It is characteristic of the hysteric attack that the patient does not lose consciousness, a fact that is rarely admitted by the patient, but commonly capable of convincing proof. Usually the fact that the patient is conscious during the attack is self-evident. The patient never hurts herself and betrays by her actions and by her subsequent statements a knowledge of her environment. The sphincter control is never lost, nor is there ever any biting of the tongue, as in epilepsy. A case repeatedly questioned, however, and acquiring the idea that loss of sphincter control is expected to be present, may at a subsequent attack wet her clothes. Similarly, she will froth at the mouth or even produce from her gums a tinge of blood.

Instead of subsiding, a hysteric convulsion may pass into a phase in which the patient acts as though she hears voices, sees visions, and in which she utters phrases, is exalted, depressed, erotic, obscene; or, such a phase may make its appearance without being preceded by a convulsion.

Contrasted with a real **delirium**, *e.g.*, one due to an infection or intoxication, a crass difference becomes apparent. The visions which the patient sees and which she dramatically addresses give the bystander the impression of being assumed, not genuine. The illusions of persons and objects are frequently exhibited in such a way as to give rise to the same conviction; thus, the moment after having called a relative by a strange name, the patient may betray that she knows exactly who the designated person is. Again, neither the incoherence nor the delusions recall those of delirium proper. Long sentences and long phrases, at all times with a rich emotional content, replace the unrelated fragments uttered in the genuine affection.

At times, instead of having a delirium the patient acts as though she were confused. At other times, her conduct suggests that of **somnambulism,** the condition simulating the somnambulism of hypnosis. In this state the patient may perform various acts often complex in their nature, requiring considerable time and bearing no relation to the occasion or to the environment in which the patient happens to be placed. During this performance the patient acts as though she were oblivious to her surroundings. This condition may persist for some time—even days or longer—and has given rise to the theory of "double personality." The patient usually returns to her normal state quite suddenly and claims that she has no recollection of what has occurred. As has already been indicated, the parallelism between hysteria and hypnosis is complete. The state of hypnosis is merely a phase of hysteria artificially induced. The "good" hypnotic subject is already the victim of hysteria before the hypnotist begins, just as the patient is already the victim of hysteria before suggestion is made or before an accident occurs.

Occasionally **sleep disturbances** are complained of or are observed in hysteria. At times the patient complains of insomnia, making, it may be, incredible statements as to the absence of sleep. Again, the patient may sleep excessively or may fall asleep suddenly. Narcolepsy may thus be of hysteric origin. Sleep may come on as a hysteric convulsion subsides or it may come on spontaneously. The duration of such an attack extends over a fraction of an hour or it may be over many hours. Several days of sleep have, indeed, been reported. The sleep, however, resembles the sleep of hypnosis; it does not seem either genuine or complete. On the other hand, it has seemed at times to be so deep as to suggest the use by the earlier writers of the term hysteric coma. Again, instead of sleep, the patient may pass into a state of ecstasy or of catalepsy. These phenomena present so obviously the features of hysteria and, further, are at the present day so rarely seen that we will not pause to consider them.

That, at times, a delirium or a confusion is simulated we have already seen; that, at others, actual insanity is claimed is not surprising. Always, however, the symptoms bear the stamp of their spurious character. No conduct is too absurd, no statement too grotesque or impossible. It must be frankly admitted that a hysteric person will, under given conditions, do anything to attract attention, anything to excite sympathy, anything to keep herself in the center of the stage. She will practise gross deceptions, simulate anuria, rise of temperature, undergo severe procedures, face painful operations, all under the autosuggestion of the genuineness of her symptoms (?) or in the voluntary and determined effort to convince physicians and others. It must also be conceded, that every now and then physicians are found who are only too ready to accept as true statements bordering on the marvelous. Physicians should bear in mind that the impossible occurs only in hysteria.

The **general nutrition** of the patient may be excellent; the weight may be up to normal or above and the surface of the body may present a healthy or even a heightened color. Indeed, the physical appearance of the patient is often in striking contrast with the serious illness from which she is supposed to be suffering. On the other hand, many patients, because of the unphysiological lives which they lead, show a more or less marked deterioration in their general health. Quite commonly, the hysteric patient does not eat properly—does not eat either the character of food nor at the times she should. As a rule, too, she is indifferent to the usual hours of sleep, disregards the rules of living, is self-willed and extreme in all that she does. If she develops special symptoms, such as vomiting or anorexia, she may lose decidedly in weight; indeed, cases are met with in which under such circumstances the reduction in weight is extreme. On the other hand, as has already been pointed out, in spite of almost incredible statements as to abstinence from food, the patient may be in excellent nutrition, evidently obtaining food surreptitiously.

Again, other symptoms that she adopts, such as paraplegia or hemiplegia, may of necessity lead to her spending her time indoors, or, still worse, of assuming the rôle for many weeks or months of a bedridden invalid. That under such circumstances the patient often becomes thin and pale, weak and flabby, is not surprising. Further, if the patient presents the history of frequent convulsive seizures, presents extensive local spasms or contractures, or adopts other symptoms involving persistent nervous strain—the excessive expenditure of strength—fatigue symptoms may naturally make their appearance. It is remarkable, however, how frequently in spite of the most flagrant inroads upon physiological laws, the patient remains in good condition. Under these circumstances, but one conclusion is possible, namely, that the patient when not under observation ceases her manifestations, reserving her dramatic exhibitions for such occasions when audiences are sure to be present. This conclusion, it need hardly be added, observation abundantly confirms.

THE APPLICATION OF REST TO HYSTERIA

The considerations of hysteria presented in the foregoing pages show that the problem of treatment is both manifold and complex. We have as the underlying basis of the manifestations which the patient presents an innate neuropathy, one of the chief characteristics of which is a feebleness of resistance to impressions received from without. Without the recognition of this fact little or no success in treatment is possible. It becomes evident at once that in order to cope successfully with the symptoms, it will be necessary to be in control of the environment of the patient. Such control can only be secured by some method of isolation. Again, as we have seen, the patient, because of her unphysiological method of living, because of the unphysiological habits she has acquired, and because of the strain to which the mere maintenance of her symptoms has subjected her, suffers from a general impairment of health; sometimes there are present the symptoms of nervous exhaustion. Under these circumstances an application of the principles of rest combined with isolation naturally suggests itself. Partial rest methods such as are suitable for the milder forms of neurasthenia, are not equally applicable to hysteria; the accompanying supervision is altogether inadequate. The patient's emotional instability and inordinate susceptibility to suggestion, together with the great possibilities of harm-doing by well-meaning friends and relatives, indicate at once the necessity for isolation. Efficient isolation can rarely, if ever, be attained in the patient's own home, and in cases which are at all pronounced, **rest treatment** must be carried out in a systematic and radical manner.

It is of the utmost importance that the physician should exercise the very greatest care in studying cases of suspected hysteria. In the first place, the history of the patient's illness, should so far as possible be elicited from the relatives or friends of the patient and in the patient's absence. As regards the personal study of the case, the diagnosis can as a rule be readily made without making examinations that are prolonged or elaborate. How powerful for harm **medical examinations** are in hysteria we have already pointed out; how commonly the symptoms are the artefacts of the physician's methods and procedures, we have already seen.

Quite commonly the symptoms are sufficiently obvious for the general diagnosis to be made and it certainly confers no benefit to a patient to develop areas of anesthesia, contractures of the visual field or other stigmata. Again, many patients present themselves after having been previously examined by other physicians, or in whom the symptoms have resulted from the suggestions of friends or from other incidental factors of the patient's environment. Such patients may present a full-fledged group of stigmata, but even here studies in which, for instance, an anesthetic area is mapped out in great detail, or in which palsies or contractures are elaborately studied, do infinite harm to the patient. A special reserve should be exercised in the study of supposedly painful areas. It is unnecessary to study such areas in detail. The superficial (and unreal) character of the pain is easily recognized. It is only when the pain is doubtful in character and when the possibility of underlying visceral disease exists, that elaborate examinations are justified. Even here, if the case be really one of hysteria, it is usually easy to exclude visceral disease, and the fact that such an examination results negatively can be made the basis for very **valuable suggestions** to the patient's mind. It is needless to say in this connection that the very manner in which an examination is made may give rise to suggestions beneficial to the patient. Such suggestions need not necessarily be made in words; and while the physician is careful not to deny

the existence of the various symptoms which the patient obviously
and often dramatically displays, he can reveal in his manner that
he does not consider them serious; or he may remark that he has
often met with similar symptoms, and has always seen them,
under proper treatment, disappear. On the other hand, a
hysteric patient is frequently jealous of her symptoms, and is
anxious that the physician shall be impressed both with their
severity and their reality, and it is, therefore, a mistake, at a first
interview, to minimize them unduly. Otherwise, the patient will
come to the conclusion that the physician does not understand
her case, that he does not appreciate her condition, or that he
has no sympathy with her or feeling for her, and thus her confidence may be shattered at the very beginning. The proper
examination of a hysteric person requires infinite tact, as
much so, indeed, as does the subsequent treatment. Every
such patient is anxious to detail her symptoms fully to the physician, and although the latter may already have obtained a
full history of the case from the relatives, it is important that he
should assume, at the first examination, the rôle of an interested
and sympathetic listener. An increasing experience has convinced
me of the importance of making a success of the first interview
and the patient must be allowed to talk freely, long, and uninterruptedly. Very gently, questions of a general character can
finally be asked, and little by little the patient can be led up to the
point of the medical examination. This should be conducted
especially from the standpoint of internal medicine, as this diverts
the patient's attention from the nervous features of her case.
Knowing as we do that hysteria frequently complicates and masks
organic disease, the medical part of the examination also assumes
a practical importance.

The attitude which is adopted by the physician in the beginning of the case, namely, that of friend and kind adviser, should be
maintained throughout the course of the treatment. Except in
the rare instances in which such a course shall deliberately be
predetermined upon for special reasons, his suggestions as to the
unimportant character of the nervous symptoms should not be
made too directly. As far as possible, they should be indirect

and allusive; and they should be repeated at subsequent visits. They can, of course, be made in various and numerous ways, by word and by action, by silence and by inattention. After a time, as the treatment progresses, it is often wise to appear to ignore the existence of the various symptoms altogether; this is especially true of the sensory stigmata. Suggestions made too directly or too frequently may constantly keep the symptoms before the patient's mind and thus defeat the physician's object. On the other hand, the appearance of indifference must be avoided. The exact course applicable in a given case must depend upon the individual judgment, good sense, and tact of the physician. Of one thing, however, he should make certain, and that is that every visit that he makes to his patient leaves her with the impression that she is getting better and that she will inevitably be well.

The **nurse,** as in the case of neurasthenia, should be well trained in massage, in the various forms of special exercise, in the giving of baths, and in the administration of electricity; but for the successful management of hysteria, she must possess other important qualities. No matter how well she is trained or how great her experience, the physician should always, before introducing her to the patient, explain the nature of the case and to some extent enter into the details of the symptoms which are present. The nurse should not attempt suddenly to suppress or dissipate the symptoms; argument and forceful methods are equally disastrous and objectionable. She should merely endeavor by her demeanor and general conduct, as well as in her conversation, to keep up gently, day by day, the impression that the patient will get well. On the other hand, she should not play the rôle of a sympathizing, pitying, or affectionate friend. How disastrous such a course is, need hardly be pointed out. Her mental attitude should be that of a calm, quiet, and cheerful companion, whose business it is to carry out faithfully and without modification the instructions of the physician. As can be inferred, the success of a given case depends largely upon the nurse. Even when the latter is educated, she is sometimes deficient in tact and, therefore, useless. The qualites which make a nurse successful in

hysteria are often inborn; many nurses are incapable of acquiring
them.   Thus, some patients need a little sympathy; they cannot
get along without it, and will not improve without it.   In others
even the slightest show of sympathy destroys utterly the influence
of the nurse and her control over her patient.   Intimacy, personal
conversations, and the undue exchange of confidences, are equally
subversive of the discipline of the sick-room.

The necessity for isolation is, as has already been pointed out,
imperative—much more so, indeed, than in simple neurasthenia.
All communications with friends or relatives, whether by letter or
indirectly by cards, flowers, or gifts, should cease.   No matter
with what precautions such communications with the sick are
surrounded, they inevitably do harm.   Especially is this the case
in the early part of the treatment; later, when convalescence has
been firmly established, flowers, books, and the like, may perhaps
be permitted.

The patient having been suitably isolated, **radical rest measures** should be instituted.   The methods which have been elaborately detailed with regard to the treatment of neurasthenia by
rest in bed (see p. 40) should be followed closely; that is to say, in
addition to rest in bed, we are to employ, in various degrees,
massage, bathing, electricity, exercise, and **feeding.**   To these
measures we must add, as has already been sufficiently indicated,
another—namely, **psychotherapy.**   This measure plays a large
rôle in the successful treatment of hysteria.   Indeed, without it
the most elaborate rest methods may fail.   Psychotherapy is
considered in detail in Part III of this book.   Suffice it to say
here, that in the treatment of hysteria ordinarily, simple suggestion, direct and indirect, usually proves abundantly sufficient.
Much, of course, depends upon the personality of the physician.
His attitude and general demeanor toward the patient have already been discussed, and here the caution must be repeated that
the physician should not be too aggressive with his suggestions,
especially in the beginning.   Indeed, his attitude should be that
of accepting the illness and symptoms of the patient as a matter
of course.   The mere institution of rest and the various physiological procedures, is a proof to the patient of the sincerity of the

massage, they will frequently yield to alternate cold and hot douching.

Electricity also may prove of much value in given cases, as it is in the treatment of neurasthenia. It is to be employed in a similar manner. The slowly interrupted faradaic current is conveniently used to stimulate the flexor and extensor muscles of the limbs and the muscles of the trunk; it promotes the general nutrition and increases the general level of the muscular tone. The rapidly interrupted faradaic current is sometimes used as a local stimulant, and is often very efficacious in dispersing painful stigmata. At other times the constant galvanic current may be used for this purpose, the anode being applied over the painful area. Again, in cases in which these areas persist, they sometimes disappear rapidly under static electricity, high-frequency or other modes of electrical application. Electricity, of course, acts under these circumstances by suggestion. We should remember, however, that sometimes electricity is as suggestive of harm as it is of good. After an incautious electric application, the patient may complain of various obscure or painful sensations, declaring that she has been made much worse, or perhaps has new symptoms, *e.g.*, a palsy or a contracture, symptoms from which she may believe she will never recover. At other times, even when an exceedingly mild current is used, she will complain excessively of pain; indeed, she will not infrequently do this when the electrodes are not even connected with the battery. Further, the effect of an imposing apparatus is as likely to be bad as good. In respect to this, as to all other elements of the treatment, therefore, the question becomes finally one of good judgment in the individual case.

The foregoing outline of rest treatment in hysteria embodies merely a general sketch of the methods that may be employed; the variations may be as numerous as the vagaries of individual patients. It should here be emphasized, however, that it is greatly to the advantage of the patient if the treatment be restricted to comparatively simple means; over-elaboration in treatment, as in examination, defeats the physician's object. Indeed, other than simple means are rarely necessary for the successful treatment of even grave and long-standing cases.

Treatment of Special Symptoms

Special symptoms often complicate and retard the progress of the case. The patient seems at times to center her thoughts on a single feature of her case—a palsy, a painful area, nausea, or retention of urine—and the skilful treatment of such a symptom becomes the key to success or failure. As a rule, the special symptoms become less marked or disappear as the general health of the patient improves. One by one they fade away under the combined influence of an increasing sense of physical well-being and skilful and constantly repeated suggestion. The fact, however, that certain stigmata are more prominent than others, makes it wise at times to give them special attention.

We have already considered the treatment of the painful sensory areas by massage, by hot and cold douching, and by various applications of electricity. They yield, as a rule, to these measures, especially if the latter be accompanied with the frequent and repeated suggestion that the pain and tenderness will pass away. Difficulties are occasionally presented by clavus, and at times by areas in the inguinal region or adjacent iliac fossa. While clavus usually yields to ordinary measures, we not infrequently find that medicines which act by suggestion are of value. A capsule containing a small quantity of starch or of boric acid, if administered with the statement that the pain will yield promptly, often proves efficient. Inguinal pain, because of the mental association between the surface pain and possible disease of the ovary or other structures, is at times exceedingly difficult to remove. Especially is this the case when the pain affects the right inguinal region or right iliac fossa. A vague knowledge of appendicitis is widely diffused through the community, and not infrequently a patient believes that he has appendicitis and insists upon operation. In such cases, the attitude of actual organic disease may be assumed, the patient lying upon the back with the thighs, especially the right, drawn well up toward the abdomen, while pain and tenderness are often exceedingly persistent. "Hysteric appendicitis," however, gradually disappears, though a number of weeks may elapse before either the superficial tenderness is gone or before the patient abandons its false interpretation.

If **paralysis** be present, the patient should be encouraged, as much as possible, to try to move the paralyzed member. As a rule the mental effort, even with the best intentions, is grossly insufficient, and the limb fails to move at all. Later on, perhaps under the stimulating suggestion that there is a manifest gain in strength and that the muscles are improving, the limb begins to be moved slightly. At times it is advisable, while the patient is making an effort, to say that the limb is actually stirring a little or that the fingers or toes are being slightly moved. At times the recovery of movement is quite sudden and complete after a skilfully made suggestion. The slowly interrupted faradaic current or other form of electric application may aid in convincing the patient that there is really nothing of consequence the matter with the muscles themselves. In this connection it is well to recall the fact that, owing to disuse, the response of a muscle to electric stimulation is sometimes diminished as compared with the corresponding muscles of the opposite limb. However, the muscles respond promptly, and this in itself acts as a powerful suggestion upon the patient. The benefit of massage and of passive movements need not be pointed out here. It is rarely necessary, or indeed justifiable, in order to reinforce a suggestion, to threaten the patient with operative interference or with unusual or cruel procedures. Indeed, such methods often confirm the patient in her belief that the paralysis from which she suffers is very serious or heroic measures would not be thought of.

Contractures occasionally present considerable difficulty. They are to be combated by massage, by passive movements, and by the continuous galvanic current—of course with suggestion.

The **visceral symptoms** of hysteria are now and then extremely obstinate, becoming veritable obstacles to recovery. Of these, loss of appetite, nausea, and vomiting—**anorexia nervosa**—are the most serious. The patient may manifest an extreme repugnance to food; often she can be prevailed upon to take it only in exceedingly small quantities, or she limits herself to some special article of diet, which she takes very sparingly. Should the symptom persist for any length of time, marked diminution of weight may result; but while such loss of flesh may be decided, it is rarely sufficient to threaten life. The difficulty is augmented by the fact that not only food, but medicines increase the nausea, or are followed by retching, eructations, the evolution of great quantities of gas, and distention of the stomach; it is frequently necessary to administer the medicines by stealth. Curiously enough, morphin in small quantities is, as a rule, well borne under these circumstances; it can be given with a few drops of brandy or a few teaspoonfuls of iced champagne. Better than any other remedy at our command, it relieves the nervous tension from which the patient is suffering. It should be given in doses of one-thirty-second of a grain (two milligrams), repeated at intervals of from one-half to two hours. Gradually the nervousness and anxiety of the patient are allayed, and the retching and vomiting are brought under control. Small quantities of food—peptonized milk, predigested beef, or some similar preparation—can now be given. Little by little the patient's confidence in her ability to take food becomes restored, and day by day the quantity of the latter can gradually be increased. At first, however, we should be content with exceedingly small quantities; a teaspoonful or a tablespoonful of some liquid food every hour or two being sufficient. A start having been made, the amount can be gradually increased until after a few weeks very full feeding is reached. The approach to solid food should, of course, be cautious. Electric applications may be made to the epigastrium; and in suitable cases this measure acts powerfully by suggestion. Either the rapidly interrupted faradaic current or a mild galvanic current should be used, the strength in either case not being sufficient to produce muscular contraction; for the latter would suggest and favor emesis. The current should be merely strong enough, and the duration of the application merely long enough, to produce a little redness of the skin. The patient believes that some special and beneficial procedure is being practised and often becomes mentally entirely satisfied.

Occasionally, the expedient of giving minute doses of morphin fails or proves impracticable. In such case opium suppositories, of sufficient strength to make an impression—e.g., one grain of the aqueous extract—should be employed. Usually in about twenty to thirty minutes the stomach has become tolerant. Advantage should now be taken of this fact to administer—not food—but a dose of twenty to thirty grains of ammonium bromid. It is of advantage to associate with the bromid, fifteen or twenty drops of aromatic spirit of ammonia, and to employ as a vehicle some aromatic water, as peppermint or spearmint. Further, the dose should be given iced and well diluted. The bromid serves the double purpose of preventing the after-nausea of the opium and of decidedly diminishing the nervous and gastric hyperexcitability. Later, small quantities of food can be given.

It is rarely necessary to resort to **rectal feeding** in anorexia nervosa. If tried, it should be persisted in for a short time only, as its moral effect is bad, the patient being confirmed in her opinion that there is something serious the matter with her stomach. In cases in which the trouble appears to be due to difficulty in swallowing or to esophagismus, it may be wise to give one or two feedings by the stomach-tube (see under *Forcible Feeding*, p. 184). As a rule, it is not necessary to resort to this expedient more than once; the mere preparation for the procedure is frequently sufficient to stimulate the patient to take food naturally.

Hypodermic medication should be avoided save in exceptional instances. Relief is given very promptly, but this relief is temporary only, and the patient soon insists upon a repetition of the dose. Finally, it is unnecessary to point out that drugs should be used as emergency measures only.

In the average case of anorexia nervosa, the difficulty of administering food is not, however, so profound as is implied in the foregoing paragraphs. Most frequently the patient objects strenuously to some special articles of diet; strangely enough— or perhaps not strangely—they are frequently the very articles that the physician most desires to give. This difficulty may be met in a number of ways. When possible, the endeavor should be made to bring about in the patient an autosuggestion favoring the dietary it is desirable to prescribe. This must, of course, be accomplished by indirect means. Thus, the article of food, most often milk, is emphatically forbidden in the presence of the nurse, or the matter of the milk is treated as of no consequence or its mention ignored by a shrug of the shoulders. Not infrequently the patient, finding that milk is not being forced upon her, or not even being mentioned in her presence, will ask the physician whether he never prescribes milk, and whether a trial in her case might not prove beneficial. Especially is this likely to come to pass if the amount of other food has been so limited as to be grossly insufficient. The advantage gained is exceedingly great, and if followed up in the proper manner, will prove of enormous utility in the final determination of a successful issue. Very much must, of course, be left to the tact of the physician and his comprehension of the mental make-up of the patient.

In **intestinal distress** and hysteric **distention,** general or limited (**phantom tumors**), the methods already detailed—massage and the suggestive use of electricity—are of value. We have already alluded to the local areas of painful hyperesthesia, at times developed in the rectum. If very persistent, such areas may be dispersed by rectal massage. **Vaginismus,** a condition similar in character, is often very difficult to treat. For obvious reasons, massage cannot here be employed, while such measures as injections, the use of vaginal electrodes—the anode with very mild galvanic current—tampons, and glass plugs, etc., are of little use. The symptom does, however, yield when the hysteria as a whole is relieved, and every energy should be directed to the general measures coupled with properly made suggestion.

Retention of urine is not, as a rule, a serious complication. The physician can rest assured that rupture of the bladder will never take place in hysteric retention; nor is even disastrous distention likely to result. The placing of the patient upon the vessel at regular but not too frequent intervals, with the suggestive sound of running water and the withdrawal of the nurse from the room at the time, are among the expedients to be employed. Occasionally, when the distention of the bladder becomes exceedingly uncomfortable to the patient, she may suddenly leave the bed and evacuate the bladder upon the floor. Patients will rarely go to the extent of wetting the bed. The catheter is to be used only as a last resort, and then not regularly. The physician should, of course, be cautioned against the possibility of mistaking a case of organic retention for one of hysteric retention, and if there be any doubt regarding this point, the catheter should be used promptly. A physical examination will, it need hardly be said, at any time reveal whether the distention of the bladder has reached a serious point. The fact that hysteria so often complicates actual organic disease should make the physician especially careful regarding this matter.

Polyuria can usually be ignored. **Anuria,** on the other hand, demands investigation. As we have seen, when it has been seemingly absolute for long periods of time, the conclusion is, of course, inevitable that the anuria is not real but spurious, the patient passing urine at times when she is not under immediate observation. Anuria is, of course, to be treated by the ingestion of large quantities of liquid and the giving of simple diuretics. It is, as has already been stated, not accompanied by the alarming symptoms that attend true anuria. In a hysteric patient, an exceedingly small quantity of urine may be voided, and yet it may be very concentrated and contain a large percentage of waste products.

Insomnia is only infrequently a marked symptom of hysteria. When present, it often yields with surprising ease to the administration of placebos. A capsule of amylum is my favorite prescription for such cases, and I have found it wonderfully efficacious.

The emotional instability, the introspection, and the **autosuggestion,** that are such prominent features of practically all cases, are to be met by the general methods already detailed. The attitude to be adopted by the physician must depend in large degree upon the mental make-up of the patient. The whole gamut of human motives—pride, ambition, self-love, filial, parental, or conjugal affection, the sense of right and wrong—may, as occasion requires, be played upon to aid the patient's recovery.

The **hysteric paroxysm** is, as a rule, entirely averted by the general rest measures. In a patient who has had frequent seizures, the latter will usually cease to recur so soon as treatment by rest in bed and isolation has been instituted. In cases in which a recurrence takes place, notwithstanding, or in which its development seems probable, the bromids may be used as a measure of exigency, but their administration is rarely necessary over a long period. It is hardly in place to discuss the management of the hysteric paroxysm in detail. Suffice it to say that if it be mild, it should be treated as of little consequence. Quite often it can be aborted by a prompt command on the part of the nurse, by a dash of cold water in the face, by a hypodermic injection of cold water, a placebo administered by the mouth, or by any other measure that makes a decided and vigorous impression. Other things equal, the symptoms of the attack should be minimized. The nurse should declare that it was mild, and also that the patient deserves credit for having controlled it so well! The last-mentioned expedient constitutes an entering wedge by means of which the patient is sooner or later stimulated to control the attacks. By the tactful use of a little praise, even when undeserved, the will-power and morale of the patient can frequently be enormously reinforced. It is a mistake, as a rule, to scold the patient; to say to her that she is to blame for the seizure, and that, but for her own wilfulness, it would not have occurred. Indeed, the influence of the nurse or the physician may be hopelessly destroyed by such a course. If, in spite of all the measures taken to prevent or minimize it, a severe attack should occur, the nurse should refrain from making comments which would lead the patient to infer that the symptoms observed are at all unusual. Indeed, it may be tactful for the nurse to say that she is very glad to have had the opportunity of observing the seizure; that she is now able to report the exact nature of the symptoms to the physician, and both the nurse and the physician should assure the patient that the attacks are not epileptic; that persons always get well of seizures such as the one which the patient experienced, and that it is quite certain that they will not recur, or, if so, only in a very mild and modified form. In any event, the patient should learn that the attack makes but little impression upon the nurse and upon the physician, that it evokes no sympathy and leads to no modification of the stringency of the treatment. Vigorous hydrotherapy in the intervals of the paroxysms is a useful adjuvant; it not only improves the general physical tone, but aids powerfully in the way of suggestion. The fact, too, that cold douches, sprays, and the like are not always pleasant to the patient, acts as a powerful stimulus to the latter's self-control.

Somnolence, allied sleep disturbances, and cataleptoid phenomena do not merit special discussion. We should remember that the treatment of the special symptoms of hysteria is the treatment of the hysteria itself. Gradually, as the effects of full feeding, absolute quiet, and rest become manifest, and as the patient's general sense of well-being increases, so will the symptoms, special as well as general, subside.

When convalescence has been well established, the patient should, as in the treatment of neurasthenia, gradually be gotten out of bed; and, little by little, physical exercise—Swedish movements, and, later, exercises in the open air—should be instituted. The amount of time devoted to exercise should gradually be increased until it is sufficient to induce healthy normal fatigue daily. The fatigue, as in neurasthenia, should be well within physiologic limits. Because of the great predominance of the psychic factors, it is important that the patient be prevailed upon to adopt some healthy mental occupation, no matter what her position in life. Mental exercise is absolutely indispensable to mental health, and the methods already discussed in connection with the convalescent period of neurasthenia apply equally here—light household duties, a course of reading or study, art instruction, music, lecture courses, social service work, stenography, secretaryship, librarian's work, employment in an office or a business in which the patient comes in contact with persons of healthy mental make-up, are among the occupations that may be suggested. Idleness is fruitful of ill health, and especially is this true in hysteria.

Home Treatment

From the foregoing consideration it is quite clear that the number of cases of hysteria which can be treated successfully at the patient's home is quite small. Such a course can be ventured upon only in mild and exceptional instances, and not then, unless the efficient and intelligent coöperation of the other members of the household can be obtained. Home treatment is more frequently useful in the hysteria of children than in the hysteria of adults.

A nurse trained in the special management of such cases should be placed in charge of the patient. Occasionally, when the signs of general ill health are slight, so that massage and the various forms of special exercise with which trained nurses are familiar are not indicated, a companion, who has been carefully instructed by the physician as to her duties, may answer the purpose. However, in the great majority of even mild cases of hysteria, a properly trained nurse is indispensable. Suitable surroundings having been provided, **partial rest** methods may be applied. As in the management of mild neurasthenia, the number of hours devoted to rest in bed should be increased. The patient should be instructed to retire early, to rise late, and to rest during the middle of the day. At the same time a **complementary exercise** should be instituted. This, as in neurasthenia, should take place in the open air, and should at first be exceedingly limited in amount; for instance, a short walk twice daily—of course, in the company of the nurse. Gradually this walk should be increased in extent and its direction varied daily. If possible, a definite object should be given to the walk, a certain place visited, some one thing accomplished. **Massage** may be instituted according to the judgment of the physician. It is not only of benefit physically, but has also a good moral effect. At the same time, the **diet** of the patient should be regulated, and here the general principles already indicated should be followed. As a rule, it will be found of advantage to diminish the amount of starchy foods and sweets, to limit the amount of the red meats consumed, and to add milk to the diet. Usually the white meats, succulent vegetables, and fruit can be used freely. Milk, it need hardly be added, should be given systematically, that is, with meals, between meals, and at bedtime; the quantity prescribed being in direct proportion to the physical needs of the patient. If she be below weight and her nutrition obviously depressed, the milk should be prescribed in gradually increasing quantities until full feeding is reached. The daily **bath**, so beneficial in the treatment of neurasthenia, should also be instituted here. It may consist of the daily sponge bathing, together with occasional bathing in the tub.

All things considered, and as already insisted upon, the **mental** or

moral management of the patient is of greater importance than all of the other measures discussed. The time in the intervals of the treatment should, as far as possible, be filled with a healthful mental occupation that will divert the patient's thoughts from herself —sewing, reading, games, increasing exercise in the open air, driving, riding, and, when the physical condition of the patient permits of it, even swimming. In attempting to apply partial rest methods to hysteria we should, however, remember that they are applicable to a very limited number of cases only, even when the patient is placed under favorable conditions. Inasmuch as hysteria is a disease that from slight beginnings sometimes develops into an exceedingly troublesome affection, it is not only in severe cases, but also in others, the best plan to institute treatment by rest in bed. Indeed, in cases of any gravity whatever, radical rest with absolute isolation is the only plan that promises success.

The **hysteria of litigants** claiming compensation for alleged injuries differs widely from ordinary hysteria in the absolute and entire dependence of the symptoms on the factor of the expected compensation. Space will not permit a detailed consideration of this form of hysteria.* Suffice it to say, that the hysteria observed in litigants is provoked not by trauma, not by fright, but is the direct result of the psychology of compensation; namely, of the recognition by the plaintiff that the success of his claim for compensation depends upon the existence and persistence of symptoms. For this reason treatment, no matter of what character, is without avail. The plaintiff neither gets well nor improves, and this situation may continue indefinitely, sometimes for years; indeed so long as any hope of settlement persists in the plaintiff's mind. However, all medical attendance ceases with the settlement. The symptoms disappear, the plaintiff forgetting all about them. The immediate absence of the plaintiff from physicians' offices and hospital clinics, the moment the money has been paid him, is one of the notorious and striking facts of compensation hysteria.

---

*See Dercum, "Hysteria and Accident Compensation," The George T. Bisel Co., Philadelphia, 1916.

CHAPTER V

HYPOCHONDRIA

Differentiation of Hypochondria from Other Neuroses—An Important but Much Neglected Subject. Character of the Symptoms; Special Forms of Hypochondria; Residual Hypochondria. Prognosis. Treatment—Rest, Exercise, Diet, Bathing, Massage, Electricity, Suggestion; Return to Business; Hygienic Life. Special Indications in Treatment; Management of Children.

THE NATURE OF HYPOCHONDRIA

In considering the subject of neurasthenia, I took occasion to point out that so early as 1765 Robert Whyte, of Edinburgh, had clearly distinguished between neurasthenia, hysteria, and hypochondria. Since his day much has, of course, been written upon functional nervous disorders. Especially is this the case as regards neurasthenia and hysteria; volumes and monographs without number have appeared upon these subjects, more particularly in later years. On the other hand, the subject of hypochondria has received scant attention. Our knowledge of neurasthenia and hysteria is now well advanced, and it is, to say the least, remarkable that the same statement cannot be made for hypochondria; and yet hypochondria is a neurosis which, though not so common as neurasthenia or hysteria, is frequently met with by the general practitioner. It well merits detailed consideration at our hands. Physicians frequently confound it with neurasthenia and at times with melancholia. Not infrequently also, cases of hypochondria are dubbed hysteria when not a single stigma of the latter affection exists. There are, moreover, no difficulties of diagnosis. The symptomatology of hypochondria differs in essential features from that of the affections just mentioned. Thus, the clinical picture of neurasthenia, as we have seen, is that of chronic and exaggerated fatigue, while the psychic and somatic stigmata of hysteria are so characteristic as to permit of no error. We are not, however, to relegate all cases that do not conform to neurasthenia or hysteria to the field of hypochondria. We are carefully to exclude the various neurasthenoid states and neurasthenia symptomatica (see pp. 81 and 84). These conditions, as has been pointed out, can in their turn readily be differentiated by the symptoms they present; the neurasthenoid states are, besides, dependent upon hereditary or acquired neuropathic conditions, and neurasthenia symptomatica upon actual visceral lesions.

Clinical Picture.—Moreover, hypochondria presents a characteristic clinical picture which hardly permits of error. In order that we may form a clear conception as to its essential features, a few general considerations are necessary. There is present in the organism, in addition to the special sensations evoked by the various stimuli of the external world, a generalized sensation derived from the body. In technical literature it is known as the "coenæsthesis." This generalized organic sense embraces, so to speak, a total of all of the somatic impressions. In the normal man, the various nutritive processes in the tissues and the functional changes of the various viscera do not, under normal conditions, impress themselves vividly upon the field of consciousness. Nevertheless, the sense of physical or organic well-being directly affects the psychic state of the individual—it dominates, as it were, his mental tone. So long as the sum total of the organic impressions is normal, an average degree of well-being is experienced. In this condition the mental attitude is objective. When, however, the organic sense is disturbed, so that a feeling of ill-being is produced, the mental attitude becomes subjective and the individual becomes introspective. In hypochondria this organic or somatic sense is always profoundly disturbed. This disturbance, however, is not accompanied, as in actual visceral or other physical disease, by discoverable lesions, and, should functional changes be present, these are so slight and unessential as to offer no explanation of the patient's condition. The patient experiences a sense of not being well, a sense sometimes slight, but more frequently so vivid as to dominate, for the time being, his life and actions. He usually seeks for an explanation of his condition in disease of one or more organs. Most frequently he complains of manifold symptoms, vague and distressing.

Hypochondria should not be confounded with melancholia. Melancholia we now know to be but a part of the symptom-complex of a more extensive disorder—melancholia-mania. The latter is a disease, hereditary in character, in which periods of emotional depression or exaltation extend over months of time and recur in successive waves during the lifetime of the individual. During the melancholic phase of such a wave, the picture is presented of intense psychic depression associated with ideas of sinfulness, spiritual ruin, or moral unworthiness. There is the great agony of the lost soul, the hopelessness of a wasted past, or the belief in some crime never to be atoned. In hypochondria, on the other hand, the patient's ideas relate solely to conditions of the body. It is the somatic state and somatic impressions with which he is concerned.

Not infrequently hypochondria is hereditary, and when an actual history of hypochondria is not present in one or more ancestors, other neuropathic factors may be noted. Hypochondria is more frequently met with among men than among women, and is more common among those who are unmarried. It makes its appearance, as a rule, before middle life, being more frequent before forty than afterward.

All causes which depress the nervous nutrition, as well as all methods of unphysiologic living, favor its evolution—sedentary occupation, excessive or insufficient food, idleness, physical indulgence, the abuse of alcohol and tobacco and other nerve-stimulants. Many cases occur among clerks, students, and professional people who lead inactive lives. It occurs not infrequently among persons who are much in contact with disease—as physicians, and, more especially, medical students. While it is common among those who lead quiet and restricted lives, it now and then is met with among individuals who live out-of-doors—as farmers, laborers, or other persons who make their living by manual work. Here the monotomy of life, the daily sameness of existence, the absence of all stimulus of change, may be the active cause. Again, idleness, the want of occupation, the absence of a definite purpose in life, are powerful factors in the production of hypochondria. The latter is common among the unoccupied wealthy and well-to-do. It is seen very frequently, also, in persons who, having led active lives up to a certain point of their existence and having accumulated means, suddenly abandon themselves to a life of ease. A professional man or a business man who has worked under pressure for many years and who suddenly abandons his calling, is in great danger of lapsing into hypochondria. The stimulus of work no longer determines his mental tone; slight disturbances of function, indigestion, constipation—the result of his lessened activity— furnish the groundwork of a nosophobia. Ere long a superstructure of imaginary ills is added, and sooner or later he becomes the victim of a confirmed hypochondria.

The underlying neuropathy of hypochondria is now and then revealed in the person of the patient. Thus, he may be delicate and neurotic in appearance. As often, however, his physical development is fine; he is large of limb and great of stature, and his appearance is in crass contradiction with the grave illness of which he complains. Again, he may be talented or may manifest ability in certain directions. It is characteristic of the hypochondriac, however, that he lacks the ability or the energy to finish work that he has begun—he lacks the momentum to carry his projects to a successful termination. Frequently such persons are in their early lives quite successful. It is only with the onset of the hypochondria that they become incapables. The neuropathic constitution is also frequently indicated by unnatural diffidence, extreme reserve, or excessive egotism. Intellectual development, it should be added, has nothing whatever to do with hypochondria, for the latter occurs alike among laborers and scholars.

The tendency to hypochondria is not infrequently noted in childhood. A child, for instance, betrays unusual fear of illness or makes an excessive ado about trivial accidents, slight wounds or bruises. Very often such a child screams, not at the moment an injury is received, but only some minutes later, after he has had time to reflect that he has been hurt. As adult life is reached, such a person may become unduly mindful of his health; he is constantly afraid of catching cold, of acquiring serious disease of the chest, or, it may be, of the bowels. It is quite a common experience for such patients to present themselves to a physician for examination while wearing an excessive amount of clothing. Layer after layer of underclothing, chest protectors, abdominal binders, and what not, have to be removed before a physical examination can be made. As often, these patients are peculiar as regards the food they eat. Not infrequently they adopt a special dietary, to which, however, they usually adhere for a limited period of time only. Thus, a patient may adopt an exclusive vegetable diet, or, on the other hand, a diet containing a disproportionate amount of meat. Most frequently it is a special dish or class of foods which is affected or excluded. Thus, cereals, breakfast foods, the special kinds of bread are greatly favored, or fruits and vegetables are declared an absolute necessity; at another time, the same articles may be strictly tabooed. At times tea, coffee, or alcoholic stimulants are rigidly excluded, only to be resumed later. At other times, water is taken in certain ways, or in fixed quantities at definite times. Very frequently, also, the patient affects the various table-waters; first one and then another is lauded for its virtues.

Along with the excessive care and fear that the hypochondriac manifests, he complains of various local symptoms. Thus, he complains of pressure about the head; his head feels as though there were an iron weight pressing upon the top, or iron bands about the temples or the back of the head. He complains of pains in his limbs; the limbs ache, they burn, or they are the seat of fine, vibratory trembling or numb sensations. He complains frequently of backache and of pain beneath the shoulder-blades. He has fulness and pressure over the stomach; the abdomen is distended and flatulent. He has distressing sensations which he refers to the liver or to his kidneys. He complains of palpitation of the heart, of pulsating sensations in the epigastrium or in the abdomen, or of other vague sensations, which he does not or cannot adequately describe.

An examination fails to reveal physical signs of moment. Not infrequently the muscles are well developed and the muscular strength is fully up to normal. There is no change in the reflexes, in the pupillary reactions, or in any of the movements executed by the patient. There is very infrequently a coated tongue and some evidences of gastro-intestinal atony and catarrh, together with constipation; these symptoms may, however, be but slightly, if at all, marked. Not infrequently, slight catarrh of the head and of the throat is noted, and when a knowledge of such a catarrh is possessed by the patient, it becomes a fruitful source of hypochondriac ideas. The patient, for instance, may believe that he is developing consumption or other frightful and serious disease from which he will never recover. More frequently, he bases upon slight gastric catarrh and constipation, ideas of serious disease of the stomach or bowels.

Beyond the indigestion and constipation, no visceral or somatic sign can, as a rule, be detected. Now and then a coldness of the hands and feet, slight lividity of the surface or other evidence of feebleness of the peripheral circulation is noticed.

True to his fear of being ill, the hypochondriac patient constantly observes his functions. Atonic indigestion and constipation offer him abundant opportunity. He may note carefully the character of the bowel movements, observing the most minute details with regard to the forms, size, color, and other qualities of the evacuations. Less frequently, he observes the urine. Now and then, however, if it be phosphatic, it is in turn carefully studied, and becomes a fruitful source of nosophobia, the patient not infrequently believing that he has spermatorrhea.

Very often hypochondriac patients keep careful records of their symptoms. It is a common experience to have them enter the physician's office, seat themselves, and then draw forth little slips of paper on which they have noted a multiplicity of symptoms, usually subjective, always trivial and unimportant, and generally incapable of verification. In manner and bearing, the hypochondriac suggests a person gravely oppressed by illness. He frequently presents the history of having visited physician after physician in the vain attempt to obtain satisfaction as to his condition. The varying diagnoses that are formed from time to time are all carefully noted by him, and all serve to convince him that he is really a very sick man. Not infrequently, he delves into medical books, increases his nosophobia, and subsequently displays a superficial knowledge of medical terms in speaking of his case. Later on he begins to make his own diagnoses, and then goes to this or that physician with his diagnosis fully prepared. Finding little satisfaction or obtaining little relief from physicians, he not infrequently begins to treat himself, and he finds in the numerous quack and patent medicines, so extensively advertised in this country, a rich field for the gratification of his nosophobia. Bottle after bottle is consumed, first of this and then of that nostrum. Pills, powders, liniments, and salves follow in their turn, and the mantle and closets of his room are not infrequently laden with empty or half-empty bottles and boxes. One of the features of marked hypochondria is that the patient is always taking medicine, of some kind or other; it may be a tonic, a laxative, or some special drug. His diagnoses vary from week to week, or often from day to day. To-day he has disease of the stomach, to-morrow disease of the liver; upon another occasion it is disease of the kidneys, or of all of these organs combined. Slight palpitation of the heart convinces him that he has fatal heart disease; a pulsating sensation in the epigastrium convinces him that he has an aneurysm.

It is noticeable that such patients frequently present an appearance of health not at all in keeping with the symptoms of which they complain. Thus, a man who believes that he has serious disease of the stomach or liver not infrequently has an excellent appetite and eats with evident comfort and enjoyment. He may show excellent judgment in the selection of his dishes and may even be an epicure in his taste. He more frequently eats too much than too little; indeed, the quantity is not infrequently excessive.

Very often we find that the hypochondriac, among other things, has extreme views or extreme habits as regards physical exercise. He has read, perhaps, that physical exercise is necessary to health, and he now begins to devote himself to this method of treatment. One system of exercise after another is taken up, and for a time he may exercise excessively. Long walks may be taken, or fatiguing runs on the bicycle. Most frequently he is devoted to room exercises, and he buys apparatus of various kinds, which after a few weeks of desultory use are allowed to become covered with dust. Extreme forms or odd forms of exercise, respiratory gymnastics, the special "system" of some athlete, exhibitor, trainer or advertising "Professor," are affected by him. At other times he takes grossly insufficient exercise, is fearful of the slightest exertion, may lie down for many hours of the day, or, believing himself to be ill, may actually go to bed.

Often he entertains absurd views in regard to ventilation, sleeping next to open windows; or, on the other hand, admitting an insufficient amount of air into his room. Equally absurd may be his habits as to bathing. Frequently he bathes excessively. Every form of douche, spray, shower, steam, or hot-air bath is tried; or he bathes in cold or in hot water daily, insists upon his plunges, or, sad to relate, very frequently manifests an excessive fear of water and does not bathe at all. No procedure is too absurd, too inconvenient, or too unpleasant for him to adopt. Any passing fad for the time being satisfies his longing for treatment. To-day it is some new form of exercise, but to-morrow it is bowel irrigation, and he now becomes a disciple of the high enema. Later "faith cure," "mental healing," or some mystic practice, claims his fealty (see Part III).

It occasionally happens that a patient becomes suddenly alarmed by some new symptom or by some trivial accident. On such occasions he may present all the signs of an acute attack of fright. The latter may be attended by palpitation of the heart, by pallor of the face, and by coldness of the extremities. Such attacks differ radically from the attacks of fear, which occur spontaneously and without special exciting cause, in neurasthenia. Furthermore, the fear is always generalized in character and never assumes the special forms seen in neurasthenia, such, for instance, as agoraphobia or claustrophobia. The fright, as a rule, does not last long, the patient being for the time reassured by those about him or by the physician whose advice he seeks. The previously existing nosophobia, it need hardly be added, is apt to be much worse afterward.

Hypochondriac patients also suffer at times from **sleep disturb-ances.** These do not, however, usually take the form of an in-somnia. As a rule, also, it is found that their statements regarding loss of sleep are grossly exaggerated. The sleep may, however, be broken, and may be disturbed by unpleasant dreams. As a gen-eral rule, however, the hypochondriac sleeps quite well.

Course.—The onset of hypochondria is, as I have indicated, extremely gradual and its course is essentially chronic. Occasion-ally its evolution is hurried by some intercurrent illness, such as an attack of acute indigestion or perhaps an acute febrile attack. As a rule, it pursues a course extending over many years. It does not, however, usually pursue an even course. Its symptoms are at times more pronounced and at times less pronounced. Indeed, they may disappear altogether for a period, a true remission setting in, which persists for months or years. The remission may come on spontaneously, or it may follow some strong emotional reaction or some acute bodily disease. Quite commonly the symptoms recur and the patient passes through another hypochondriacal period. In other cases, again, a permanent recovery may take place, no recurrence ever being manifested. In many cases also, the hypochondria fades with increasing years and ultimately dis-appears; especially is this the case with the hypochondria that has its inception in youth and early adult life. Young hypochondriacs offer a relatively favorable prognosis. This does not apply, how-ever, to cases in which the neurosis is already evident in childhood. Here, neuropathic factors are frequently present. It need hardly be said that cases with a family history of hypochondriasis are ex-ceedingly unfavorable. Equally is this true of cases presenting a history of insanity or other nervous degeneration in the ancestry. In the acquired form of hypochondria, the prognosis is somewhat better, provided the etiologic factors, such as the sedentary habits, abuse of nerve-stimulants, and the like, can be corrected. In cases in which hypochondria makes its appearance relatively late—*i.e.*, toward forty or between forty and fifty years of age—the progno-sis is relatively unfavorable, though even here as old age is ap-proached, it fades away. Rarely it merges into a mild senile dementia. It is a remarkable fact that throughout the course of hypochondria the general mental faculties are clear and well preserved.

In very many cases the symptoms remain, with slight fluctuations, practically stationary for years. In other cases, however, the affection is progressive. The patient gradually becomes depressed and the depression gradually increases. Outside matters no longer interest him; affairs of family and friends no longer concern him. He avoids others, is solitary, undecided, weak of will and unfitted for any regular occupation. Little by little his nutrition begins to suffer. He grows thin, gray, and sallow. His skin and mucous membranes are dry. He no longer sweats readily. The bowel movements are dry. Constipation becomes more marked than ever, and often there are excessive discharges of mucus. His ideas are now exclusively concerned with himself. His liver, and the condition of his bowels, are the principal topics of his conversation. The taking of pills or the use of injections constitutes the all-important business of his daily life.

Of course, the greater the duration of hypochondria, the more unfavorable is the outlook as regards recovery. Even in young persons the prognosis is unfavorable after marked hypochondria has persisted uninterruptedly for a number of years, say three or four.

Special Forms of Hypochondria

While hypochondria usually presents itself in the generalized form above described, it not infrequently assumes a special form; that is, the clinical picture is dominated by a special set of symptoms. The two special forms most commonly met with are, respectively, the gastro-intestinal form and the sexual form.

In the **gastro-intestinal form,** the patient complains of various vague and distressing sensations referred to the abdomen or to the digestive tract, and while there is usually present some atonic indigestion, perhaps also slight gastric catarrh and constipation, the statements of the patient as to his sufferings are out of all proportion to the symptoms. He observes himself most closely. A slightly coated tongue, or a fancied or unusual feature of the bowel movements, alarms him, while slight indigestion may be accompanied by great sinking sensations and sudden fright. These are the patients who adopt extreme diets or curious rules as to eating, who exhaust the catalog of laxatives, and who find great satisfaction in the use of injections, kneading the abdomen, special exercises, etc., and who, in their zeal for each newly discovered dietary, medicine, or procedure, advise it for their friends and sound its praises among their acquaintances. Such cases are frequently wrongly classed as "nervous dyspepsia." Mentally, these patients are, as a rule, extremely impressionable. One who was for a time under my observation, happened to hear that an acquaintance had been operated upon for appendicitis. He became greatly frightened, at once went to bed, and sent for his physician. The fright induced a number of loose bowel movements, which further confirmed him in the belief that he too had something serious the matter with him. It was with difficulty that he was persuaded to leave his bed and to go to his business, which, however, he finally did.

The **sexual form** of hypochondria is one of the most common; so common, indeed, as not to merit a detailed description. Its victims frequently believe themselves to be impotent. Quite commonly they are young men who have never attempted the sexual act; not infrequently they are engaged to be married. As a rule, when marriage takes place, they prove to be entirely competent. Every now and then, however, this is not the case, the fear, the nervousness, and especially the belief that impotence exists, leading to failure. The sexual organs are, it is unnecessary to say, perfectly normal to physical examination. Such cases are correctly classified as cases of "psychic" impotence. Sexual hypochondria is more common in early youth; and not infrequently the belief in sexual deficiency or impotence is based upon a previous masturbation, even when the latter has been slight and insignificant. Quite commonly the occurrence of seminal emissions forms the nucleus around which the hypochondria centers. This is equally the case whether the emissions are excessive or whether they are merely normal in their frequency.

Residual Hypochondria.—A third form of hypochondria which is quite frequently met with and not always recognized, is that which every now and then follows in the wake of some other illness. It is not uncommonly a sequel of some disease of an exhausting character, such as typhoid fever or other acute and profoundly debilitating affection. Occasionally, it follows a neurasthenia which has perhaps been severe, but from which the patient has made a complete recovery; yet, notwithstanding the recovery, the patient for weeks and months afterward still believes himself to be ill. This form of hypochondria may also follow acute mental affections. It is not rare after an attack of severe delirium or after confusional insanity. It is quite frequently met with as a sequel of middle-life melancholia.

I propose for this form of hypochondria, the term **residual hypochondria.** The patient, even after having made a recovery from some acute affection, persists for many weeks, or it may be many months, in believing himself to be ill. Upon all occasions he talks about his illness; he never tires of recounting his sufferings and his harrowing experience. Not only does he disclose his feelings to the members of his family and intimate friends, but even to entire strangers. He firmly believes that no one has ever been quite so ill as himself. So firmly is he convinced of this idea that he cannot but believe that he is still somewhat ill—that it would not take much to bring about a serious recurrence, and that it would be easy to endanger his life. He declares that he is weak, that he is nervous, that he is easily upset, gives various accounts of pains or other distressing sensations in the limbs, the back, or the head. He insists time and again that he is not well, and that he must take the utmost care of himself. He acquires peculiar habits with regard to his clothing, the ventilation of his room at night, the number of covers on his bed, the character and amount of his food and of his bowel movements; he presents, on the whole, a train of symptoms very similar to those met with in ordinary hypochondria. In my experience, however, these patients complain less frequently of gastro-intestinal troubles; they are more apt to lay especial stress upon the occurrence of vague pains and distressing sensations in the head, the back, and the limbs. Indeed, their statements regarding the pains they suffer are often grossly and transparently exaggerated. Not infrequently they assert that their suffering is exquisite and excruciating, and yet the unsubstantial character of the pain is proved by the fact that it is often relieved by placebos. A starch capsule is frequently elevated to the rank of a powerful therapeutic agent. Similar is it with the persistent and distressing insomnia of which these persons complain. It is frequently relieved by placebos or by absurdly small doses of some hypnotic, as fifteen drops of paraldehyd. As in ordinary hypochondria, the patient is very fond of taking medicine. Indeed, he never tires of it. A simple physiologic plan of treatment does not satisfy him; he must have prescriptions.

We should carefully distinguish between the affection, simple hypochrondia, as it is here pictured, and the **hypochondriacal stage** observed in the developmental period of **various psychoses**. Simple hypochondria is a well-defined neurosis in which the conduct, views, and opinions of the patient are dominated by an all-convincing sense of illness. **True qualitative mental changes** are, however, absent. Different is it in the developmental period met with in some of the insanities. Here the patient may pass through a hypochondriacal period, as in paranoia and melancholia; but, in addition, specific mental changes sooner or later make their appearance. Hallucinations of sight and hearing, especially the latter, are striking features. The patient tells us of voices or of apparitions, and as the disease progresses these special sense hallucinations form the foundations of delusions. At times also hallucinations exist, which are referred to the viscera. They are not interpreted, however, as indicating disease of the liver, indigestion, Bright's disease, spermatorrhea, etc., as in simple hypochondria, but, in insanity, they form the basis sooner or later of some grossly delusional belief, such as the presence of snakes in the stomach, loss of the viscera, absolute closure of the bowel, absence of the mouth, etc. Simple or true hypochondria is a well-defined affection and is not prodromal to any other. Its symptoms constitute a clinical whole, which frequently persists for years with little change; indeed, it may last an entire lifetime.

PHYSIOLOGIC METHODS OF TREATMENT IN HYPOCHONDRIA

An analysis of the symptoms of hypochondria throws but little light upon the pathology of the affection. However, it is a legitimate inference that the affection occurs essentially in persons of a neuropathic or psychopathic constitution. The neuropathy, as proved by the family history, is frequently hereditary; it may, however, be acquired. The prognosis, we need hardly point out, is much more favorable when hereditary factors are not prominent. The indications as to treatment are unfortunately not so clear as in the case of neurasthenia and hysteria. The physician realizes that it will not suffice to make merely the diagnosis of hypochondria and then to state to the patient that the latter suffers from a purely imaginary disease, that he is not ill, but merely believes himself to be ill. As a matter of fact, the patient is really ill—indeed, ill from a very troublesome affection. There is some underlying cause for the disordered and exaggerated cœnesthetic impressions of the patient—probably some obscure disturbance of metabolism —and merely to deny the existence of the condition is as unscientific as it is inconclusive. The wisest course is not to dispute the reality of the condition, but to point out to the patient clearly the functional character of the symptoms and the entire absence of organic disease. Especially is this course valuable if, previous to the expression of the opinion, the physician has made an elaborate physical examination. Hypochondriacs like to be examined, and one of their most common grievances is that nobody will listen to their symptoms, no one will take the time to examine them properly. These cases are among the most troublesome with which the physician has to deal and their successful management requires endless tact and judgment.

The problem of treatment resolves itself, first, into the application of physiologic measures; and, secondly, the correction of special symptoms.

Rest and Exercise

At the outset we are confronted by the question of rest. Shall a hypochondriac patient be rested? and if so, how much and for

how long a period? Rest, especially absolute rest, is not without
its dangers (see p. '45). Particularly is this true in hypochondria,
and, as a general rule, treatment by systematic rest in bed should
not be employed in this disease. Exception, however, should be
made in cases in which there is a marked impairment of the general
health, decided lowering of nervous and muscular tone, or special
symptoms so marked as to justify placing the patient in bed. In
the majority of cases rest, if employed at all, should be **partial**
only. The obvious aim of our treatment should be to raise the
activity of the various functions of the patient to so high a level
that there will be substituted for the general feeling of ill-being
from which he suffers, a sense of well-being. It is essentially a
problem of physiologic living and physiologic therapeutics that
confronts us.

We should first carefully regulate the patient's **manner of living.**
We should insist upon an increase of the number of hours devoted
to **rest,** but at the same time we should institute a systematic form
of **exercise.** We should more than ever bear in mind the physiologic truism that the preservation of a function depends upon its
exercise; and as the patient's general health improves, the time
devoted to exercise must be increased; we must exact from the
patient, also, the meeting of every business or professional obliga-
tion. Cases of hypochondria do best when they are under the
full pressure of work. Work, mental and physical, means the active stimulation of function, and this means a relatively higher
level of health. Work, further, necessitates an **objective mental
attitude,** and in favorable cases, the patient devotes less and less
time to the consideration of his symptoms. It is not necessary
here to say that, in addition to rest and work, we should apply
the other physiologic measures at our command as they seem indicated. Especially valuable is **hydrotherapy,** whether applied by
simple or elaborate methods. The stimulating and beneficial
effects of bathing in its various forms, in hypochondria, are sufficiently obvious, nor need we dwell here upon the value of **massage**
as a method of stimulating nutrition. Massage is especially
indicated if the patient be unduly fatigued by exercise, or if fatigue-
pains and aches are present. Electricity also is of value, active

general faradization or active treatment with the static machine being most effective. Indeed, the use of electricity, and especially of static electricity, is now and then followed by most satisfactory results. Sometimes the improvement is very rapid and even brilliant, static electricity acting powerfully by suggestion. Unfortunately recurrences sooner or later ensue.

Not infrequently we meet with cases of hypochondria which have been of such long duration and are so profound that nothing can be accomplished by partial rest methods. It is usually impossible to bring such patients under the beneficial discipline of a prescribed method of living, and under these circumstances, it is an excellent plan to place the patient for a short period on **absolute rest in bed**; for the physician is then, for the time being, master of the situation. A well-instructed nurse, of the same sex as the patient, is an indispensable aid. Elaborate physiologic methods should then be instituted, not only for the beneficial effects of the discipline and routine involved, but also for the therapeutic effects of the measures themselves. They should invariably, of course, be administered along with the suggestion of returning health. By their means—especially by massage and bathing—indigestion, constipation, and sleep disturbances can be decidedly alleviated or entirely corrected. The plan to be adopted is, in general, that which has been detailed in the application of rest to neurasthenia. It must especially be borne in mind, however, that the patient should not be allowed to have much leisure time for thinking, but that the various physiologic methods employed should be so adjusted as to fill in the day as much as possible. As in the treatment of neurasthenia, **massage** should be begun gently and should not at first be given for too prolonged a period. The **bath** should, as in the treatment of neurasthenia, be limited at first to a warm sponge bath between blankets. Later on, cold sponging, alternate hot and cold douching, or the drip sheet bath vigorously applied should be substituted. **Electricity** also should, at first, be confined in its application to the slowly interrupted faradaic current applied to the muscles of the limbs and the extensor muscles of the back. Later, the application of electricity may be made more vigorous, general faradization may be em-

ployed, and further on, during the out-of-bed period, static electricity can be substituted. As a rule, the patient begins to improve.
Indeed, he is apt to show improvement early in the treatment, but
we must not expect the improvement to be so great as in the case
of neurasthenia or hysteria.   The novelty of the treatment, which
makes so favorable an impression at first, soon wears off, and it
is, therefore, a good plan not to pursue the expedient of rest in bed
for too long a time.   Just as soon as a profound physical and mental impression has been made, and while the novelty of the various
measures employed is still in full force, the patient should be gotten
out of bed and **active exercise** instituted; the latter should be very
slight at first, but should be steadily increased in vigor until a
maximum amount is attained.   In many cases, the approach
to exercise must be extremely gradual.   Many patients submit
willingly to massage, but object seriously to any attempt at active
or even extended passive movements.   It not infrequently occurs
that the massage must be associated with passive movements that
are at first extremely slight in extent, and little by little these movements are to be made more and more free until every joint in the
body is moved several times in all of its physiologic directions and
to its fullest extent.   Little by little movements with resistance are
added, until finally a full system of active movements is instituted.
Gradually other forms of exercise are employed until, as already
stated, a maximum amount is reached.   What this maximum
shall be, must depend largely upon the judgment of the physician.
Care should be exercised that pain is at no time given in making
passive movements, and especially that the patient is not exhausted or that the cardiac action be not disturbed during movements of resistance or the other active exercises.   I know of no
matter concerning which greater tact is required than in the
gradual introduction of the patient to active exercise, especially
if the victim of the hypochondria be a woman.   The time spent
in bed, should, of course, be gradually decreased as exercise is
instituted until the patient is out of bed for the entire day.

It is necessary to repeat emphatically the **caution** that the
period of absolute rest in bed should be short; say, three to six
weeks.   After this interval, the plan of treatment should gradually

be converted into one of **partial rest**, exercise being instituted at a relatively early period. Full rest methods unduly prolonged are sometimes dangerous in hypochondria; indeed, if practised unwisely, they may be followed by disastrous results. The patient learns to love the coddling care of the rest treatment and insists upon its prolongation, declines to get out of bed, and resists tenaciously exercise or activity in any form. Care also should be taken that the treatment, and especially the institution of the various physiologic methods, should not serve to confirm in the patient's mind the belief that he is seriously ill. As in hysteria, the unfailing **suggestion** should be made to the patient both by the physician and nurse, directly and indirectly, first, that he is not seriously ill, and, secondly, that he will inevitably get entirely well. Further, the patient should never be accused of being hypochondriacal. As a rule, he does not ask for a specific diagnosis, and he is readily satisfied when he is told that he is suffering from one of the forms of "nervous prostration."

It is of great importance in hypochondria not to allow too long an interval to elapse between the rest treatment and the **patient's return to his business.** Such persons, if sent away to the seashore, to the mountains, or to other health-resorts, even in the company of a nurse, are apt to relapse, and much ground that has been gained may thus be lost. It is important that the return to work be early and that a new method of living—the discipline of new habits—be rigidly maintained. The resumptiom of work should take place while the patient is still under the immediate supervision of the physician. I know of no affection in which it is so necessary to keep in active touch with the patient as in hypochondria. Every hour of the day must be filled with work, with the active interests of the patient's business, with exercise, or with various prescribed duties. The aim is, of course, to give the patient's mind as objective an attitude as possible, and to leave him little time to dwell upon his symptoms. As a rule, the patient will bear various forms of hard exercise after a rest treatment, and among these horseback-riding is one of the most beneficial. In this connection we are aided by the fact that sooner or later, if the approach be made sufficiently gradual, exercise strongly appeals to the average hypochondriac; after a time he becomes "enthused." First one method of exercise and then another is tried, and every effort should be made to interest him in an active out-of-door life. In unfavorable seasons of the year, exercise in the room or gymnasium must substitute exercise in the open air. The latter, of course, is always to be preferred when practicable.

In some cases of hypochondria, the relief to symptoms brought about by the application of physiologic methods is very great. The highest possible functional activity means for these persons the highest possible degree of health, and it is this highest possible functional activity which we must seek to establish after a course of rest treatment.

Special indications in the treatment of hypochondria must be dealt with as they arise. Especially is it important to give our attention to the digestive tract, so frequently disordered in hypochondria. Atony, catarrh, and constipation should be treated, as in the case of neurasthenia, by a suitable diet and appropriate medication. The principles already laid down (see p. 48) should be followed. We should diminish the amount of the red meats and of the starchy foods, and, other things equal, should add milk to the diet. The rôle played by a possible gouty diathesis should be borne in mind. Again, the tendency to constipation and the great amount of thought which the hypochondriac gives to the condition of his bowels suggests the necessity of adopting methods for producing easy, and, as far as possible, normal evacuations. The hypochondriac is always in better spirits when the bowels are freely moved. In the average case two movements a day are better than one.

In the sexual form of hypochondria, a general plan of treatment is, of course, to be instituted. The patient is also to be told that the occurrence of seminal emissions does not justify a belief in sexual weakness or impotence—that seminal emissions are normal phenomena. Should the latter actually occur with undue frequency, measures should, of course, be instituted to control them. Liquids late at night should be avoided lest the bladder be over-distended during sleep; the bowels should be kept freely open;

sleeping upon the back should be prevented; and, if necessary, an alkaline bromid or minute doses of hyoscin hydrobromate should be given at night. Especial emphasis is, however, to be placed upon physiologic methods, especially upon the various forms of bathing, exercise, and diet.

In children in whom a tendency to hypochondria is noted, every effort should be made to minimize the importance of affections from which they suffer or accidents through which they pass. Little attention should be paid to transient illness or slight cuts and bruises; above all, should sympathy be withheld; nothing should be said or done to create the impression in the child's mind that he is seriously ill or has been hurt. The neglect of this precaution often leads in a suitable soil to a confirmed hypochondria in later life. It is important to see that children of hypochondriacal tendencies are not put under too severe a pressure at school; they should lead hygienic lives—especially as regards food, exercise, and work. Everything should be done also to harden such children by judicious exposure. We should remember, further, that it is bad for children of hypochondriacal tendencies to live with invalids or be much in their company.

CHAPTER VI

THE APPLICATION OF REST IN CHOREA AND OTHER FUNCTIONAL NERVOUS DISEASES; AND IN ORGANIC NERVOUS DISEASES

Chorea; Epilepsy; Spasm; Paralysis Agitans; Headache—Migraine; Neuralgia; Painful Spine—Coccygodynia. Neuritis—Multiple Neuritis; Sciatica; Local Palsies. Diseases of the Spinal Cord. Diseases of the Brain.

CHOREA

Rest methods are applicable not only to the great neuroses, neurasthenia, hysteria, and hypochondria, but also to various other functional nervous diseases. Especially are they applicable to chorea. Indeed, the chorea of childhood frequently yields to simple or **partial rest** methods alone. The indications are those of increased rest, full feeding, and sponge bathing. Massage and electricity are not usually applicable—at least not until convalescence has been fully established. In the average case of Sydenham's chorea it is, of course, not necessary to place the patient continuously in bed. The child should, however, be withdrawn from school, should go to bed early in the evening, and be allowed to rise late in the morning. Exercise for variable periods in the open air should be insisted upon, as well as rest in the middle of the day.

Every now and then in **severe** cases, it is necessary to adopt **full rest** measures; indeed, when the movements are very severe, the patient is necessarily in bed, and in such cases elaborate rest methods and full feeding should be instituted. It need hardly be pointed out that in many cases it is necessary to have the headboard, footboard, and sides of the bed, covered in such a way that the patient cannot in the violence of his movements inflict any injury upon himself. Various remedies must, of course, be used in conjunction with rest in these severe cases, and I would mention especially the bromids, medinal and trional. Trional, particularly, is of value. It should be given in small doses, two to five grains, according to the age of the patient, at intervals of four hours. The employment of arsenic, iron, and other tonics need not here be dwelt upon. Rest measures, it need hardly be added, should in severe cases be continued long after convalescence has been established.

EPILEPSY

Occasionally rest, with general physiologic measures, is applicable in epilepsy. In cases made worse for the time being by unphysiologic living or by overstrain, we are able to lessen the frequency of the seizures and to diminish the amount of medicine required. Exercise, and especially open-air work, must, of course, constitute a prominent feature in any plan of treatment that is instituted. The rest should rarely be more than partial. Full rest measures are only exceptionally applicable. Their value is in direct proportion to the signs of general ill health and of loss of strength and weight that may be present. In a few instances in which such signs were very evident I have seen a truly remarkable improvement ensue upon a rest treatment followed by rigid physiologic living.

SPASM

Rest methods are also occasionally of value in functional spasms and functional tremor, though permanent results are never achieved. Every now and then, in a case of spasmodic torticollis, in which the movements are excessive in their severity, benefit can be obtained by placing the patient in bed upon full rest methods, and especially will this be the case if some motor depressor, such as conium or gelsemium, be administered coincidently. Gelsemium particularly is of value. In large doses it is, of course, a poison and its use should always be attended with care. It may be given in the form of the fluid extract, beginning with five drops and with intervals of several hours. Four hours is a convenient interval, as the effect of a single dose lasts from three to four hours.

Gradually the dose should be increased to ten, fifteen, or even twenty drops. Twenty drops, indeed, should be considered the maximum dose, and should not under ordinary circumstances be exceeded. During its administration, the patient should be watched, and if ocular symptoms, such as double vision, make their appearance, the drug should, for a time, be discontinued. During the use of this agent the spasm diminishes to a very great extent, and in some cases almost ceases, though I believe it has never been known to do so entirely. However, so pronounced is the amelioration that it affords, especially if its administration be attended by the employment of full rest measures, that the patient is very materially benefited.

The application of rest to the tics is considered in Part II.

PARALYSIS AGITANS

In discussing the application of rest in functional nervous diseases, it is important especially to point out that in at least one of these affections **rest methods are never applicable**; namely, paralysis agitans. Cases of paralysis agitans are not only not benefited, but are sometimes made worse, by full rest treatment. Rest favors the tendency to fixation and rigidity, a tendency which is sooner or later a prominent feature of the disease. Systematic **exercise** is indicated in paralysis agitans. From the very nature of the disease, the patient usually tends to remain quiet, and it is exercise, gentle in character, to which he must be urged. The exercise may be passive or active. The movements should be modeled after those devised by Fraenkel for the treatment of locomotor ataxia; that is, they should be movements of precision. The patient feels relatively comfortable when he is in motion. Even such purely passive motion as is obtained by riding in a carriage or in a railway train gives some comfort. No attempt should be made to treat the tremor. Certain drugs, such as hyoscin hydrobromate and parathyroid extract, will lessen it, but their use over long periods is objectionable.

It should be added that **massage** is, as a rule, badly borne by patients with paralysis agitans. This is true likewise of **electricity**.

Bathing is also best limited to relatively simple procedures. Simple hygienic measures, in which partial rest plays a minor rôle, together with general tonic medication, is the plan of treatment which should be followed in this disease.

HEADACHE

Many forms of headache are relieved by systematic rest in bed, and it becomes of importance to select cases suited to this mode of treatment. Everything necessarily depends upon the cause of the pain. Rest methods are, of course, most successful in those cases in which the headache is merely part of the symptom-group of a neurasthenia. However, even when the headache is due to some local cause, such as eye-strain, rest methods are often of inestimable value. Time and again we find that after the eyes have been corrected by proper glassing, the headache persists. Frequently relief is only obtained by giving the nervous system as a whole a more or less prolonged rest. This is true also of the headaches that result from visceral disturbances, as of the stomach. Frequently the latter depend upon a simple atony and can best be treated by rest in bed. In cases in which the headache appears to be due to a diathetic cause, such as gout, or what is vaguely called rheumatism, we must combine with the rest a suitable dietetic treatment and the thorough administration of salicylates and allied remedies. The advantages of hydrotherapy need not here be pointed out, as they have been sufficiently dwelt upon in discussing the treatment of neurasthenia.

Migraine

Other forms of headache, such as migraine, can also be greatly benefited by rest methods. In obstinate and persistent migraine, rest methods constitute the only means of bringing about decided improvement in the patient. The rest should be absolute, and the details should be carried out as elaborately as possible. It is not necessary here to point out the great importance of the dietetic treatment, especially the exclusion of red meats and of starchy foods and sugars, nor to dwell upon the great value of milk. Free use also should be made of bathing. Everything should be done to stimulate the elimination of uric acid and its salts and the group of allied toxins. Liquids should be administered freely. At various times, the salicylates and alkaline waters should be given freely. In other words, the treatment should consist in rest, combined with judiciously applied diathetic and eliminative measures. As a rule, it will be found that the intervals between the paroxysms of headache gradually increase, and also that the attacks themselves become much less severe. If the treatment be carefully carried out, the improvement is usually very great, so much so as in many instances to amount to a practical cure. The patient also gains in weight and strength, while the general nutrition is greatly improved.

NEURALGIA

It is not necessary here to enter into the details of the treatment required by individual cases of neuralgia, save to point out the great value of massive doses of strychnin in trigeminal neuralgia. The initial dose should be one-thirtieth of a grain (2 milligrams) at intervals of four hours. In the course of twenty-four to forty-eight hours, the interval should be lessened to three hours. After another twenty-four or forty-eight hours, the dose should be increased to one-twentieth of a grain, and later on, if the pain has not been relieved, the interval may be shortened to two and a half hours. In the large majority of cases, the drug is well borne, and the toxic action of strychnin, as evidenced by sensations of stiffness about the jaws or back of the neck, is absent. It is of the utmost importance that as far as possible rest be carried out during the period of medication; indeed, in many cases the treatment will fail unless rest and full feeding be employed.

The importance of dietetic measures in other forms of neuralgia, and especially the value of the salicylates and allied remedies in cases in which a gouty or an alloxuric diathesis is present, is quite evident. Finally, in cases of brachialgia, sciatica, or other local forms of the disorder, rest methods should, as far as possible, form an integral part of the treatment.

The importance of rest in neuralgia need not here be pointed out. Patients usually discover for themselves the fact that rest and quiet diminish their suffering. If the nerves affected be situated in the upper limb, as in **brachial neuralgia,** absolute rest should be secured by placing the arm in a **splint,** as in the treatment of a neuritis (see p. 162); if the neuralgia exist in a leg, as in sciatica, absolute rest in bed should be insisted upon (see p. 166); often the treatment will fail unless a splint be applied. As a rule, even in chronic cases, either complete recovery or marked improvement follows these simple expedients.

PAINFUL SPINE; COCCYGODYNIA

Painful spine is usually a part of the symptom-group of neurasthenia. No matter in what portion of the spine the pain may be situated, it is made much worse by fatigue, mental or physical. As may be inferred, it is usually diminished by rest. The proper treatment is a more or less thorough course of rest cure combined especially with **hydrotherapy.** Absolute rest, with hot and cold douching, gentle or vigorous according to circumstances, yields the best results. Electricity also is of value in many cases, more especially the constant galvanic current. The condition is sometimes exceedingly persistent, and success depends largely upon the detailed methods pursued. As a rule, a patient with painful spine presents numerous neurasthenic symptoms, with or without a complicating hysteria, and it is the neurasthenia to which treatment should primarily be directed, rather than to the local condition. In all severe cases little can be expected from any course of treatment other than absolute rest for a prolonged period. The methods which have already been detailed (see pp. 40 and 118) should be followed. Massage should be resorted to as in ordinary rest treatment, the masseur having been instructed, however, to avoid in the beginning the painful areas. Gradually, however, the latter should be included in the rubbing, at first gently and later more and more vigorously. Associated with spontaneous pain in the spine, there is usually hyperesthesia of the overlying tissues, and the pain produced by pressure or contact of any kind may be exquisite. However, as the general condition of the patient im-

11

proves, massage can be applied freely. A few writers recommend counterirritation by the actual cautery in the more severe cases. However, if a thorough and radical system of rest treatment be carried out, such measures are wholly unnecessary. Internally, tonics, cod-liver oil, and other nutrients may be administered. If a gouty or a rheumatic diathesis be suspected, a course of the salicylates should be instituted.

When the pain is situated in the coccyx, we should not lose sight of the fact that actual disease of the bone may be present. Such cases occasionally necessitate surgical interference.

REST IN ORGANIC NERVOUS DISEASES

Rest in the treatment of organic nervous diseases assumes a special and peculiar importance. It is necessary that we consider rest, first, in relation to diseases of the **nerves**; secondly, in relation to diseases of the **spinal cord**; and, thirdly, in relation to diseases of the **brain.**

NEURITIS

The first indication of treatment in neuritis, no matter what the cause of the inflammation, is **rest.** If the affected nerve be situated in a limb, this can be accomplished by the use of a well-padded **splint,** the limb being fixed in such a position as to place the nerve, together with the muscles and other contiguous structures, in a state of relaxation. The position of moderate flexion is usually the one in which this result can best be attained. A fixed position is to be maintained and tension is to be relieved as far as possible. It is remarkable how rapidly relief of pain follows the institution of this simple expedient, and in the average case the recovery, unless there be special causes at work, dates from the application of the rest.

Other measures should, of course, also be employed. It is of advantage, for instance, in most cases, especially if the neuritis be **acute,** to make local applications of **heat.** The heat can be either dry or moist. If the nerve be superficial—as, for example, the ulnar at the elbow—moist heat can be applied with benefit. In the majority of cases, however, dry heat will answer our purpose best, as it interferes less with the dressing. The temperature of the application must be regulated by the effect produced; in some cases a moderate degree of warmth, in others a relatively high temperature, gives the best results. Occasionally, though rarely, applications of cold assist in the relief of pain. Counterirritation by blisters or sinapisms, especially if the neuritis be acute and the result of trauma or other physical cause, does more harm than good, and should, except in special cases, be avoided. If there be a febrile reaction, as is sometimes the case, it may be advisable to make use of general measures, such as rest in bed, free sweating, and purgation.

When the acute stage has passed away, a **subacute** condition remains which is due to the incomplete subsidence of the inflammation. **Rest** is to be continued, and if pain and tenderness persist unduly, **counterirritation** may now be employed though it is rarely necessary. In special regions, such as the axilla, counterirritation is best avoided altogether. In inflammation of the brachial plexus or of the nerves of the arm, gentle inunctions with ichthyol ointment, one part to four, may be employed. It is exceedingly probable that some of the benefit derived is the result of the local massage which the proper application of the inunctions necessitates. After a stage has been reached in which pain has largely or entirely subsided, massage is of the utmost utility. Its employment is indicated at a period when all inflammation has subsided and only the sequels of the latter persist. It should be applied daily in such a manner as to exert an effect upon both nerves and muscles.

The **galvanic current** is occasionally of use in diminishing the pain of neuritis in the chronic stage. The constant current should be employed, the anode being applied over the painful portion of the nerve-trunk and the cathode at some indifferent point. The application should be continued for several minutes—from five to fifteen, according to circumstances. A very weak current should be used at first, its strength being increased little by little. If the tenderness of the nerve-trunk has altogether disappeared, faradaic electricity or the interrupted galvanic current is indicated. Both are useful not only as affording information of the quantity and quality of the changes that the nerve and the muscles supplied by it have undergone, but also as a direct means of stimulating the nutrition of these structures. Regarding the choice of the current, the rule should be followed, other things equal, that that current be employed which excites the greatest degree of response in the muscles with the least pain or distress to the patient. If the neuritis has been marked, reaction of degeneration is usually present, and this may, in severe cases, advance to such a degree that the muscles fail to respond at all. Electricity is then for the time being useless, and our main reliance should be placed upon massage.

If it appear from the history that the neuritis is the outcome of a localized rheumatism or gout, appropriate remedies should be given internally. More than to allude to the salicylates, the various alkalies, lycetol, piperazin, atophan or colchicum, is hardly necessary here. As a rule, the salicylates should be used either in the form of some salt of salicylic acid, or salophen or aspirin, in the early part of the treatment. The dose should be relatively large and should be continued for a number of days—a week or more. If the trouble persists unduly, small doses of some alterative, such as potassium iodid or corrosive sublimate, may be given. The administration of the iodid or mercury can be continued for a relatively long period, but the doses should, of course, be small.

It is of the utmost importance that local rest should not be maintained too long. So soon as the acute symptoms have subsided and pain is under good control, the splint should be removed and passive movements should be instituted along with massage. It is not necessary to speak of the harm done by keeping a limb upon a splint too long—of the fixation of the joints, the atrophy of the muscles, and the general impairment of nutrition of the limb. We should bear in mind that there is no greater stimulus to the nutrition of a limb than the exercise of its function, and just so soon as it is practicable, the patient should be instructed to use the limb. After a neuritis, patients are apt to nurse the limb—for instance, an arm—for too long a period. They should be encouraged to use it gently at first and to exercise it vigorously later on.

Multiple Neuritis

In all forms of multiple neuritis, whatever the origin, absolute rest in bed is imperative. In most cases, indeed, the loss of power in the limbs is so pronounced that the patient is already in bed when the physician arrives. This is especially true of the toxic cases, notably those due to alcohol. In other cases, as those that follow infectious fevers, the patient, not knowing the seriousness of his condition, may remain up and around unless advised to the contrary. Absolute rest in bed, let us repeat, is imperative. The limbs should be so placed as to be neither excessively flexed nor unduly extended, and should be supported upon soft pillows, or, better still, if they be very painful, upon cotton batting kept in position by flannel bandages. In other cases flannel bandages alone, if not too firmly applied, give considerable comfort.

It is best, if possible, to avoid the administration of analgesics. Only when the pain is not relieved by the rest and the position of the limbs, should these drugs be used. Morphin, in small doses, may be employed in severe cases. The various coal-tar products are best avoided. It is not necessary to say that the etiology of a given case will necessarily influence the treatment. If alcohol be the cause, its withdrawal must constitute the first step in the treatment. If, on the other hand, a diathetic factor, such as rheumatism, be established, anti-rheumatic medication must be instituted. Salicylic acid and its salts are, as a rule, not well borne by the stomach. Synthetic substitutes, as salophen, and especially aspirin, are much more useful. The advantages of lycetol, atophan and piperazin need not be pointed out. These remedies, however, are of little value unless associated with the rest methods. After the pain has subsided, or has been brought in a very large measure under control, massage and passive movements may gradually be instituted. Later on, the patient may also be treated by electricity. The slowly interrupted faradaic or galvanic current may be used in order gently to stimulate the muscles and nerves.

The treatment of multiple neuritis is essentially a treatment by "rest-cure" methods, and it is remarkable how much can be accomplished by these methods in the ordinary case. Even in patients that have been bedridden and in whom contractures have

appeared in the limbs, it is possible, by the systematic employment of massage, passive and active movements, and electricity,
to bring about a remarkable degree of improvement and even entire recovery.

Sciatica

The treatment of sciatica may be considered under two heads:
(1) the treatment of acute or recent sciatica; and (2) the treatment
of the chronic or established form.

The first indication in the treatment of acute or recent sciatica
is absolute rest.   This can be attained only by putting the patient
to bed.   The limb should be well protected by flannel bandages and
fixed upon a well-padded splint in a position of moderate extension.
Next, the bowels should be opened freely by a saline purge, and,
inasmuch as leaving the bed is impossible without disarranging the
dressing, a bed-pan should be used.   Usually, the fixation of the
limb upon a splint diminishes the pain very decidedly.   Hypodermic injections of morphin are rarely needed if this expedient be
adopted.   When pain persists after the application of the splint,
the patient, if his heart be strong, may be relieved by doses of antipyrin, from ten to twenty grains (0.65 to 1.3 gram); the other coal-
tar analgesics are also of use, and permissible when the heart presents no contraindication.

As a rule, it is of decided advantage to administer freely one of
the salicylates.   The dose should be sufficient to evoke evidences
of the physiologic action of the drug, such as fulness in the head
and ringing in the ears.   To accomplish this end, ten to twenty
grains (1.3 gram) of sodium salicylate in solution, largely diluted,
should be administered every four hours.   The unpleasant effects
may to some extent be mitigated by associating with it equal doses
of sodium bromid, or moderate doses—one to three grains (0.065
to 0.2 gram)—of caffein citrate.   Later on, small doses of the
iodids and mercurials may be substituted for the salicylate.   However, it cannot be too emphatically impressed upon the mind of the
reader that rest and not drugs must be the essential principle of
the treatment of sciatica.   General rest in bed should be persisted

in for a time—several days or weeks—after the pain has entirely subsided.

The larger number of patients suffering with sciatica apply for treatment after the affection has become established as a **chronic** condition. In such cases the hopelessness of temporizing methods should be pointed out to the patient, and his consent to a prolonged period of rest treatment, extending over six or eight weeks or longer, should be obtained. The first indication is, as in acute sciatica, to place the patient **absolutely at rest,** and, at the same time, to fix the limb upon a **splint** in a position of moderate extension. While the patient is in bed, the principles embodied in the general application of rest should also be followed. General massage and, as soon as the pain in the limb permits it, local massage should be employed. This is also true of electricity. At the same time a suitable diet, from which red meats, starches, and sweets are excluded, should be instituted, while full feeding should be brought about by the addition of milk in a steadily increasing quantity. The treatment should extend over a period of from six to ten weeks.

Local Palsies

Local palsies, no matter what their origin, demand, in addition to massage and electric treatment, **rest of the muscles.** This rest is of the utmost importance, and upon its proper institution depends, in a large number of cases, recovery. For instance, a **deltoid muscle** which has been paralyzed by a blow, may refuse for weeks and months to improve. The arm in such a case hangs helpless at the side of the trunk. Owing to the relaxed condition of the muscle and the weight of the arm, the humerus may drop so much that it becomes possible to insert the finger between the head of the humerus and the acromion process. The muscle is not only suffering from the effect of the paralysis, but is being constantly overstretched by the weight of the arm. Under such circumstances recovery may be greatly delayed or may not ensue at all. Just so soon, however, as the weight of the arm is taken off the muscle by a bandage or sling which holds the humerus well up in its socket, the muscle is placed in a condition favorable to improvement. I have repeatedly seen persistent failure follow the neglect of this simple expedient. When the limb is properly supported, the muscle is no longer in a state of tension, but is relaxed, and now usually responds to treatment by massage and electricity. Another instance is seen in footdrop; the power to flex the foot upon the leg may be very slight or altogether lost, but if the weight of the foot be taken off the muscles by a "rubber-muscle" or other device, recovery is greatly favored. The necessity of placing a paralyzed muscle in a position of relaxation is not sufficiently recognized. By this expedient the muscle is placed in a position of relative rest. Not only do massage and electricity prove more efficacious under these conditions, but voluntary efforts at exercising the muscle are much more likely to yield favorable results at an earlier period.

DISEASES OF THE SPINAL CORD

Rest is of great service in various diseases of the spinal cord. Much judgment is required in the selection of cases and in the degree of rest which is to be applied. Patients suffering from acute affections of the cord, such as acute myelitis and trauma, are of necessity in bed, and in them the very nature of the affection veils the possible benefit that may ensue from rest. In patients, however, who suffer from chronic affections of the cord but who are still able to walk, rest, if judiciously applied, is often followed by decided improvement. For instance, we now and then meet with patients suffering from syphilis of the cord who, in spite of the judicious employment of intravenous injections of salvarsan, intraspinous administration of salvarsanized serum, of spinal drainage, of the iodids and mercurials, fail to improve. Not infrequently if, in addition to antisyphilitic treatment, such patients be placed in bed with full rest methods, improvement gradually becomes manifest, and in time virtual recovery may ensue. The rest methods greatly stimulate nutrition, and perhaps also facilitate the action of the remedies. I have repeatedly observed favorable results in cases otherwise persistent and obstinate.

Rest methods are also of value in organic diseases of the cord, such as chronic myelitis and the various system degenerations, such as amyotrophic lateral sclerosis, ataxic paraplegia, and

tabes. A word of **warning** is here indicated. Complete and continuous rest in bed often results in an alarming increase of the paraplegia or other motor disturbances present. In a case of myelitis, in which the patient is still able to walk, continuous rest in bed for even a short period may greatly impair the power to walk or even to stand, and this is equally true of absolute rest in other organic cord affections. In tabes, especially, full rest methods are of the utmost value and during their continuance the various special methods of treatment in vogue, spinal drainage, intravenous and intraspinous injections and anti-syphilitic remedies generally, may be employed to the best advantage (see section on treatment of paresis and tabes, Part II). It is important to add, however, that full rest methods should not be applied to other chronic diseases of the cord; in the latter the degree of rest should never be absolute. Rest should always be combined with **exercise,** and the success attained in a given case depends entirely upon the relative proportion of these measures. While the patient is resting, the rest should be absolute, *i.e.*, in bed; but from the very beginning of the treatment, exercise, especially standing and walking, should be systematically carried out at definite intervals during the day. As a rule, very little exercise suffices in the beginning, and its amount should be increased only very gradually and with the greatest care.

The exercise should assume in all cases the form of **movements of precision,** such as have been introduced by Fraenkel in the treatment of locomotor ataxia. A large number of different movements of precision may be employed; more depends, however, upon the proper application of the principle than upon the employment of any one movement. The principle of precision being adhered to, much may be left to the ingenuity and skill of the nurse or masseur superintending the exercise. In the beginning, a relatively simple plan answers best. Thus, the patient should be instructed, as in the special instance of **tabes,** to place his feet carefully in walking upon a given line or stripe upon the floor, to follow with his feet special points in the pattern of the carpet, to walk forward, to walk backward, to turn first to the right and then to the left, to walk in a circle, to walk in figures of eight, and, finally to walk up and down steps. In performing each movement, he is to be guided as much as possible by the criticisms of the attendant. Frequent repetition and the employment of the vision constantly to correct the errors of movement, lead in many cases to a decided improvement—a kind of reëducation of movement. In cases of beginning **amyotrophic lateral sclerosis,** or of **chronic myelitis,** the patient should be instructed to make a special effort to raise the thighs in walking so that the toes do not strike the ground and are not dragged. As far as possible by voluntary effort, the patient should be encouraged to imitate the normal action of the leg and foot, even if the result can be attained only by grossly exaggerating the movements or certain phases of the movements. A gesture of the leg and foot which is often of especial value, is one which exaggerates the *"Paradeschritt"* of the German soldier, or the goose-step. By special effort the thigh is well flexed upon the abdomen, next the leg is extended, and finally the whole limb is thrown forward and the foot gently brought to the ground. Numerous variations of these gestures may be devised according to the special symptoms or weaknesses present in a given case.

The exercises, it need hardly be stated, should not be limited to walking, but may consist of complex movements of the foot and leg while the patient is seated upon a chair or lying upon his back. Appropriate exercises of the arms and trunk should likewise be instituted.

The improvement that follows the careful application of these exercises, especially if disease be not far advanced, is frequently remarkable. In tabes it is often striking, and in cases of chronic myelitis and amyotrophic lateral sclerosis, very decided improvement may also be noted. Of course, in cases in which organic disease is far advanced, so that there is present extreme ataxia, excessive spasticity, or great weakness, little can be gained. In the early stages, however, much can frequently be accomplished. A cardinal principle should always be borne in mind, namely, that gymnastic procedures should be employed only as a part of a plan of treatment in which rest in bed plays the greater rôle. Further, the exercise should always stop short of fatigue. We should remember that in organic disease of the cord we deal with neurones which are enfeebled or are undergoing degeneration, and that if they be overtaxed, harm and not benefit will ensue.

Other measures may also be instituted. Massage, for instance, is often of decided value and should always be employed. In combination with passive movements or with slight resistive movements, it is a good adjuvant to or preparation for more active exercise. Electricity is also of service in some cases. It should be used especially in the form of the slowly interrupted faradaic or galvanic current in such a way as to bring about a limited number of distinct contractions in the flexor and extensor groups. In spastic conditions, for obvious reasons, it should be avoided.

By every means in our power, the general nutrition should be raised to as high a level as possible, and to this end, in addition to the physiologic procedures here detailed, various medicines may be employed. These include the ordinary tonics and alteratives. Little that is tangible can, it is true, be traced to their administration—at least as regards the special symptoms presented by the cord; nevertheless, they may prove of general benefit. Again, it is important in syphilitic cases to follow the specific treatment by some preparation of iron or arsenic or possibly by cod-liver oil. Strychnin is also of value, but should not be employed indiscriminately. It is rather as a general tonic that it is of service and not because of its specific action on the cord. When spasticity and contracture are present, it should for obvious reasons be avoided.

DISEASES OF THE BRAIN

The application of rest in diseases of the brain I have already largely considered in the discussion of such functional disorders as neurasthenia, hysteria, and hypochondria. That rest is of benefit in various chronic organic conditions, such as brain syphilis and other subacute affections, there can be no doubt. The question of its application is always to be decided by the symptoms present in each individual case. It is also largely influenced by the general condition of the patient. Applied in organic brain affections, it cannot, of course, be regarded as curative, but merely as placing the patient under circumstances most conducive to recovery when recovery is possible.   The application of rest in the treatment of **paresis** and of **mental disorders** generally is considered in the following chapters.   Suffice it to say here, that rest and full feeding stimulate the defensive resources of the organism as do no other procedures.

PART II

THERAPEUTICS OF MENTAL DISEASES

PART II.—THERAPEUTICS OF MENTAL DISEASES

CHAPTER I

THE PREVENTION OF INSANITY AND THE GENERAL PRINCIPLES OF THE TREATMENT OF THE INSANE

The Prevention of Insanity; Marriage and Insanity. General Principles underlying the Treatment of the Insane; Rest, Isolation, Commitment to Asylum. Details of Management—Hygiene; Food, Forcible Feeding; Massage; Electricity; Bathing; Medication; Hypnotism and Suggestion; Restraint; Treatment of Bed-sores. Physician and Patient.

A discussion of the therapeutics of mental diseases resolves itself into a consideration, first, of the prevention of insanity, and, secondly, of its treatment.

The Prevention of Insanity

The prevention of insanity is one of the most serious problems confronting mankind. Insanity occurs among the biologically defective and aberrant. Save in that relatively small proportion in whom it is acquired as result of intoxications and disease affecting the individual, it is expressive of a hereditary neuropathy. This neuropathy is the result of the various morbid influences to which the stock has been exposed, perhaps for generations. It is a deterioration the result of such causes as syphilis, alcoholism, tuberculosis, the infections and intoxications generally, privation and unhygienic living and surroundings. Under such circumstances the organism becomes structurally impaired while its nutritive, *i.e.*, its metabolic processes, become alike aberrant and deficient. Among the causes enumerated, an overwhelming rôle must be assigned to syphilis and alcoholism; contrasted with these factors, all others—even tuberculosis—play a relatively insignificant part. Clearly in the battle against insanity, humanity must strive especially for the prevention, control and gradual elimination of syphilis and alcoholism, and for the education of the community in the principles of hygienic living generally.

Among the various drastic measures that have from time to time been advocated, is sterilization of the insane. This procedure to which there seems to be no valid objection is, however, far from meeting with general approval and at present there is no other way of dealing with the problem than that of institutional isolation. The baneful effects on the community from the free propagation of insane, defective and criminal stocks is so well recognized that it seems hardly necessary to point out that isolation should be carried out as effectively as possible.

The prevention of the marriage of insane persons is another problem that likewise has not yet been satisfactorily solved. In this matter the physician can exercise a salutary influence only if his advice be sought, and this is but rarely the case. Save in special instances, he should when the opportunity presents itself, advise strongly against marriage. It would, however, be both unjust and unscientific to maintain that *all* persons who have suffered from a mental disorder should not marry. Various factors should be taken into consideration. Mental diseases, as has been indicated, can be divided roughly into two groups—those which are, and those which are not, essentially neuropathic and hereditary. In the **hereditary** group we have the well-known degenerative psychoses; to wit, the various forms of arrest, imbecility, dementia precox, mania, melancholia, circular insanity, paranoia, and the neurasthenic-neuropathic insanities. They all present marked neuropathic and hereditary factors, and it is the duty of the physician to advise strongly against the marriage of a person who has suffered from any of these affections. It is otherwise, however, with regard to insanities that depend for their occurrence upon accidental poisons or upon infection. Surely a person who has had, say, a prolonged delirium or a confusional insanity, following typhoid fever, ought not, for this reason alone, to be forbidden marriage. So it is with mental disorders following other infectious or exhausting diseases. Should such a patient, however, in addition present a neuropathic family history, this fact should weigh against marriage. That many persons who become insane in consequence of infectious diseases, visceral disorders, and exhausting affections of various kinds present also a family history of insanity, is well known. However, it is equally true that the factor of heredity may be entirely wanting, and in these cases there is no ground on which marriage can be forbidden.

Marriage in relation to insanity presents also another aspect; in persons of feeble and neurotic constitution, marriage may of itself prove a cause of insanity. The new functions assumed, the strain of pregnancy, child-birth, or lactation, may in women of feeble constitution, as is well known, result in alienation. The factors on which an opinion can be based are not often presented to the physician, and he will rarely have an opportunity of giving advice. We should remember, on the other hand, that marriage, entailing as it does a physiologic method of living, may in itself be beneficial. This is true, not because of any special virtue in the marital relation as preservative of health, but because of the regularity of living which married life imposes upon men, on the one hand, and the functions of pregnancy and motherhood it confers upon women on the other. The living together of the sexes in the married state is the normal relation, and one conducive, other things equal, alike to mental and physical health. In men the aberrations, dissipations, and irregularities of youth are brought to an end, and in their place come wholesome responsibilities. In women, married life entails the physiologic stimulus of child-bearing and lactation, while the care of children and of household directs the mental activities into normal channels. After all, the question as to the advisability of a marriage can be decided only upon the facts presented by each individual case. No general rule can be formulated.

While the physician can do but little to prevent the marriage of neuropathic persons, he has, at least, frequently the opportunity of giving important advice as regards their children. His first duty, whenever possible, is to impress the parents with the necessity of rearing the child according to the elementary principles of physiology and hygiene. Neither the objects of this volume nor space will permit us to enter into a discussion of the physiology of childhood. How vast a field there is for care in the clothing, the feeding, and the training of the child need not here be pointed out. How greatly this field is neglected can be instanced by calling to mind the remark of Herbert Spencer that greater attention is sometimes given to the feeding of the horses in a gentleman's stable than to the feeding of the children in the nursery. Children are quite commonly given food which not only gives rise to serious digestive disturbances, but which is altogether unsuited for the proper development of their bodies, and, at an all too early age, they are permitted the use of stimulants. Suitable clothing, out-of-door life, and exercise are also frequently neglected, and due attention is not paid to the education and general upbringing of the child. A child, otherwise healthy, is often brought up so loosely, is so indulged in every whim and caprice, is so pampered and petted, so thoroughly "spoiled," that when circumstances force the grown-up lad or adult woman to face the serious questions of life, energy, will-power, judgment, self-control—nervous strength in all its forms, is sadly lacking. On the other hand, children who are brought up harshly or too rigidly, who are denied the ordinary pleasures of childhood and youth, and upon whom a too close application to study, and, perhaps, to physical labor, has been forced, are likely to develop sooner or later various nervous disorders. Again, an education that provides a child simply with desk instruction, with books, to the exclusion of physical exercise; or an education that taxes a child too much in one direction, such as music, is also attended by grave dangers. The absurd and often cruel custom of forcing prolonged musical training, requiring many hours of daily practice, upon children who have no special or natural musical talent, and who have, in addition, all the other tasks of school, is only too common in this country. That under these circumstances hereditary neuropathies should come to the surface, is not surprising. Children are easily fatigued nervously, and we should remember, besides, that nervous fatigue is more readily induced in some children than in others. Especially is this true of the children of neuropathic parents. Unusual readiness of fatigue in a child is a symptom which should always demand serious consideration. Not infrequently children are inattentive at school, not from any wilful fault, but because they are incapable of sustained attention for a prolonged period. The inattention of children at school is, in the vast majority of cases, a fatigue symptom, and should be so regarded. A child is often treated as wilfully bad, stupid, or vicious, merely because it is fatigued. How injudicious punishment is under such circumstances, how much it favors both mental and moral degradation, it is not necessary to dwell upon. Again, the pressure of school, especially at the period of puberty, is especially injurious. Not infrequently a child is precocious, learns with ease and but little effort in the years immediately preceding puberty, but during the time that puberty is being established, becomes slow, inattentive, acquires only with effort, and makes but little progress. These changes are symptoms. Such a child should be watched with the utmost care and the hours of mental and nervous work diminished; if not, for a time, abolished.

It is not possible to enter here into the details of the wants of childhood, and it must suffice to point out that all influences tending to lessen physical vigor or to interfere with nutrition—in a word, all infringements upon physiologic living—are to be guarded against. Especially during the developmental period between childhood and youth, sleep, exercise, and food should be well proportioned, and the use of all stimulants, such as tea and coffee, and especially alcohol and tobacco, should be prohibited absolutely.

THE GENERAL PRINCIPLES UNDERLYING THE TREATMENT OF INSANITY

The treatment of insanity, after it has become established, resolves itself, into first, and especially, the application of physiologic methods; and, secondarily, the use of medicines. At the outset, let me point out that physiologic methods, which are so powerful in comparatively simple nervous disturbances, such as neurasthenia and hysteria, are much less productive of results in mental diseases. Nevertheless, they should in some form be rigidly applied. In the management of mental disease, the first and cardinal principle is rest. Rest is often enforced by the nature of the illness; the patient's condition is such that he is of necessity in bed, or his condition is such as to compel his removal to and his isolation in a hospital for the insane. In general terms it should be stated that so soon as a mental disorder has been recognized, mental and physical rest should, as much as possible, be enforced. In all of the acute psychoses, the patient fares best if it be possible to place him in bed. Cases of melancholia and other depressive forms of insanity can, as a rule, be placed in bed and remain there with but little resistance. Otherwise is it, however, with the various excited forms. Here the patient can only exceptionally be induced to lie down. Whenever possible, however, the patient should be placed in bed and a method of treatment instituted which in a degree approximates a so-called rest treatment. Even when the patient is restless and can be induced to remain in bed for comparatively short periods of time only, much good results.

In order to secure rest and quiet, or to bring about some diminution in the excitement, it is important to remove the patient from his own home. The well-meant but mistaken ministrations or officious interference of relatives and friends keep up the patient's excitement or intensify his depression. Isolation can, of course, be secured by commitment to an asylum. In the milder and non-asylum cases, it can be secured by removal to a private hospital or sanatorium, or by sending the patient, under the care of one or more nurses, to the seashore, to the mountains, or to some other available health-resort. Isolation from friends is, as a rule, quite as imperative in mental diseases as it is in neurasthenia and hysteria. It is not, however, absolutely necessary in all cases. As I have already pointed out in considering the treatment of neurasthenia, isolation is an expedient powerful for good; but it is sometimes powerful for ill—especially if it be too rigidly enforced or too long maintained. The benefits of isolation are so obvious in severe cases as to make a detailed discussion unnecessary. Time and again the opportunity occurs of observing patients who have been very much disturbed at home, rapidly becoming quiet under the isolation of a hospital. It is also observed, as a rule, that patients, who may be improving, are disturbed and upset, sometimes seriously, by the communications and visits of friends. Other patients, however, become depressed or have their depression increased if visits and communications be cut off entirely. They may believe that their friends have deserted them; or that their relatives no longer care for them. Especially is this untoward result apt to take place in the milder forms of melancholia which do not justify asylum commitment.

The question of the proper isolation of the patient is also intimately connected with his personal safety and with the safety of others. The danger of suicide, assault, or injury should never be lost sight of, and if the treatment of a patient whose symptoms are not so pronounced as to justify asylum commitment be undertaken at his own home or elsewhere, he should be surrounded with every precaution and safeguard; the incessant care and watchfulness of attendants must replace the locks and protections of the institution.

In a large number of cases, the necessity of commitment to an asylum is so obvious, both from the nature of the illness and from the violence of the symptoms, as to admit of no discussion. In another and not inconsiderable group of cases, however, the symptoms neither necessitate nor justify asylum commitment and the treatment must be conducted elsewhere. The factors entering into commitment will be discussed in detail in considering the management and treatment of the various mental diseases. It is necessary here only to formulate the following general rules:

First, commitment should be advised whenever the patient is dangerous to himself or to others.

Second, commitment should be advised when it is evident that the treatment cannot be carried on satisfactorily outside of an institution.

Third, in all cases the physician should take sufficient time to satisfy himself thoroughly both as to the actual existence of insanity and as to the advisability and necessity of commitment.

Lastly, we should invariably decline to commit, whenever any doubt, no matter how slight, arises. The legal responsibility of physicians in making hasty or improper commitments should always be borne in mind.

The commitment of the patient to an asylum or his proper placing elsewhere having been determined, we are next confronted by the details of treatment. These consist of the general care and feeding, of the employment of physiologic methods, and of the administration of medicines. The importance of correct hygiene need not be dwelt upon, save to point out that in the care of the insane, owing to the long duration of the illness, careful hygiene is imperative. Air and sunlight, cleanliness and liberal feeding, are simple and yet essential physiologic measures.

The application of full or radical rest methods is, of course, indicated and feasible, in but a limited proportion of the insane, and these again are mainly cases of recent origin. Naturally, too, full rest treatment is especially practicable and most readily carried out in the milder and less disturbed cases. Many patients are kept in bed with difficulty, others again take to their beds willingly or spontaneously. However, whenever practicable, the indications for radical rest are very clear. The patient in addition to the special mental features which characterize his case, frequently presents in a more or less marked degree the evidences of weakness and exhaustion; the more thorough, therefore, the rest the better.

The indications for full feeding are likewise clear and even more imperative than in simple and uncomplicated neurasthenic states. Hypernutrition not only adds to the substance of the body but profoundly modifies metabolism. In excessive feeding, for instance, protein substances which have been only partially reduced, gain access not only to the portal circulation but even pass through the liver. Once in the blood, the latter assumes the function of completing the digestion. It would appear that all the cells of the body in addition to the special function imposed upon them by the special organs or tissues of which they are component parts, also retain the primitive function of digestion and it would appear that in no tissue is this function better preserved than in the blood. Here the various leucocytes, the plasma and even the ery-throcytes and the blood plaques play a rôle. Abderhalden found, in accordance with this truth, that ferments make their appearance in the blood when the intestinal tract is overfilled with protein, peptones or carbohydrates. Not only is the ferment-producing power of the blood stimulated in hyperfeeding, but the lipoid sub-stances also are largely increased in amount and lipoids, as we know, play a most important rôle in the formation of antibodies.

The problem that confronts us in insanity is not only one of exhaustion but also of intoxication, and hypernutrition assumes here a special significance and importance. The intoxications to which the organism is subject may be roughly divided into two groups. Some poisons exercise but a short tenure; that is, the intoxications which result from them are of short duration. In such instances, the organism successfully resists and disposes of the poisons speedily and promptly. The poisons are successively submitted to the defensive action of the gastro-intestinal juices, the defensive action of the liver and other glands, are variously changed chemically, and finally destroyed or eliminated; but these are not the poisons nor the processes which usually concern us. The poisons with which we deal in mental diseases are mainly those of long tenure, those which are not destroyed by the various glands and other defensive structures, and which consequently influence the metabolism of the organism for long periods of time, usually many months. Not only is this true of the poisons present in mental diseases which are essentially neuropathic and heredi-tary, such as the manic-depressive group and the group of dementia præcox and paranoia, but also of those in which the poi-soning is primarily of extraneous origin. Thus, when prolonged insanities ensue after acute infections, the poisons at work have their origin in a secondary disturbance of function of the liver, of the thyroid, of the kidney, of the adrenals and of other glands and tissues. The fact of such involvement is based on indisputable clinical and pathological evidence. Consequently a disorder of metabolism ensues which constitutes of itself an autointoxication, an autointoxication secondary to the original infection. However, whatever the character or the source of the intoxication, nature is forced to fight the battle by the gradual formation of antibodies, *i.e.*, by the continued effort at immunization.

As will appear in the subsequent discussion of the subject, many of the patients take food willingly and readily. Others, again, must be urged to eat, and others still must be fed by artificial means; that is, so-called **forcible feeding** must be resorted to. Frequently, it is of the utmost importance to give food in large quantities. As a rule, a generous, mixed diet is indicated. It is neither necessary nor practicable in the larger number of cases to institute special dietaries. Occasionally, however, it is important to diminish the amount of starchy foods, the amount of sweets, or the amount of red meats. This is especially the case when there is marked atony or catarrh of the stomach or other digestive disturbance, or when the illness is of such a nature that the patient exercises but little. Milk, as in neurasthenia and hysteria, is a valuable adjuvant to the other foods, and whenever forcible feeding is attempted, it is indispensable. The indications for forcible feeding will be considered in detail in the following pages. It can be accomplished by **passing a stomach-tube** through the mouth. The tube, having a funnel-shaped extremity, should be warmed, well oiled, and, having been passed into the esophagus—not the larynx—liquid food in any desired quantity can readily be administered. As a matter of fact, however, feeding by passing the tube through the mouth is rarely practised. The patient frequently keeps his mouth closed and teeth clenched, and the mere effort of the operator to force open the jaws usually induces resistance and struggling on the part of the patient. The serious and exhausting effects of all measures involving violence need not be commented on; besides, the teeth of the patient may be broken or other injury may be done. Far easier is it, as a rule, to make use of the **nasal passages.** Almost always the tube can readily be passed through the nose. The tube should, as before, be warmed and oiled and the attempt made to pass it first in a horizontal direction along the floor of the nose. If obstruction be met with, the tube should be withdrawn and the other nasal chamber should be tried. The nasal septum is usually deflected to one side and but little difficulty is, as a rule, experienced. While passing the tube, it is wise gently to depress the chin, as by this expedient the tube is much less likely to enter the larynx. If the patient be permitted to throw his head backward, the tube may even pass around the soft palate and enter the mouth, where it may curl upon itself or protrude between the lips. As a rule, little or no difficulty is encountered in properly introducing the tube. As it enters the pharynx, the patient may gag or possibly cough. The operator should wait quietly until these symptoms have subsided, when, the tube being passed on a little, a reflex act of swallowing occurs and it safely enters the esophagus. Generally fourteen to sixteen inches are passed into the nose before the stomach is reached. The fact that the tube is really in the stomach may be verified by gently percussing the stomach while the operator holds the free or funnel-shaped end of the tube near his ear. The tube having been properly placed, a pint or more of milk, with or without raw eggs and perhaps with necessary medicines, is poured slowly and gently into the funnel-shaped end. After the feeding has been completed, the tube should be withdrawn slowly. Especial care should be taken to see that the tube is entirely empty, so that no milk or other material used in the feeding may enter the larynx. The entrance of food into the larynx and bronchial tubes leads to very serious results. It may find its way into the smaller air-passages and give rise to a fatal broncho-pneumonia—an inspiration pneumonia. The fact that the pharyngeal and laryngeal reflexes are frequently lessened and sensibility obtunded, renders care imperative. If the operator during the passage of the tube should feel some doubt as to the course it is taking, he can instantly detect the entrance of respiratory air into the tube by applying his ear to the funnel-shaped extremity. However, nasal feeding is commonly attended with but little danger and can often be practised for many weeks or even months. Whenever nasal feeding, or, for that matter, feeding through the tube by the mouth, is attempted for the first time, at least two assistants should be present. The patient may be seated in a chair or lie upon his bed. A nurse should be stationed upon each side of the patient, so as to control the arms and legs. Occasionally, another nurse is required to hold the head. The tube should then be carefully passed by the operator and the feeding accomplished. The majority of patients in whom forcible feeding is necessary, offer but little resistance; they soon learn to adapt themselves to the procedure so that it can usually be carried out expeditiously and with but little trouble. Artificial feeding should be practised at least twice in the twenty-four hours, though in given cases it is necessary to resort to it more frequently. The tube should always be cleansed scrupulously. The nostril should also be carefully inspected afterward and a little liquid petrolatum applied. We should remember that too frequent or awkward introduction of the tube may irritate or inflame the mucous membrane.

If organic obstruction of the esophagus be suspected, or if the tube has been passed with difficulty, so that the operator has reason to fear that it has become folded or bent upon itself, it should be withdrawn and another attempt made to introduce it. Sometimes it answers the purpose better to insert near the funnel-shaped extremity of the tube a piece of glass tubing through which the flowing of the liquid food can be observed. It is important to add that no force should at any time be used, either in the passage of the tube through the nasal chamber, or in its subsequent course through the esophagus into the stomach. The quantity of food administered must depend upon the case. It should be relatively small at first, especially if the stomach be irritable or vomiting seem likely.

Other forms of forcible feeding may also be attempted. Thus, a patient may be placed upon his back, the arms and head firmly held, while small quantities of liquid food may be slowly fed into the nose by means of a spoon, a feeding-cup, or a funnel. The food trickles back into the pharynx and is swallowed. Such procedures as these, however, are not often necessary, the nasal tube furnishing a much more satisfactory method.

Such physiologic measures as massage, electricity, and bathing, although of demonstrated value in the treatment of neurasthenia and hysteria, have only a limited application in the treatment of insanity. This is true especially of electricity, and to a somewhat less extent of massage and hydrotherapy.

Massage, in general so useful when patients are kept at rest, is impracticable in a large number of cases of insanity because of the extreme restlessness of the patient. In many of the depressive forms, the necessary handling and manipulation irritate and annoy the patient and often do more harm than good, while with disturbed and excited persons, it is out of the question. Massage is, nevertheless, of distinct value in the milder forms of mental disease, especially mild melancholia, and during the convalescent periods of various other affections.

Electricity also has a very restricted field, much more restricted, indeed, than that of massage. Like massage, it frequently irritates and distresses the patient instead of benefiting him. It may, however, be employed to a moderate degree in some of the mild depressive cases. The slowly interrupted faradaic current, of sufficient strength to induce contractions of the various groups of muscles of the trunk and extremities, may be of benefit, just as in neurasthenia. Occasionally static electricity is employed; the static breeze to the head, general electrization, and sparking of the trunk and limbs are believed to act as stimulants. The application of static electricity in the treatment of insanity is, however, in my experience exceedingly limited.

In **bathing** we have a measure of undoubted value, and one which can usually be employed without much difficulty. In most cases of melancholia, for example, the patient will submit quietly to a bath in bed. Other patients, again, can be bathed very readily in the tub. The bath, it should be remembered, is not for purposes of cleanliness but for its direct sedative or stimulating action. It is as a nervous sedative and calmative that it is of most value. An expedient practised extensively for many years past in Germany, especially by Kraepelin, and of late years in this country, consists in the use of the **prolonged warm immersion bath.** The patient is placed in a bath of a temperature of 95°F. (35°C.), and allowed to remain in the tub for one or two hours, several days, several weeks, or, it may be, for months. The procedure is especially adapted to active deliria, to acute mania, to the excited periods of dementia præcox and to other acute disturbances.

If the patient is struggling and difficult to place in the bath, Kraepelin may give him a full dose of sulphonal several hours before the procedure is attempted. Sometimes a hypodermic injection of scopolamin given shortly before quiets the patient sufficiently. A better plan is to give a hypodermic injection of morphin sulphate, one-eighth or one-fourth grain, together with scopolamin, one two-hundredth or one one-hundredth grain. This usually quiets the patient decidedly and does no harm while it greatly diminishes the chances of injury in very violent cases. Most frequently, it should be added, disturbed cases can be placed successfully in the bath without previous medication.

The patient who has been noisy and struggling, having been placed in the bath, soon becomes quieted. The warm water has a calmative and relaxing influence. He is resting lightly on broad canvas strips, and the fact that he is half floating in the warm water, the freedom of restraint resulting from the absence of clothing, and the fact that no resistance is offered to his movements, soon bring about a cessation of his struggling. At the same time elimination by the skin is greatly stimulated; there is a rapid fall of blood-pressure, due to dilatation of the peripheral vessels; and probably there is also a corresponding lessening of tension and fulness of the cerebral vessels. The pulse rate, respiration and bodily temperature reveal no changes of moment.

If the patient continues to struggle or to be restless in the bath, Kraepelin does not force him to remain in it, but renews the attempt after an interval. Sooner or later, the patient gets used to the procedure and is placed in the bath without difficulty. The patient may go to sleep in the bath or upon being removed to his bed. As indicated above, he may be permitted to remain in the bath, according to circumstances, for an indefinite period. The desire for food is much increased, and, as a rule, the patient is fed very readily. The nourishment should, just as in the case of a patient in bed, be given at regular intervals and, if necessary, night and day. The bowel movements and urine are discharged directly into the water and are carried off by the discharging pipe; the advantages of this in filthy cases needs no comment. Bed-sores are prevented, or, if they have already occurred, are kept ideally clean.

Finally, the occurrence of menstruation offers no obstacle to the treatment.

Obviously, a warm bath such as above described can only be given in institutions properly equipped and is out of the question in the emergencies of private practice. Under these circumstances recourse may be had to a warm wet pack and, indeed, with the most gratifying results. The sheet in which the patient is wrapped should be dipped in *warm* water, 95°F. or more and the patient thoroughly wrapped in blankets in addition. Soon free sweating and relaxation set in. The result is greatly hastened and enhanced if we give the patient an eighth or a quarter of a grain of pilocarpin muriate hypodermically. Should the application of the pack be attended by much struggling, it is proper to give a hypodermic injection of morphin and scopolamin, though this is usually not necessary. The patient should be allowed to remain in the pack for about two hours. It should be added that in melancholia, neither the continuous warm tub-bath nor the warm pack are indicated. If, however, there is much agitation in a case of melancholia, the warm pack may prove of value.

Cold baths and douches are rarely of use in the insane, except, perhaps, in the case of convalescents. Patients with depressive insanity do not react well to cold, while in disturbed cases, the risk is incurred of increasing the excitement.

Other methods of hydrotherapy do not call for consideration. There is one procedure, however, which deserves special mention and which in given instances is of great value, and this is **hypodermoclysis.** Hypodermoclysis in certain toxic cases, for instance, in the toxicity of defective elimination, greatly stimulates the latter function and is often productive of the very best results. A more radical expedient is the direct introduction of salt solution into the veins. Here, of course, free venesection should precede the introduction of the salt solution. The effect on the mental condition of the patient, for the time being, is under given circumstances surprisingly good.

Obviously, however, there are narrow limits to the success attending our efforts to bring about elimination; and this arises from the nature of the intoxication present. When we consider the nature of this intoxication, the facts prove to be extremely interesting and important. We know that the poisons in insanity are not mineral salts and also that they are not leukomains. Thus, there are no facts of chemistry to indicate that either the mineral salts or the leukomains are the toxic factors, and, secondly, both of these groups of substances are readily eliminated—readily discharged from the organism—while the toxins of insanity are either eliminated very badly or not at all. Indeed, the position of the toxins of insanity is exactly like the position of the toxins of infection, for example, of typhoid fever. No amount of purging, diuresis, or sweating enables us to get rid of the toxins in typhoid fever. The latter are protein bodies, the injurious character of which nature combats by the process of immunization, a process long and tedious. In insanity the poisons are likewise protein substances, which nature endeavors to combat by the formation of antibodies. The parallel between the behavior of infection and the course of mental diseases is more than suggestive; indeed, in the manic-depressive group this parallel appears to be complete. It appears also to be complete in the secondary autointoxications resulting from the infections, and equally, though less clearly so, in the secondary autointoxications following poisons introduced from without. In all forms of secondary autointoxication, it may be safely claimed, the tendency is to a restitution of the normal condition.

What can we do here to assist nature? In what way can we favor the production of immune bodies? Evidently the resources of the organism are increased by adding to its substance, and the first indication is to give an abundance of nourishment, to practice full feeding just as we do in tuberculosis and in states of depressed nutrition generally. Full feeding does more than to add to the weight of the body and to encourage the repair of exhausted tissues; it distinctly favors the formation of lipoid substances, substances which we now know play a most important rôle both as antigens and antibodies. The practical results of full feeding, and at times of massive feeding, are so well known as not to call for comment. That these results are due not only to a general improvement in nutrition, but also to the more liberal and readier formation of antibodies, is a most important fact for us to recognize.

Medication.—One of the special indications in the treatment of mental cases is the production of sleep. There can be no doubt that this is one of the most important indications presented, and one that is often very imperfectly and half-heartedly met. Simple physiologic methods of inducing sleep, such as exercise, bathing, massage, the drip sheet, the taking of food, of hot milk, suggestion, placebos, may all fail and, indeed, do fail in a large number of cases. If the patient secures some sleep, say four or five hours out of the twenty-four, we may be justified, other things equal, in withholding sedatives. If, however, the insomnia is very pronounced and persistent, grave danger both to the physical and mental condition of the patient may ensue. The mental symptoms may become more pronounced and grave exhaustion may supervene. Indeed, patients have been known to die from want of sleep and the accompanying exhaustion. Further, a long experience with the milder forms of mental disease, such as are treated outside of institutions, as well as with the early periods of the more pronounced forms, has convinced me that the tarmpt correction of sleep disturbances is of the utmost imporprnce. Many patients in whom this matter is neglected, become rapidly and markedly worse. Others, again, in whom it receives prompt attention, are often spared a prolonged or a grave attack. As we have just seen, physiologic methods often fail to induce sleep; what then are we to do, especially when the patient's need is urgent?

Of late years a prejudice has grown up in the mind of physicians as to the use of **sedatives.** This prejudice is often so strong, especially in institutions, as to lead to an utterly inadequate use of these remedies or even to their entire exclusion. This prejudice, I am convinced, has its origin in the following causes: first, it is a reaction against a former somewhat too free use of these remedies; secondly, it has its origin in an insufficient and often mistaken knowledge of their mode of action, and in an exaggerated fear of their harmful effects; thirdly, the prejudice has been distinctly fostered by the attitude of the lay public, and especially the lay press. The word "dope" a slang word of the slums, has in large degree replaced such words as "medicine" and "remedy." The word "dope" is used not only by the laity and the lay press, but, I am sorry to add, even by some physicians. The latter have, in a degree, encouraged an **unscientific attitude** toward sedatives that has worked injury to their patients. Drug habits cannot and do not ensue if the physician exercises a reasonable precaution. This may, in private practice, entail some difficulty, not, however, in institutions, for here the administration of the remedy given is completely under the control of the physician. Physicians in private practice are, in my observation, habitually exceedingly careful in prescribing sedatives. Many physicians do not prescribe them at all unless the medicine is to be given by a nurse to whose hands the control of the remedy is thus confided. Whatever may be said as to these details, however, there cannot be any doubt as to the necessity or propriety of the use of sedatives under given conditions. To withhold them under given conditions is equivalent to withholding nitrous oxid during the extraction of a tooth or denying a patient the sleep of ether during a surgical operation. Further, just as skill and judgment are required in the giving of an anesthetic, so are skill and judgment required in the administration of sedatives.

Space will not permit us to consider more than a few general principles. An ideal remedy would be one which would induce a sleep approximating the normal sleep and which would be followed neither by physical depression nor other unpleasant symptoms. A large number of sedatives are at present at our disposal and many of them fulfil, approximately at least, the above conditions. Recently Dr. Richard Eager* of the Devon County Asylum, at Exminster, England, has carefully reviewed the use of sedatives. He points out the necessity of procuring sleep in certain cases, and that physiologic methods often fail completely. He points out, especially, the necessity of procuring sleep in cases with depression that threaten to be cases of melancholia, and further, that many

---

*Eager, Richard: "Journal Mental Sc.," July, 1914, p. 461.

of the hypnotics that are used induce sleep which is like the natural sleep and are not attended by depression or unphysiologic effects; and he insists that patients every now and then die from the exhaustion which the want of sleep induces. Some medicines are comparatively harmless; others have cumulative effects. Some do not conduce to the formation of drug habits; others still are liable to do so, especially if prescribed recklessly.

Of course, all physicians recognize that sedatives should not, save exceptionally, be used over long periods of time. Their obvious application is to secure the immediate relief of a distressing insomnia. Frequently, after such relief has been secured the patient continues sleeping without the medicine, or under the influence of a placebo. In given cases, should this not be the result, the remedy should, notwithstanding, be from time to time suspended, and, if later a sedative again becomes necessary, an entirely different one should be given.

Insomnia as met with both in the neurasthenic states and in the course of the various mental diseases, is unquestionably toxic in its origin and is but one of the many symptoms expressive of the toxicity from which the patient suffers. Compared with this toxicity the action of sedatives is evanescent. Their effect on the nervous tissue is merely transient and no harm can come from their judicious application; indeed, incalculable benefit often follows their use.

Further, another and most important point remains to be considered. When drugs are used habitually, tolerance to their use, as we all know, is sooner or later established and an increasing dose is required to produce an effect. The establishment of this tolerance doubtless depends on the formation of **antibodies**; in the case of some drugs, for example, morphin, the formation of an antitoxin has been definitely proved.* This fact has, however, an added significance. Justschenko and other writers point out that under the use of sedatives, lipoid substances are increased in amount. Justschenko declares that biochemical investigations have shown that under the influence of sedatives, for example, in

*Hirschlaff: "Riedel's Berichte," 1904, p. 27; also "Abstr., Jahresbericht f. Neurologie u. Psychiatrie," 1904, p. 1228.

13

severe melancholias, there is an increase of cholesterin in the blood, and cholesterin is, as is well known, a powerful antitoxic and anti-hemolytic body. In other words, sedatives directly stimulate the formation of antibodies, and there can be no doubt that in their judicious use we have, in given instances, a valuable means of aiding in the recovery of our patients.

A few general statements in regard to hypnotics will prove of value. Personally I never use—or very rarely—the **alcohol group of sedatives,** which includes, among other things, alcohol, paraldehyd, amylene hydrate, chloral hydrate, and butyl chloral hydrate. Alcohol is sometimes given to promote sleep in persons suffering from neurasthenia; more especially in the form of beer or ale. The sleep so induced, however, is not apt to be prolonged, and besides the wisdom of prescribing alcoholic beverages for neurasthenics may well be questioned; and I have rarely so employed them. In the therapeutics of fully developed mental disease, alcohol plays no rôle whatever. Of the other sedatives belonging to the alcohol group, all may be dismissed as no longer necessary since they have of recent years been displaced by other and more serviceable remedies. Perhaps an exception should be made in favor of paraldehyd. The latter has the great advantage of acting with the utmost promptness and certainty and at the same time of acting as a stimulant and not as a depressant. Its unpleasant odor and taste, however, make it difficult of administration save in alcoholic subjects, who take it very readily when it is suspended in whiskey. It is, therefore, especially adapted to procuring a first sleep in alcoholic delirium and, because the sleep induced is short, some other and more slowly acting remedy may be given at the same time.

The **sulphonal group** presents several valuable sedatives, each of which has special advantages. Trional, ten to thirty grains, acts kindly and without depression or subsequent unpleasant after-effects. Sulphonal, ten to twenty grains, acts slowly and is of special advantage when it is desired to procure a prolonged sleep. Like trional, its action is not accompanied by depression, but, because it is slowly eliminated, some hebetude may persist for a time after awakening following full doses. Tetronal closely resembles trional. Porphyruria, said to follow the too free administration of the sulphonal group, I have not met with.

The group of veronal, medinal, luminal and adalin appears to be especially valuable. Veronal is usually given in five to ten grain doses; if given too freely, it gives rise to a sleep that is too prolonged and is in some instances followed by heaviness and hebetude. Medinal (veronal sodium), five to fifteen grains, is eliminated with great readiness; it acts very promptly, the sleep approximates the normal, there is no depression and no unpleasant after-effect. Luminal, one and one-half to five grains, much lauded by Eager, has proved in my hands to be very valuable. Adalin appears to be an almost perfect hypnotic. The sleep induced is light and gentle and unattended by any concomitant or subsequent effects. It has the further advantage of being efficacious in relatively small dose, e.g., five grains; although not infrequently fifteen grains are required.

The bromid group can be dismissed with the statement that the bromids are not suitable for prolonged administration and not as valuable, as hypnotics, as other remedies in our possession. Opium and its alkaloids also appear to have a very restricted application. Opium, however, is especially recommended by Eager in agitated melancholia. No drug habit follows its use in such cases, even when the administration is prolonged. Scopolamin is a drug of undoubted value. It is efficacious in producing quiet and sleep in even so small a dose as one four-hundredth grain, though commonly one two-hundredth or one one-hundredth of a grain are required. It has of late attracted renewed attention through its use in the production of the so-called "twilight sleep" in the obstetric clinic at Freiburg. Administered hypodermically together with morphin (one one-hundredth of a grain of scopolamin and one-eighth of a grain of morphin) rapid sedation and sleep follow. The sleep is not profound, but the patient can be handled and submitted to various procedures without the slightest difficulty. If scopolamin be used alone in large dose, it may be followed by dryness of the mucous membranes. Hallucinations and even delirium are also said to follow its too free use. This, I am convinced, is rare. Finally, it should be added that such a thing as a scopolamin habit is unknown.

In considering the **administration of sedatives** to the insane, preference should always be given to the milder remedies. It is also an important point to remember that it is not wise to continue the administration of the same drug or the same combination of drugs continuously night after night. It is an excellent plan, also, to **alternate** the medicines; thus, veronal can be given upon one evening and sulphonal upon another.

From an *à priori* standpoint, all narcotics are objectionable. However, the deterioration and demoralization of the patient from continued loss of sleep and unrest is worse; so that it is wisest in given cases to use them. They should always be used with judgment and with discretion, but if used at all, they should be given in sufficient doses to do the work intended. The amount required by the patient can, as a rule, be determined by a careful trial. Moderate doses should be given first, and, if necessary, larger doses later.

The **alterative** remedies, the iodids and mercurials save in specific cases, are at the present day comparatively little used in asylums for the insane. If brain syphilis be present, they are, of course, of value. They are also employed for varying periods of time in the majority of cases of paresis, usually alternating or in connection with the use of salvarsan and salvarsanized serum (see Chapter II). Cases of dementia resulting from gross diseases of the membranes and vessels of the brain also offer a field for their use. The details of their administration will be considered later on.

The various **tonic** remedies may be employed as indications arise. The so-called nerve tonics are of little value. Strychnin is of decided benefit in cases with marked depression of the circulation. Its action upon the nervous system in mental diseases is unimportant. Digitalis, strophanthus and nitroglycerin are also useful, at times, if there be cardiac weakness.

The bitter tonics possess a limited field of usefulness only. Of themselves, they rarely induce an insane patient to eat. Occasionally iron is of value, notably in cases in which there is anemia.

The same is true of arsenic. The administration of these medicines does not, however, have any effect upon the mental disease itself.

Laxatives must be employed in quite a large number of cases of insanity. Here special indications must determine the choice of individual remedies. These it is not necessary to discuss in detail. Because of the atonic condition of the intestinal tract in so many of the patients, it is often advisable to use cascara; and because of the catarrhal conditions present in so many others, it is at times advisable to use sodium phosphate, Carlsbad salts, or other saline.

Thyroid extract is a useful remedy in a limited number of cases. Its value in myxedematous dementia and cretinism is beyond question. It is also of value, occasionally, in some of the depressive forms of insanity, though this value is limited (see Chapter II).

Hypnotism and Suggestion.—So far as my own experience goes, **hypnotism** plays no rôle in the treatment of insanity. **Suggestion,** however, without hypnotism, is undoubtedly useful in some cases. Especially are suggestions of returning health and happiness valuable in the convalescent stages of the depressive affections; for instance, in the convalescence from melancholia. Suggestions made under these circumstances have a distinctly bracing and stimulating effect. Under their influence, the patient eats better, sleeps better, and suffers less. However, suggestion, even of this kind, is applicable only in a limited number of cases.

Sometimes psychotherapy is of value in the neurasthenic-neuropathic group of mental disorders, *i.e.*, in psychasthenia. **Psychanalysis** is discussed in Part III of this book.

Restraint.—At times, the question of restraint presents itself In modern asylums with their manifold precautions for safety, and especially with the large number of attendants, physical restraint has almost entirely disappeared. Camisoles, anklets, and wristlets are rarely required and still more rarely justified. However, in exceptional instances, restraint is not only justified, but imperative. Thus, the patient may be constantly endeavoring to injure his own person or is engaged in a constant and exhausting struggle with his surroundings and attendants. Again, restraint may be imperative in a patient who has suffered from a serious surgical injury, such as a fracture of a limb, and this applies, of course, also to a patient upon whom some surgical operation has been performed necessitating absolute quiet thereafter. Usually a sheet properly applied answers every purpose. At other times, a camisole—a canvas shirt with long, closed sleeves and laced up the back—may be used. If restraint be applied, the patient should be none the less carefully watched. Patients frequently make renewed attempts to struggle, and if not watched may, in spite of the restraint, injure themselves. We should remember also that if restraint alone be depended upon to quiet a patient, the continuous struggling likely to ensue greatly favors exhaustion. It is wisest, therefore, in some cases to give nervous sedatives or hypnotics at the same time.

The most efficient and humane form of restraint yet devised is the continued **warm bath** described in the preceding pages (see p. 187). It is also the most physiologic form of restraint. Similar remarks apply to the **warm pack.** Here, as in the bath, the warmth and moisture not only conduce to the relaxation and the quieting of the patient, but the pack is at the same time an efficient and kindly restraint.

Treatment of Bed-sores.—When bed-sores supervene in the insane, they should, of course, be treated surgically. The importance of cleanliness cannot be too strongly insisted upon, though the difficulty of securing this in cases in which there is involvement of the sphincters is obvious. The danger of septic infection is always present and should as much as possible be guarded against. Caution must be exercised not to use sublimate, permanganate or antiseptics too freely. After a first thorough surgical cleansing, it may suffice to use a ten or twenty per cent. solution of alcohol and subsequently protecting the ulcer as thoroughly as possible.

Physician and Patient.

It is necessary to consider briefly the personal relations of the physician to the patient. It should not be necessary to state that the physician's attitude should be one of kindly interest, and that as far as possible his conduct should be such as to inspire confidence. While he may never be able to enter into close relation with some patients, it is quite possible to establish friendly relations and confidence in others. It is, in my opinion, always essential that the physician should not deceive the patient, nor should he allow any deception to be practised upon the latter by others. Patients not infrequently become aware of intended deceptions and it becomes correspondingly difficult to gain their confidence. In regard to the delusions of the patient, the physician should prove himself a quiet listener. While he should be careful not to agree with the patient, nor even to appear to accept the delusions in any way, he should in a large number of cases avoid an open contradiction. Direct and flat contradiction of the patient's belief sometimes greatly disturbs him and may bring on attacks of marked excitement. Besides, in most cases, such a course is for the time being useless. Altercations and discussions are to be deprecated. Passive resistance to the patient's delusions is a far more effectual method of dealing with the situation. In many cases unnecessary talking should be avoided. Threats should never be indulged in. Attempts at discipline or punishment are equally reprehensible.

CHAPTER II

THE TREATMENT OF THE SPECIAL FORMS OF MENTAL DISEASE

Clinical Grouping of Mental Diseases. Delirium, Confusion and Stupor; Melancholia, Mania, and Circular Insanity; The Heboid-Paranoid Group. The Neurasthenic-neuropathic Insanities; Simple Dementia; Paresis; Insanities of Intoxication and the Drug Habits.

As I have elsewhere pointed out, mental diseases readily arrange themselves in five great groups, as follows:

I. Delirium, Confusion, and Stupor.

II. Melancholia, Mania, and Circular Insanity (Manic-depressive Insanity).

III. The Heboid-Paranoid Group (Dementia Præcox, Paranoia).

IV. The Neurasthenic-neuropathic Insanities. (Psychasthenia).

V. Dementia.

It will be most convenient to consider the treatment of the various mental affections in the order in which they are enumerated.

DELIRIUM, CONFUSION, AND STUPOR

Delirium

It is necessary first to review some of the elementary facts in relation to delirium.

As I have elsewhere shown, the various forms of delirium separate themselves clinically into three types: First, **simple febrile delirium**; that is, the delirium which is a symptom and accompaniment of the various exanthemata, infectious fevers and acute visceral diseases. Secondly, **specific febrile delirium**; that is, the delirium which is variously known as *delirium grave*, typho-mania, acute delirious mania, Bell's delirium, or acute delirium. This type of delirium is probably a specific clinical entity. It is very active, is characterized by a febrile state, the rise of temperature being generally quite high, while there are not present any surface lesions such as are found in the exanthemata, nor any sign of visceral involvement as in pneumonia or meningitis. It would seem, therefore, to be due to a specific infection, the bacteria or toxins of which expend their action upon the brain, without giving rise to lesions of the cutaneous surface or of the viscera. The third form of delirium is **afebrile delirium**; this type frequently makes its appearance as a sequel of acute exhaustion or of acute infectious diseases and intoxications. It is not accompanied by fever, but by all the signs of profound asthenia. Every now and then it ensues during the post-febrile period of one of the exanthemata, for example, typhoid fever. It is a not infrequent sequel of influenza. At times it follows trauma, surgical operations, or the shock and infection of labor. Exhaustion, infection, or intoxication appear always to be prominent factors. As examples of afebrile delirium following the action of poisons, we may instance the delirium from alcohol, from lead, from the prolonged misuse of drugs.

The **symptoms of delirium**, no matter what its origin, are always the same: illusions, hallucinations, confusion and hurry of thought, fleeting and fragmentary, unsystematized delusions; incoherence. The same elements are always present. This is true whether the delirium occurs in a young person or an old person; whether it be mild or whether it be furious; or whether it follows typhoid fever, pneumonia, or erysipelas, on the one hand, or alcoholic, plumbic, or other intoxication, on the other. It should be added also that the deliria are always relatively short in duration —a few hours, a few days, or, at most, a week or two.

Treatment.—The treatment of delirium is based upon general principles. When occurring as simple febrile delirium and when mild and purely symptomatic in character, delirium can in practice be entirely ignored. Its treatment in such cases is essentially the treatment of the underlying disease. Every now and then, however, the delirium accompanying the infections—for example, typhoid fever—is so grave as to necessitate some modification of the treatment. Especially, when occurring early in the course of the disease, it is of evil omen, indicating that the nerve-centers have been overwhelmed by the invasion of the bacteria or their resulting toxins, and that grave exhaustion has supervened. Two factors must, therefore, be taken into account: first, the direct toxic action upon the nervous system, due to the infection; and, secondly, the exhaustion. Similar factors doubtless play the essential rôle in specific febrile delirium, while in the afebrile form we deal with the late toxins of infection or other poisons, and likewise with exhaustion.

Obviously, in the treatment three indications must be considered: first, the elimination of the poisons; secondly, the allaying of the excitement; and, thirdly, the maintenance of the nervous strength. So far as possible, these indications must be met promptly and simultaneously. The means at our command consist in the administration of liquids in large quantities, in the free use of baths, in the free administration of nourishment, and, according to indications, in the use of cardiac stimulants and nervous sedatives.

Liquids in large quantities, of course, act as diuretics, while the action of the skin can be profoundly stimulated by hydrotherapy in various forms. When fever is present, cold sponging, cold sprinkling, and other forms of cold bathing are applicable. In the afebrile forms of delirium—i.e., those which come on in the post-febrile or convalescent period of infectious diseases, as typhoid fever, or which result from drug intoxications, as alcohol—the most effective form of hydrotherapy is the prolonged warm immersion bath. The temperature of the bath should range from 90° to 95°F. (32.2° to 35°C.). In household practice an immersion bath is not often applicable, because a bath tub is not always convenient or because the patient struggles too violently. Much more available, and in many cases more efficacious, is the warm wet pack. This can be given in the ordinary way, save that the sheet, instead of being dipped in cold water, is dipped in warm water (see p. 189). The patient having been thoroughly and closely wrapped, blankets are applied over the sheet and the patient allowed to remain in the pack for upwards of an hour and under given circumstances even longer. As a rule, profuse diaphoresis results with marked diminution of the excitement. This effect may be greatly enhanced, as has already been pointed out, by the hypodermic use of pilocarpin. In delirium of marked severity, however, both the wet pack and the immersion bath have, in private practice, serious drawbacks. The necessary manipulations of the pack or bath may add greatly to the fright and confusion from which the patient is suffering and may greatly aggravate his exhaustion. Under these circumstances recourse may be had, as already indicated, to hypodermic injections of scopolamin and morphin. The wet pack should not be repeated frequently. Especially is this caution necessary in cases of prolonged delirium and in those in which exhaustion is a marked factor. The depression from the excessive sweating induced by the wet pack should in this connection, especially, be borne in mind.

It is obviously of the utmost importance, especially if the delirium be at all violent and the patient be expending much strength in his struggles, to administer **sedatives** of various kinds. No well-founded objection can be made to their judicious administration. The quiet and the sleep produced are of the utmost benefit to the patient. As a rule, the milder hypnotics discussed in the preceding chapter prove efficacious. Recourse may be had to medinal or sulphonal. These drugs can be administered advantageously in combination; for instance, ten grains of medinal with ten or fifteen grains of sulphonal. Even when the excitement is intense, such a combination frequently induces sleep of many hours' duration. Luminal, three to five grains, often proves of great value. So valuable are these remedies that every possible effort should be made to administer them. Many delirious patients, especially alcoholics, will swallow readily everything that is offered them, and in such cases bromids or other medicines can be given. Regarding the bromids, the depressing action of the large and repeated doses usually necessary should not be lost sight of; above all should they be avoided in patients whose cardiac action is weakened. Paraldehyd, a remedy of undoubted value, is rejected in most cases of active delirium, and yet is by some patients, notably the alcoholics, greedily accepted, especially when administered in whisky. The paraldehyd has the great advantage of producing profound sleep within a few minutes, though the sleep may be of only two or three hours' duration. It is a valuable adjuvant when medicines of the veronal or sulphonal group have been given; for it hastens the sleep which ensues upon these drugs only after a decided interval of time. In non-alcoholic cases, because of its nauseous taste and disagreeable odor, and doubtless also because of the hallucinations and illusions of taste already present, it cannot be administered, and we must resort to other measures.

Regarding the choice of hypnotics in delirium, or the method of administration, no hard and fast rule can be formulated. General principles alone can be indicated. It should be borne in mind, other things equal, that the best results are obtained in cases in which they are used promptly; even in patients who are treated by sponging, warm baths, or wet pack, some hypnotic should be administered early and in sufficient dose; the effect of the bath is thereby enhanced and prolonged. Furthermore, patients who struggle so violently that a bath is out of the question may, as has been indicated, become amenable to the wet pack or other hydrotherapeutic procedure after hypnotics have been administered.

In addition to our efforts to allay the excitement, restlessness, and struggles of the patient, measures should so far as possible be instituted to maintain his strength. In all cases of delirium in which the symptoms are at all pronounced, there is danger of exhaustion. Indeed, exhaustion always supervenes in the grave forms, and here constitutes, barring accident or injury, the one source of danger. In specific febrile delirium (Bell's delirium), so commonly fatal, it is the usual cause of death. It behooves us, therefore, to make every effort not only to combat the impending exhaustion, but if possible to anticipate it. Liquid food, milk, eggs, beef preparations of various kinds, should be administered in as large quantities as possible. Feeding in delirium is often excessively difficult; the excitement, the confusion, and the struggles of the patient may be so pronounced that for a time it may become impracticable to administer nourishment in the ordinary way. Frequently the attention of the patient cannot be attracted, or, if attracted, it can be held only for very short periods of time. At other times he cannot be made cognizant of the food; he may believe that it is poisoned, or he may regard it as some offensive or disgusting substance. Notwithstanding the difficulties, every effort should be made to administer food. As a rule, it is possible to get down sufficient for the immediate necessities of the patient, though the total amount for the twenty-four hours may be small. **Rectal feeding** may become necessary; under ordinary circumstances it is not practicable to resort to **forcible feeding** with the tube. In cases so severe as to suggest it, forcible feeding is very difficult. In practice it should be resorted to only with patients who subsequently to the excitement become exhausted and stuporous.

If loss of strength be pronounced, recourse should be had to **heart tonics** and **stimulants.** In this connection strychnin, digitalis, strophanthus, nitroglycerin, cocain, and perhaps adrenalin should be borne in mind. The general principles underlying the application of these drugs in other asthenic states apply equally here. Strychnin in doses of a fortieth, a thirtieth, or even a twentieth of a grain every four hours; digitalis in half-ounce doses of the infusion at similar intervals, are in many cases urgently indicated, especially if cardiac weakness be marked. The value of cocain, both as a cardiac and nervous stimulant, should in cases of this kind not be forgotten. Hypodermic injections of a sixth or a fourth of a grain at four-hour intervals are often of the greatest value. Alcohol also may be employed with advantage, being administered very much as in the asthenic states of the continued fevers. Not only does it have a favorable influence upon the circulation, but also a calmative and sedative effect upon the nervous system.

By far the greater number of the cases of delirium which make their appearance during the post-febrile period of the infectious fevers, *i.e.*, the afebrile deliria, terminate in recovery. As a rule, a subsidence of symptoms is noticeable in a few days, and it then remains to treat the case by simple supporting measures. If marked asthenia supervenes, **rest treatment** with massage and perhaps other physiologic measures should be instituted and maintained until recovery is complete.

Simple febrile delirium runs a course dependent upon the disease of which it is symptomatic, and no special comment as to its subsequent management is necessary. Specific febrile delirium (Bell's delirium), however, usually offers an exceedingly grave prognosis, and in cases of recovery the convalescence is exceedingly tedious. Supporting and tonic measures are, therefore, especially indicated throughout.

Confusion

Confusion, confusional insanity, amentia, or *Verwirrtheit*, as it is variously termed, presents an etiology similar to that of the afebrile deliria. Like the latter, it frequently comes on during the post-febrile period of the acute infectious diseases, for example, typhoid fever. It is seen typically in the confusion which so often follows influenza or which may make its appearance after erysipelas, acute articular rheumatism, the puerperium, profound exhaustion, trauma, surgical shock, etc. Like the afebrile deliria, it may also follow the prolonged abuse of drugs and stimulants. Into its causation there enter, as in delirium, two factors: first, the toxins of infection, or other poisons; and, secondly, persistent exhaustion. Confusion differs from delirium not only in the less violent, less acute character of its symptoms, but also in its duration. As a rule, when once established it lasts many weeks, three or four months being a not uncommon period. There are present, as in delirium, hallucinations and illusions, confusion of thought, and incoherence; hurry of thought is also present, though cerebral activity is never aroused to the same pitch as in delirium.

Treatment.—Because of the profound exhaustion, it is of the very greatest importance to place the patient in bed. In many asylums, cases of confusional insanity are permitted to be up and about the wards. Better progress by far, however, is made when they are placed in bed. As a rule, food is administered more easily in cases of confusion than in cases of delirium. The patients also permit themselves to be handled and bathed more readily. Not infrequently, also, it is possible to institute, especially during the period of convalescence, massage. It is wisest to imitate, so far as possible, the strict rest methods of the full bed treatment of neurasthenia (see p. 40). The rest in bed, especially in the early stage of the affection, should be absolute. Forced feeding should be instituted, as in neurasthenia—milk, eggs, and other food being given in large quantities.

Frequently it is necessary to give scopolamin, medinal, sulphonal, or like remedies to produce sleep, although this need is not so urgent as in delirium; nor must the drugs be given in so large amounts or so frequently repeated. In this connection we should bear in mind the long duration of the affection, and restrict the use of hypnotics as much as possible. Tonic and supporting remedies are also indicated. Strychnin, digitalis, or iron may at various times be employed. The more rigid the rest, the more absolute and conservative the supporting treatment, the better will be the result and the less the necessity for medication. Time is, however, a necessary element in all cases. In the vast majority, simple physiologic methods are followed by complete recovery.

Stupor

In stupor, which is the third member of our first group of mental affections, we have a disease closely allied both to delirium and to confusion. Every now and then a case is met with, in which some infection, poisoning, or profoundly debilitating influence is followed by mental confusion, but in which the confusion is markedly tinged with dulness and hebetude, and in which little by little mental obtusion becomes more and more pronounced until finally the faculties are completely in abeyance. Such a case forms one of simple stupor, or so-called stuporous insanity, or acute dementia. Simple stupor does not make its appearance suddenly. Generally, there is a prodromal period of several days or weeks, during which, as in the beginning of confusional insanity, the patient is hallucinatory and confused; and, indeed, in the beginning the case resembles one of confusion without much excitement. Little by little mental obtusion becomes more and more pronounced and the power to appreciate the surroundings less and less, until finally the patient lies motionless in bed, oblivious to everything about him. Care should, of course, be taken not to confound simple stupor with the stupor of catatonia or melancholia.

Treatment.—The treatment of stupor is essentially **supporting** in character. Like confusion, the disease is of long duration; many weeks, perhaps several months, pass by before convalescence is fully established, and during this time as much food as possible must be given to the patient. Feeding does not usually offer much difficulty; frequently it is possible to administer very large amounts of milk and raw eggs—even as much as three quarts of milk and six to eight eggs daily, with other food in addition. Now and then stupor is so profound as to necessitate a resort to **forcible feeding**.

Supporting drugs are occasionally necessary, especially when there is marked feebleness of the heart and general depression of the circulation, as shown by coldness, moisture, and lividity of the extremities. The general principles of **rest** treatment should be rigidly applied. **Massage,** among other measures, should also be used. We should remember, however, that, as in confusion, massage may not be well borne. It may irritate and annoy the patient.

As might be supposed, quieting remedies are rarely indicated. However, every now and then stupor is associated with a certain amount of physical restlessness; and in this case, small doses of some gentle hypnotic may be employed. The management of stupor is essentially that of confusion, and, as in confusion, the more strict the application of rest and supporting measures, the better the general result.

Considerations of Management Common to Delirium, Confusion, and Stupor

The foregoing paragraphs show that delirium, confusion, and stupor present much that is common, not only in their symptoms, but also in their treatment. They should likewise be dealt with in common from a general point of view. Thus, hallucinations, illusions, and distressing delusions being prominent symptoms, this fact should be considered both in the surroundings and in the method of dealing with the patient.

The patient having been placed in bed, all objects that might favor the production of delusions or multiply hallucinations and illusions—such as pictures on the wall, dark and suggestive ornaments, striking furniture, fur mats, and similar articles—should be removed from the room. The room should be moderately darkened, but not enough to give rise to illusory shadows or to make the objects in the room indistinct. The utmost possible quiet is necessary. All persons should be excluded from the sickroom except the nurses immediately in charge of the patient. The nurses should not walk about needlessly, nor should they engage in unnecessary talking. Least of all should they carry on whispered conversations or indulge in gestures or other demonstrations before or over the patient. Some attention should be given, also, to the dress of the nurses. There is no objection, as a rule, to the ordinary white uniform, but unusual or striking articles of attire, as a black dress, a black shawl, a hood, should be avoided. In many instances, it is wise to remove the nurse's cap, as the latter sometimes impresses the patient strangely. Care should be taken not to approach the patient suddenly or in an unusual way. Especially should the nurse avoid bending over the patient from the head of the bed; the inverted face of the nurse sometimes badly frightens the patient. Attention to simple details, such as are here hinted at, is in practice quite important.

Commitment to Asylum.—The question of the commitment to asylums of patients suffering with delirium, confusion, or stupor, must be decided by the circumstances of each individual case. Deliria are usually of short duration; and when adequate assistance can be obtained, treatment can be carried out efficiently and satisfactorily at the patient's own home. It is certainly not justifiable to commit a patient to a hospital for the insane because of an affection of which the active stage is commonly limited to a few days. In confusion, the circumstances which usually obtain do not differ, so far as nursing and medical attendance are concerned, from those surrounding a patient ill with a continued fever. The patient is,

14

as a rule, not violent, and can readily be controlled.   Two nurses, one relieving the other, are necessary in most cases, as it is not safe to leave the patient alone.   Because of the long duration of confusion, the expense involved by trained nursing and medical attendance outside of a hospital, necessitates, in many instances, the commitment of the patient to an asylum.   In other cases the violence of the symptoms and unusual difficulty of management may also determine commitment.   Similar remarks apply to stupor.   Stupor can be treated with every chance of success by skilled nursing and medical attendance outside of the asylum. Occasionally the undue prolongation of the symptoms and the continued expense may necessitate the patient's commitment.

Special Indications.—When any of the members of this group —delirium, confusion, and stupor—are related to or accompany special pathologic conditions, as rheumatism, gout, diabetes, alcoholic or metallic poisoning—for example, plumbism—this relationship must, of necessity, be considered in the treatment. In addition to the physiologic and symptomatic measures described, special remedies and measures are to be directed against the underlying condition.   These it is unnecessary to detail here.   Similarly, when mental symptoms accompany tuberculosis, malaria, malignant or other visceral affections, the treatment of the insanity must necessarily include the treatment of the physical disease from which the patient is suffering.   In all of these affections, the mental symptoms assume the form of more or less well-defined delirium, confusion, or stupor.   It is true that special phenomena predominate in certain of these diseases.   Thus, in **diabetes** the tendency is toward confusion with depression resembling melancholia; at other times stupor or coma supervenes.   In **gout,** active delirium or active confusion dominates the picture; while in **rheumatism,** delirium, confusion, and stupor appear in practically an equal number of cases.   In **malaria,** confusion or a stuporous state sometimes spoken of as pseudo-paresis, is most frequently present. In **tuberculosis,** confusion, with depressive and persecutory ideas, is not rarely met with; while in malignant and other **visceral affections,** delirium, confusion, or stupor may characterize the picture in varying degrees. Here, confusion is rather the more common form of mental disturbance, and it is, as a rule, accompanied by painful and depressive hallucinations and delusions. A similar mental state may be met with in pregnancy or may ensue during the period of lactation. It is hardly necessary to add to this category the active delirium, often mistaken for mania, which may arise during the puerperium or follow shortly after. Clearly, in every case of delirium, confusion, or stupor, the etiology of the affection should be diligently inquired into and as far as possible the underlying pathologic cause determined. That this may have a most important bearing upon the treatment, local or general, is self-evident. On the whole, however, the treatment must be based upon the general principles previously outlined.

MELANCHOLIA, MANIA, AND CIRCULAR INSANITY

The second group of mental diseases in the classification that I have adopted is made up of melancholia, mania, and circular insanity. Just as the members of the first group, delirium, confusion, and stupor, are closely related to one another, so are melancholia, mania, and circular insanity closely allied forms. Indeed, the view is now held that melancholia and mania are but different phases of one and the same disease. We have to deal with a degenerative affection, manifesting itself in two kindred though distinct and clinically opposite phases. The identity of the etiology of melancholia and mania; the great rôle played by heredity (estimated by Kraepelin at 80 per cent.); the fact that both affections occur especially in persons of the emotional and excitable, the poetic and artistic temperament; that they both occur by preference in early adult life; that they both present similar prodromal factors; that each runs a course of gradual increase, maximum intensity, and final subsidence; that each presents in its course a phase which is the complement of the other; that in each the emotional state dominates the entire picture; that they both tend in their individual attacks to recovery; that each tends to recur; that opposite phases of melancholia and mania are found in the same individual; and, finally, that cases are met with in

which the elements of both phases are present at the same time
(the so-called "mixed-form" of Kraepelin)—can leave no doubt as
to the close relation between the two disorders. Again, as has
already been pointed out (see p. 183) the facts of etiology indicate
that in these affections we have to deal with a toxic state autogenous in its nature; further, the symptoms and course strongly suggest
that the recovery from the individual attacks is due to the successful battle of the organism with this toxicity—possibly by the formation of antibodies, or by such a restitution of function on the part
of ductless glands or other structures that the poison is no longer
produced or is replaced by normal substances. While at present
it is impossible for us to interfere actively by means of serological
or other biochemical methods, we can at least favor and probably
at times hasten a restitution to the normal by the use of physiologic methods of treatment.

Inasmuch as our knowledge of these affections is almost exclusively clinical, our treatment must necessarily be general and
symptomatic. For this reason also, notwithstanding the close
clinical relationship between melancholia and mania, their treatment is best considered separately.

Melancholia

Melancholia, as is well known, presents itself in a variety of
forms; first, the **simple acute melancholia**; second, melancholia of
mild intensity and subacute course, **hypomelancholia**; third, **melancholia without delusions**; and, fourth, **melancholia with stupor.**
Melancholia agitata does not merit separate consideration, at least
not from the viewpoint of treatment; for the management of cases
with prolonged agitation does not differ from that of ordinary
acute melancholia with episodes of agitation. Melancholia of
irregular course and **chronic melancholia** will be touched upon in
the discussion of the treatment, so far as seems necessary.

In a large number of cases of melancholia, we are confronted at
the outset by the question of **commitment to an asylum.** Quite
commonly the surroundings of the patient are such as to preclude
proper care at home. In such cases, if the symptoms be at all
pronounced, commitment should be urgently recommended.

Especially should the danger of suicide, and the necessity for the protection afforded by institution management, be clearly pointed out to the relatives.   However, there is a very large group of cases in which the melancholia is either so mild in degree (hypomelancholia) or in which the patient is so lucid, suffering neither from hallucinations nor from delusions (melancholia without delusions) that commitment to an asylum is neither necessary nor justified. Such cases can be treated effectually by rest methods elsewhere. It is always incumbent, however, for the physician to see that the patient is supplied with a capable nurse or attendant and that other provision is taken to safeguard the patient against the possibility of suicide.   While the tendency to self-destruction is not pronounced in all cases of melancholia, the physician should, as a matter of precaution, regard it as a possibility in every case, no matter how mild the melancholia may appear to be.   We should remember that even in apparently mild cases, the psychic pain from which the patient suffers may at any time become so accentuated, or the delusion of the unpardonable sin become so vivid and overwhelming, that suicide may unexpectedly be attempted. The further fact, also, that patients every now and then make attempts upon the lives of those about them, as a mother upon her children, forms an additional reason why care should be taken. In cases of frank and typical acute melancholia, the question of commitment is often decided by the intensity of the symptoms and the surroundings of the patient, and the danger of self-destruction is thus averted.   In the milder or extra-mural cases, it is best to consider the danger of suicide as always present; not that it is so in reality, but because we are unable to foretell in a given case when, or whether the danger will or will not become actual and acute.   In a very large number of the mild cases, the management of the patient is exceedingly simple and can be carried out with comparatively little trouble, provided the nurse is watchful and notifies the physician at once of any undue accentuation of symptoms.   If episodes of increased intensity occur, the vigilance of those about the patient should of course be redoubled. Suicide in extra-mural cases is, on the whole, infrequent and readily preventable. It is not so much an actual, as a possible, danger; none the less it should be constantly guarded against.

The question of commitment or non-commitment having been determined, it becomes necessary to consider the question of management. To begin, the patient should be isolated, especially from the members of his family and from his immediate circle of friends. Much harm is done by the association of the patient with his relatives. Their mere presence is a constant reminder of his changed condition; their sympathy and solicitude accentuate his suffering and, as a rule, emphasize his delusions. The patient always fares best if he be isolated for a more or less prolonged period. Isolation does good; it rarely does harm, unless, indeed, it be unnecessarily prolonged. If it be continued during the period of convalescence, the patient may feel that he is being neglected by his relatives, and this in turn may serve as a cause of depression. In cases, too, of hypomelancholia, which usually run a very prolonged course, the patient not infrequently feels, if the isolation be of great duration, that he has been abandoned by those who ought naturally to care for him, and this may in turn serve as a potent agent of harm. There can be no question, however, that in all cases of melancholia, as in neurasthenia, isolation is of the utmost benefit. How long the isolation shall last, when and how frequently it shall be broken in upon, must depend entirely upon the judgment, the tact, the good sense, of the physician. Such isolation is necessarily attained for patients who are committed to an asylum. In other cases, it is best brought about by the removal of the patient from his own home. A properly equipped pr vate hospital, a "rest house," a farmhouse in the adjacent country, where the patient is within easy access of his physician, will equally secure the desired isolation.

As a matter of course, when the patient is treated outside of an asylum, he should be provided with a trained nurse. A mere attendant will not answer. The results achieved, it need not be stated, are far better when the patient is under the care of an intelligent and well-trained nurse, while his safety is more certain. In some extra-mural cases it is best to provide the patient with two nurses, so that he is never for an instant left alone. Later on, when convalescence is established, the vigilance may be relaxed and one nurse only will be needed. We should always remember that excess of precaution does no harm, while the lack of it may lead to the most unexpected and disastrous consequences.

Our patient having been properly placed, and supplied with a suitable nurse or nurses, treatment is to be instituted upon the following principles: In the first place, we should remember that the patient is not only in a condition of profound mental depression, usually with painful hallucinations and delusions, but also that he always presents, in addition, symptoms of profound nervous weakness. To these symptoms I have applied the term **neurasthenoid**; while they are like those of neurasthenia, they are not truly neurasthenic. The face is apt to be pale and drawn; the hands and feet are cold, often livid, and sometimes moist. The patient is also more or less emaciated, having often lost many pounds in weight, sometimes as much as thirty or more. His pulse is often soft and feeble and the impulse of the heart weak. Nervously he is easily fatigued. Save when disturbed by periods of agitation, he is apt to remain seated quietly in his chair or lying still in his bed. He speaks but little and sometimes not at all. Exertion, mental or physical, as a rule, fatigues him readily and sometimes adds greatly to his distress, often bringing on episodes of agitation. Under these circumstances it need hardly be pointed out that **rest** is urgently indicated. It is perfectly true that **relative rest** in many cases answers the purpose well. Indeed, with agitated patients, it is often difficult to institute full rest, but there can be no doubt that in all cases in which **prolonged rest in bed** can be instituted, the suffering of the patient is mitigated and the course of the disease favorably influenced. Whenever it is possible, other things being equal, radical rest in bed should be carried out. This rest should always be of many weeks' duration, just as it is in the treatment of neurasthenia. Even in cases of melancholia in which the duration of the disease is unusually prolonged, say a year or more, the patient should from time to time be submitted to periods of rest, these periods alternating, according to circumstances, with other periods of open-air and out-of-door life. The periods of rest should be adapted so far as possible to the recurring waves of increased intensity of symptoms, which waves, experience teaches us, characterize these cases of prolonged and irregular course.

Let us suppose that in a given case—an extra-mural case—rest treatment has been decided upon. It is necessary first to give some attention to the room which the patient is to occupy. If the melancholia be pronounced, or if the symptoms be such as to give rise merely to the suspicion of suicidal attempts, the precaution should be taken not only to place the patient under the supervision of one or more nurses, but also to see that he does not have access to instruments with which injury might unexpectedly be inflicted. It is not necessary to point out that a penknife, a pair of scissors, the implements of a work-basket, nail-files, or similar objects should be excluded from the room. The windows also should be protected against any sudden impulse of the patient to use them as a means of self-destruction. It is an exceedingly simple procedure to adjust screws in the frames of the windows in such a manner that the sashes cannot be lowered or raised sufficiently to permit of the egress of a human body. In other cases, an ordinary strong wire screen, fastened in the window-frame, ostensibly for the purpose of excluding flies or mosquitos, answers an equally good purpose. It need hardly be added that these various precautions should be instituted without the knowledge of the patient and never in such a way as to suggest to his mind, even remotely, the fact that self-destruction is considered as a possibility.

The patient having been placed in bed, rest methods, similar to those instituted in the full bed treatment of neurasthenia (see p. 40) should be instituted. It will soon be found, however, at least in the majority of cases, that certain modifications of method are necessary. A sponge bath should be given in bed, between blankets as usual, but the nurse will soon learn that the patient is averse to unnecessary handling; indeed, that he is frequently made irritable and nervous by such handling. Similar is it with massage, which is so efficacious in neurasthenia and hysteria. Patients with melancholia very frequently object, especially at first, to being rubbed. Rubbing that is too vigorous or too prolonged is often harmful in its immediate effects. Particularly is this true of cases with a tendency to agitation. However, in the larger number of cases, the patient sooner or later becomes accustomed, not only to the companionship of the nurse, but also to the daily bath, and little by little, especially if the nurse be tactful, to the massage. It is hardly necessary to point out that it is imperative that the massage should be given by the nurse and not by a stranger. The patient gradually learns to submit to a degree of handling and manipulation of all kinds at the hands of his nurse which would be out of all question at the hands of a stranger. A skilful nurse will usually be able, sooner or later, to establish rest methods—so far as absolute rest in bed, bathing, and massage are concerned—as thoroughly as in cases of simple neurasthenia. Electricity is, as a rule, inapplicable, especially during the height of the depression. It may, however, in most cases, be employed with advantage during the period of convalescence. In many cases, on the other hand, it can never be instituted at all.

In another respect the application of rest treatment in melancholia differs somewhat from that in neurasthenia. In melancholia there is, in the larger number of cases, not only a diminished appetite but actually disgust for food. Feeding should, therefore, be instituted with much tact and judgment, and here again much depends upon the nurse. In the larger number of cases, by tactful management, full feeding can sooner or later be brought about; the patient taking not only some solid food three times a day, but in addition large quantities of milk. It is frequently a good plan to begin with the administration of liquid food alone—especially milk; and only some time later to attempt the administration of solids. With many patients, when the dislike for food is very pronounced, we may be obliged to limit our efforts to the administration of milk or of milk and eggs, for a prolonged period. In many cases there is not only a loss of appetite, but often the patient is delusional with regard to his food. He may believe that it is poisoned or that it is foul or putrescent, or he may have formed the deliberate purpose of destroying his life by abstaining from food altogether. Much depends upon the tact and the personality of the nurse under such circumstances. Not infrequently, when the patient has refused to take food in response to persistent urging, the simple expedient of placing the glass of milk within easy reach, at his bedside, sometimes results—after a while and if the patient ostensibly be left alone—in his drinking the milk.

In the milder or extra-mural cases it is not, as a rule, necessary to resort to forcible feeding. The patient often gets along for a time upon a surprisingly small amount of food without visible or marked decrease in his strength, especially if he be resting in bed. However, when it has become impossible to administer food for two days, or at most three days, in succession, and especially if the patient's strength has notably diminished, it is necessary to institute forcible feeding. Sometimes before resorting to this expedient, a new nurse—a woman in the case of a male patient—may be brought in to urge him to take food. Sometimes, indeed, the physician himself may be successful when the nurse fails. The patient should be gently spoken to. The necessity of food should be clearly and repeatedly pointed out; every tactful method of persuasion should be instituted. Finally, the patient should be told very plainly that unless he takes food willingly, he will be fed forcibly. Not infrequently, also, when the patient is in the presence of the actual preparations for forcible feeding, he will compromise by taking a certain amount of food. The victory thus gained, it need hardly be said, should be followed up closely. A patient who has obstinately refused to eat, will sometimes swallow mechanically if the food be placed in his mouth. Patients will not infrequently allow themselves to be fed in this way with a spoon. A proportion of cases, however, remains, in which forcible feeding becomes an absolute necessity. In such instances the feeding should be performed in the manner already described (see p. 184). The quantity of food given at any one time and the frequency with which the feeding should be repeated will depend largely upon the patient. It is best at first to limit the feeding to twice daily. A mixture of milk and eggs, measuring as much as sixteen ounces, should be very slowly introduced into the stomach. If the patient tolerates this amount well and there is no vomiting or regurgitation, the quantity may gradually and very decidedly be increased. The feeding may be carried out twice, rarely three times, in the twenty-four hours. Forcible feeding may be a necessary procedure for many days and weeks—indeed for many months; and in some cases it has been carried out for a number of years.

As already stated, forcible feeding is but rarely necessary in extra-mural cases. In the latter, by tact and persuasion, quite a large amount of food can usually be administered. We should always be careful, when full feeding has been instituted, to have the nurse note the character of the evacuations, so as to observe whether the food is being well digested. If the food be not properly digested, it is wise, of course, to diminish the quantity that is given.

Among the **special symptoms** that require attention is the **insomnia** from which the patient suffers. Sometimes, but not frequently, simple expedients, such as induce sleep in neurasthenia, will induce sleep in melancholia; thus, a glass of hot milk at bedtime, or a warm sponge bath, given just before the sleeping hour. Elaborate baths are only exceptionally tolerated. Neither the drip sheet nor the wet pack can, as a rule, be employed. It is true that in some cases, especially in prolonged hypomelancholia, the wet pack affords a very valuable method of inducing sleep; in ordinary cases of melancholia, however, both the drip sheet and the necessary manipulations of the wet pack distress and annoy the patient. Notwithstanding this, hypnotics should not be resorted to unless the insomnia is troublesome and threatens the success of the treatment. The patient is frequently able to get along with comparatively little sleep or a sleep that is broken. Often he is anxious for the administration of medicine, and under ordinary circumstances it is wisest to begin with a placebo, such as a capsule of starch. In mild cases this may satisfy the patient, but, as a rule, it fails to bring about sleep. Not infrequently, hypnotics must be resorted to, and then the rules already laid down should be followed, namely, that the milder of the hypnotics should be used, that they should be used in small doses, and, finally, that they should not be continued for any length of time.

Another symptom that requires serious attention is the **suffering** and agitation of the patient. This, in some cases, may become intense in degree. When it is pronounced and is not mitigated by the rest methods, the full feeding and other measures employed, recourse should from time to time be had to sedatives and pain-allaying remedies. As a matter of experience, it is found that quite frequently small doses of the bromids decidedly lessen the patient's sufferings. In other cases the bromids are powerless or the dose required is excessive. Furthermore, the prolonged administration of the bromids, even in small doses, is liable to accentuate the physical depression which the patient already presents. A far better plan is that of using small doses of morphin or of some preparation of opium. It is not infrequently found that an exceedingly small dose of morphin, such as enters into a cough mixture, a thirty-second or a sixteenth of a grain, produces the most decided amelioration. In other cases, of course, larger doses are required. An important point, in my experience, is the superiority of small doses at short intervals over large doses at long intervals. Thus, it is better to administer, say a thirty-second of a grain of morphin six times daily, than a sixteenth of a grain three times daily. The minute doses are well tolerated and produce an even sedation extending over the entire day. In cases in which small doses of morphin do not quickly produce decided betterment, it is well to substitute a liquid preparation of opium; for example, the deodorized tincture. The quantity administered should be the minimum that will give relief. It is a remarkable fact, furthermore, and one of considerable practical importance, that opium, as well as morphin, is extremely well borne by melancholic patients. Even when decided doses are necessary, the drug rarely induces nausea and does not seem to increase the constipation; certainly the digestive tract is much less disturbed by opium in cases of melancholia than under normal conditions. It is no less remarkable that during the period of convalescence the opium can be withdrawn rapidly and easily. The patient does not appear to miss it, and there is practically no danger whatever of establishing a drug habit; unless, indeed, the drug has been given recklessly and unnecessarily. Nevertheless, opium is not to be resorted to as a routine measure; it should be reserved for cases in which the suffering is extreme and evident. Under such circumstances, however, it is merely humane to use this potent means of relief, and the drug should be given in sufficient dose to be effective. Not infrequently, codein answers every purpose, a half grain or a grain, three or four times daily, decidedly mitigating the patient's suffering. As a matter of course, opiates should not be given continuously for prolonged periods, but should be withdrawn from time to time.

Tonics may be used from time to time in the treatment of melancholia, though they do not markedly influence its course. The temptation to prescribe strychnin in all asthenic states leads also to its occasional use in melancholia. However, there are many patients by whom strychnin is badly borne and in whom it obviously increases the nervous tension, already a cause of suffering. There are times, of course, when the patient is steadily losing ground—especially if he be growing rapidly weaker or if there be evident signs of cardiac failure—when it may be wise to use the strychnin in decided doses for the moment. It should be remembered, however, that strychnin used merely as a general tonic in the course of melancholia is of little value. Iron may be given from time to time, as may also Fowler's solution. These remedies are at most, however, adjuvants to the treatment and of relatively small importance. The bitter tonics exert little influence in exciting an appetite during the height of the disease, and they are, as a rule, taken unwillingly. During the period of convalescence they may prove of value.

Cases of melancholia rarely pursue an even course. The period of maximum intensity of the disease, as well as the period of convalescence, is interrupted now and then by intervals in which the symptoms are less and then again more pronounced. Such slight periods of improvement and again of accentuation of symptoms will naturally also be observed in the patient who is being treated by full rest methods. A patient who is much improved one week may not be quite so well the next or, it may be, for a number of weeks to follow. Notwithstanding these fluctuations, the measures instituted should be resolutely and rigidly persisted in.

Even when the patient is under rigid rest treatment, it is a wise plan to allow him to sit up or exercise about the room for a few minutes twice daily. Now and then, when the rest is absolute and continuous, the patient's muscles become exceedingly relaxed, and when occasion requires that he should leave his bed, increased physical weakness may be very evident. At times this weakness is extreme. Usually such a degree of relaxation is prevented by the slight amount of exercise required in getting out of bed to move the bowels and the exercise required in sitting up while the bed is being made. In many cases, however, slight waves of exaggerated physical weakness, followed again by a return of physical tone, occur in spite of any precaution adopted in the treatment; of these, no adequate explanation can be given.

Rest methods are in mild cases of melancholia sometimes followed by striking results. Occasionally a treatment, extending over six or eight weeks, is followed by a brilliant recovery. Such an issue is not, however, common. Ordinarily, a much longer period, equivalent to that necessary in a profound case of neurasthenia, is required; namely, rest methods persisted in for three or four months. It is not necessary to add that the more rapid results are, as a rule, obtained in the melancholias of early life, while those occurring in middle age usually require a much longer period of treatment. However, that rest treatment abridges the duration of many cases of melancholia, there can be no doubt. It is not, of course, so successful as in cases of neurasthenia, but even when it does not seem to shorten the duration of the disease, it greatly ameliorates the symptoms. Suffering, nervousness, and insomnia are usually markedly lessened. Furthermore, patients who would otherwise die of exhaustion, and patients whose symptoms are unduly prolonged and tend to become chronic, are beyond all doubt saved by elaborate plans of treatment. Finally, in cases that are very prolonged—*i.e.*, cases that last two or even more years—the institution of rest methods for varying periods of time, *repeatedly* during the long course of the disease, is of undoubted value and certainly favors recovery—if recovery is to occur at all.

When, in cases of melancholia that have been submitted to full rest treatment, **convalescence** becomes established, the patient should, as in neurasthenia, be permitted to resume his relations with his friends and the outside world only very gradually. We should remember that the period of convalescence is liable to interruption by recurrence, and that these recurrences often depend directly upon undue strain and unnecessary fatigue.

Little by little, as the case progresses, the patient should be permitted to get out of bed; little by little passive movements should be added to the massage, and finally movements with resistance may be instituted. The time out of bed should gradually be increased, and very soon the patient should be permitted to exercise for short periods in the open air.

The management of the patient, subsequent to a course of rest treatment, is of even greater importance in melancholia than in neurasthenia. If possible, the patient should be sent to the seashore, to some resort in the country or in the mountains, as circumstances may dictate. Here healthful outdoor living should be followed for a number of weeks, and, if possible, for a number of months. Vigorous exercise should, of course, be the rule. Eventually the return of the patient to his occupation is to be attempted. He should be cautioned against overfatigue and against subjecting himself to any unusual strain. A simple hygienic life is imperative, and stimulants—tea, coffee, alcohol, and tobacco—are to be avoided.

It need not be pointed out that during the entire period in which a case of melancholia is under treatment, both the physician and the nurse should adopt a demeanor and speech which regard the recovery of the patient as an admitted fact. The patient will often speak deprecatingly when his recovery is alluded to; often he denies recovery as being within the range of possibility, and declares that neither his doctor nor his nurse understand his case, otherwise they would not speak of his getting well. The constant suggestion of improvement and of returning health, and of the uselessness of worrying and dwelling upon the past or some imaginary sin, does not have much effect upon the patient during the height of the disease. During the period of convalescence, however, such suggestions are not only tolerated by the patient, but, after a while, are greedily listened to. Very soon the possibility of recovery is admitted and the patient begins to ask as to when he will be well. The fact that this question is asked at all, is an augury of recovery. There can be no doubt that during the period of convalescence suggestions of returning health have a stimulating effect.

It seems wise to add a word with regard to the employment of thyroid extract in the treatment of cases of melancholia of prolonged course. In moderate doses it acts as a stimulant not only to the thyroid but to the entire chain of ductless glands and thus increases metabolism generally. In a number of instances, also, it appears to act as a cerebral stimulant. However, its action is inconstant and disappointing, and if given in decided doses, it will add to the nervousness from which the patient is already suffering. It need hardly be stated that with agitated patients it should not be used at all. I use it only occasionally in very prolonged cases and for brief periods, during waves of increased depression. On the whole, its action is disappointing.

Mania

Mania does not present so great a variety of forms as does melancholia. The variations depend rather upon the intensity and duration of the symptoms than upon their character. So far as we are concerned, the question resolves itself into the management of typical acute mania, of hypomania, and of chronic mania.

In cases of typical acute mania, the question of commitment is decided for us by the case itself. The symptoms are frequently so pronounced, the patient is so violent and noisy, so difficult of control or restraint, that the necessity for commitment is obvious not only to the physician, but also to the friends and relatives. However, when the patient is merely in a condition of mild maniacal excitement—so-called hypomania—commitment may be neither indicated nor justified. Indeed, under such circumstances, commitment is frequently resisted by the relatives. The lucidity of the patient is, as a rule, perfectly preserved, and it is only at times, when the excitement attains an unusual intensity, that commitment becomes necessary. Many cases of hypomania can be treated during the entire course of the disease outside of the asylum.

Treatment.—It is unnecessary, after what has been said relative to the treatment of melancholia, to point out here the necessities and advantages of isolation. In typical acute mania, isolation is an imperative necessity, and is, of course, insured by commitment. In hypomania, it may be attained by the removal of the patient from home, either to a private hospital or to a house in the suburbs or in the country. The special plan adopted will depend entirely upon each individual case and all the circumstances surrounding it.

The treatment of mania consists essentially in the application of physiologic methods. So far as practicable, rest should be a prominent feature. In the milder cases of mania, such as permit of extra-mural treatment—e.g., hypomania—full rest treatment can usually be instituted and carried out with great success. The patient can frequently be prevailed upon to go to bed at the outset, and by a little tactful management, together with the judicious and occasional use of sedatives, the rest in bed can be continued for a sufficiently prolonged period. The details do not differ from those adopted in neurasthenia. The patient should rest continuously in bed, should leave the bed only long enough to void the urine and empty the bowels, should be bathed in bed between blankets, and should receive massage daily. Care should, of course, be used not to add to the patient's excitement by undue handling; for this reason, massage may be for a time inapplicable, though frequently the patient submits quietly to this part of the treatment. Electricity, however, can rarely be employed, because of the excitable condition of the patient, save now and then, during the period of convalescence. Because of the duration of hypomania, the period of treatment necessary is usually quite prolonged; it frequently extends over three or four months or more.

At the outset it is wise, as a rule, to give an efficient dose of calomel, followed by a saline, so as to empty the intestinal tract. The purge itself usually acts as a sedative and prepares the patient for a subsequent course of full feeding. The diet should be practically such as is employed in ordinary neurasthenic cases. Other things equal, milk should be given with meals, between meals, and at bedtime, and in as large a quantity as the patient can take and digest. Full feeding is absolutely essential.

In cases treated by rest methods outside of the asylum, a well-trained nurse is, of course, indispensable, and if the symptoms be at all pronounced, two will be required, so that the patient shall never be left alone. Precautions similar to those instituted in cases of melancholia should be taken as regards the room which the patient is to occupy. The windows should be secured in the manner already described, while all instruments or utensils, by means of which the patient could inflict injury upon himself or others should be removed from the room. In cases of hypomania the danger, either to the patient or to those about him, is exceedingly slight. It should, however, always be guarded against.

In all cases of mania, whether treated at home or in the asylum, it is necessary to allay as far as possible the excitement and insomnia from which the patient is suffering. Whenever practicable, we should endeavor to produce quiet by some form of bathing—warm sponge bathing in bed between blankets, the warm pack, or, best of all, the prolonged immersion bath carried out in the manner already detailed (see p. 187). Usually, in ordinary acute mania, it is wisest to bring the patient partly under the influence of some sedative or hypnotic before attempting any radical procedure of hydrotherapy (see p. 188). In cases of marked severity, there is resistance to handling of all kinds, and it is only after the administration of sedatives that baths can be applied without the serious risk of exhausting the patient by useless struggling. Medinal or, better still, medinal with sulphonal (10 grains of each), may be administered; or one one-hundredth of a grain of hydrobromate of scopolamin with one-eighth of a grain of morphin, as previously described, may be employed, or such other of the hypnotics used as the circumstances of the case seem to indicate. Luminal frequently proves of the utmost value, and is by some physicians preferred to any other sedative (see p. 195). The bromids should be reserved for temporary administration only, and the like is true of chloral. The use of medinal and sulphonal, in the manner already indicated, usually answers every purpose. The patient becomes relatively quiet and frequently sleeps, or at least permits bathing and other necessary manipulations.

Occasionally, the excitement is so extreme, the struggling so incessant, and the danger of injury so great, that the patient must be physically restrained and for this purpose nothing proves so efficacious as the warm wet pack. Of course, if it is possible to place him in a permanent warm bath this is to be preferred. Sometimes mechanical restraint becomes urgently necessary in a patient who has already suffered some serious surgical injury. Restraint can be accomplished quite readily by means of ordinary bed-sheets. Thus, a sheet, loosely rolled, is passed back of the patient's neck and under both armpits. Each end is then firmly secured to either side of the bed. In a similar manner, the legs may be fastened by a sheet which encircles separately each one of the ankles and is then fastened to either side of the bed. If it be necessary to restrain the patient entirely, he can be completely rolled in a sheet, the arms being flexed over his chest, the legs extended; the ends of the sheets are then firmly secured by means of safety-pins. An excellent restraining sheet can be obtained at most surgical instrument makers. Much prejudice exists against the use of the canvas shirt, and as, a rule, it can be entirely dispensed with; however, if properly made, there can be no objection to it. It is needless to say that physical restraint in a given case should be removed as soon as possible, and I need not here repeat the caution that it is none the less necessary to watch closely a patient to whom physical restraint has been applied. He should not for a moment be left without the watchful care of his attendant.

Because of the duration of mania, caution is to be exercised in regard to the prolonged use of drugs. They are to be regarded as emergency remedies. So far as practicable, they should be varied from time to time. The efficiency of paraldehyd in overcoming sudden and intense excitement should not be forgotten. Its unpleasant taste, as has already been pointed out, may, however, prove a serious obstacle to its use. It is frequently a good plan to give medinal and sulphonal first, and if sleep does not follow after a reasonable interval, to use paraldehyd. Sleep is induced promptly and is subsequently prolonged by the action of the medinal and sulphonal.

Very soon the suitable dose of the various hypnotics required in a given case is learned, and no difficulty, as a rule, is experienced in inducing a certain amount of sleep and relative quiet; especially if bathing be also in a measure employed. Very frequently small doses of luminal, two to three grains, answer every purpose.

During the period of **convalescence**, exercise should be added to the rest methods. As far as possible, this exercise should take place for short periods of time in the open air. Tonics—iron, strychnin, arsenic, and the various bitters—may also be employed as indicated. After treatment has been completed, a considerable interval of time should elapse before the patient returns to his ordinary occupation or subjects himself to any strain of consequence. Great care should be exercised in this respect, as recurrences are not infrequently brought on by injudicious waste of the patient's nervous strength. The remarks made in regard to the management of cases of neurasthenia in the period of convalescence (see p. 56) are equally applicable here.

Circular Insanity

Circular insanity consists in an alternation of phases of depression and exaltation, the phases being in themselves indistinguishable from separate attacks of mania or melancholia. The affection, therefore, does not require special consideration here; the treatment is that of melancholia, on the one hand, and of mania on the other. It is important, however, to bear in mind that in a person who has once passed through an attack of circular insanity, there is a pronounced tendency to recurrence. The patient should, therefore, other things equal, be under more or less supervision during the intervals of his lucidity. These intervals are exceedingly variable in duration, lasting from a few weeks or months to several years. It is hardly necessary to say that during their continuance the life of the patient should be regulated by a strict adherence to simple hygienic and physiologic methods of living. It is not improbable that by such means, the intervals of lucidity can be prolonged. At any rate, the patient's health and efficiency is undoubtedly kept at a higher level under such conditions.

THE HEBOID-PARANOID GROUP (DEMENTIA PRÆCOX, PARANOIA)

As in the case of the other affections which we have thus far considered, it is necessary, first that we entertain certain basic conceptions as to the problems which confront us. The heboid-paranoid group of mental affections includes, on the one hand, the great mass of the insanities of youth and, on the other, the delusional lunacies of adult life. We have here to deal with individuals who are biologically defective, whose organization is so imperfectly or aberrantly constituted that it breaks down under the mere strain of living. The breakdown may occur early or relatively early, and then presents itself in the form of a so-called precocious dementia; or the breakdown may not occur until adult life has been reached when it presents itself in the form of a paranoia. As might be anticipated heredity plays here a very important rôle. The percentage of cases that present a neuropathic family history is very large, 80 to 90 per cent. Secondly, the patients frequently bear upon their persons the marks of morphologic arrest and deviation. These consist in peculiarities of conformation of the skull, the features, the ears, the limbs, the circulatory apparatus. These may not in themselves seem important, but in reality they are very significant. They indicate not only departures from the normal in structures accessible to observation, but of the organism as a whole.

Further, of late certain remarkable facts have been made known to us concerning metabolism in dementia præcox. Fauser, who was the first to apply the study of defensive ferments to mental disease, found in the blood of patients suffering from dementia præcox defensive ferments against the sex glands and against the cortex. Owing to an abnormality of the sex glands— probably biological in its nature—unchanged sex-gland protein enters the blood, and in the subsequent breaking up or reduction of this protein, substances are formed which are injurious to the cortex. The substance which enters the blood is, of course, the internal secretion, the hormone, not the germinal product. It is a foreign body and its presence in the blood excites the formation of a defensive ferment, which brings about not only a digestion—a lysis—of the hormone itself, but also a digestion—a lysis—of the cortical tissue. It is this latter fact to which the mental deterioration of dementia præcox is due. Pathological facts thus confirm the clinical interpretation of the disease as being an endogenous deterioration. The findings of Fauser hold good not only for the hebephrenic and catatonic forms of dementia præcox, but apparently for the paranoid forms as well. The course of dementia præcox varies much in different cases; notwithstanding, a general average obtains. There is, first, a gradually beginning onset of symptoms, usually of the character of a confusion, but sometimes possessing elements of systematization; second, there is present, in the early period of the affection, depression, hypochondriasis, exhaustion, and in the later period, expansion; third, in the great majority of cases the affection is progressive, the mental impairment steadily increases and terminates in dementia. However, this is by no means the invariable course. Thus, the patient may pass through an attack with its phases of depression and expansion and the other attendant mental phenomena, without presenting at the end of the attack any recognizable mental impairment. While this undoubtedly occurs it is distinctly the exception. Again, an increasing clinical experience has shown that the cases in which recovery had been believed to have taken place, quite frequently suffer a recurrence of symptoms, sometimes after a number of months, sometimes after several years and that after such a recurrence, the mental deterioration is usually pronounced. However, cases are met with in which recurrences are not observed. Quite commonly, some evidences of mental deterioration are noted, though it must be admitted that there are some instances in which these are practically non-existent.

The problem that confronts us is a very difficult one and yet it must be realized that the physiologic methods of treatment are the only ones that hold forth any promise. According to the case and according to circumstances, these should be employed. Everything should be done to raise the general level of the patient's health and treatment should be as intensive as possible. Rest—at times complete, at times partial—full feeding, exercise, and massage are to be variously employed. There can be no doubt that in some of the milder and non-asylum cases, the careful and persistent application of these measures, together with a general supporting treatment, is followed by an arrest of the progress of the disease, and, at times, indeed by a complete recovery. Now and then, though not often, brilliant results are achieved even in cases of marked severity. I am convinced that the percentage of recoveries is larger in dementia præcox than an observation based purely upon asylum experience would indicate.

Because of the long duration of the disease, treatment outside of an asylum is attended by very considerable expense, inasmuch as the services of a trained nurse or an attendant are necessary. Indeed, sometimes two attendants are required. The various special indications—excitement, insomnia, depression, and weakness—are to be combated as they arise. In every way the general health of the patient is to be conserved, his functions maintained, and his symptoms controlled. The relatives should always be given to understand that the disease offers an unfavorable prognosis in the majority of cases, that there is, however, a possibility either of arresting the disease, or of a more or less persistent improvement. In this connection it is well to bear in mind that catatonia affords, on the whole, a more favorable prognosis than simple hebephrenia, and that hebephrenia affords a more favorable prognosis than dementia paranoides; dementia paranoides presents a prognosis which is almost as unfavorable as that of fully developed paranoia.

Psychotherapeutics in the form of psycho-analysis is advocated by the Freudian school. This is fully discussed in Part III.

The management of the various forms of paranoia—delusional lunacy—is of the utmost importance, although the results of treatment, so far as the patient is concerned, are unsatisfactory. Paranoia is essentially a progressive degenerative disease of many years' duration, and one which is only occasionally influenced by treatment. The important practical point which the physician must face in every case is the question of commitment. The delusional lunatic is so often dangerous that, the diagnosis having been established, it is wisest, other things equal, to advise institution care. In many cases, the necessity for commitment becomes obvious to relatives and physician alike from the assaults or attempts at assaults which the patient makes and from the dangerous character of his delusions. In other cases, again, the patient's own safety demands the protection of the asylum. This is equally true whether the patient be in the persecutory or the expansive stage of the disease. The fact that patients not infrequently practise self-mutilation, and occasionally commit self-destruction, offers another reason why commitment should be insisted upon. On the other hand, it is well known that some cases of paranoia are harmless or comparatively so. Not all cases, therefore, require commitment, but the fact remains that the larger number not only demand restraint, but demand it imperatively. Experience shows that not infrequently the mild, so-called "non-asylum," cases develop dangerous symptoms, and in every case the relatives should be clearly informed as to the nature of the patient's affection. It should also be pointed out to them that the disease becomes more pronounced with time, and that some measure of supervision should always be exercised.

It is necessary, finally, to call attention to one important point in regard to the commitment of cases of paranoia, and that is, that in doubtful cases, the full concurrence of the various relatives should be procured before commitment is ventured upon. We should remember that remission of symptoms sometimes ensues under the quiet, the sleep, the good food, and the general physiologic life of the asylum. Under such circumstances the patient may subsequently declare that he has never been insane, that he has been unjustly committed, and may bring legal proceedings against the physicians who signed his commitment papers. While the danger of a successful prosecution is slight, physicians are not infrequently put to great annoyance and personal inconvenience by paranoiacs in whom, in spite of well-established lunacy, considerable mental power has been preserved. The patient is often shrewd enough to deny or to conceal his delusions, or when confronted by the undoubted evidence of their existence, to attempt some plausible explanation of them.

The **medical treatment** of cases of paranoia consists, of course, in the application of general hygienic and physiologic measures. As far as possible, life in the open air should be instituted. Whenever the nature of the case permits, the patient should be interested in some occupation. Quite a number of patients can be made busy in one way or another. Women can be employed in household duties, sewing, or fancy work. So far as possible, the occupation should be varied and should include some work in the open air, such as gardening. Men, especially, can engage in out-of-door pursuits, such as farm work and trucking. In a large number of asylums quite a percentage of patients can be occupied in this and similar ways. Rational forms of amusement should also be encouraged, e.g., music and in-door games, such as billiards and pool. The extent to which these measures can be carried, if instituted at all, depends, of course, upon the fitness of each individual case. Other things equal, work proves most beneficial.

THE NEURASTHENIC-NEUROPATHIC INSANITIES (PSYCHASTHENIA)

The neurasthenic-neuropathic insanities form a group of affections having as their basis both neurasthenia and neuropathy. That both of these factors are present in every case can, I believe, be demonstrated. When we take up the consideration of the psychic phenomena of neurasthenia, we are impressed at the very outset by the symptom of ready exhaustion—of marked diminution in the capacity for sustained intellectual effort. As is well known, nervous exhaustion may supervene in individuals who are otherwise perfectly normal. It may result from unphysiologic living, overwork, overstrain, and other factors productive of chronic exhaustion. It is thus an affection to which every one is liable, those of normal, as well as those of pathologic heredity. The symptoms of neurasthenia, as ordinarily met with, are those of chronic fatigue, and I have upon various occasions applied to it the term of the fatigue neurosis (see Part I, Chapter II). The attempt to do mental work brings on, more or less rapidly, the signs of fatigue. Soon there is difficulty in sustaining and concentrating the attention, and, at the same time, there is a marked diminution in the spontaneity of thought. When the condition is pronounced and confirmed, the patient becomes irritable, nervous, lacks confidence in himself, betrays indecision regarding trivial matters, and is often emotional to an unusual degree. His equilibrium is readily disturbed; a play at the theater or a newspaper account of a murder may move him to tears, or a trivial incident may provoke him to unusual annoyance or anger. In other words, added to the symptom of ready exhaustion we have that of deficient inhibition. His lack of confidence in himself may grow into a feeling of timidity; a man forceful and aggressive loses the readiness with which he arrives at decisions, loses in will-power, and may even become chronically afraid. Weakness, indecision, and fear are closely associated, and it is not surprising that a patient in a condition of chronic exhaustion should become morbidly afraid. How fear manifests itself in neurasthenia, it is hardly necessary to point out in detail. There may be present a vague generalized sense of being afraid, or there may occur isolated, spontaneous attacks of generalized fear—a fear accompanied by marked outward physical signs. In such attacks, the face becomes pale, the heart palpitates, the pulse is small and rapid, the respiration hurried; there may be a cold sweat upon the body, and the patient may sink from weakness upon a chair or upon the ground. Indeed, if an attack be intense, there may even be relaxation of the sphincters. In other cases the fear, instead of retaining a general character, assumes a special form. If, in addition to being neurasthenic, the patient be also neuropathic—i.e., if there be in him the elements of nervous degeneration, hereditary, congenital, or acquired—some pathologic association may be formed in his mind, so that the emotion of fear becomes linked with certain relations to the environment. This to my mind is the most probable explanation of the origin of the various phobias—agoraphobia, claustrophobia, and the like. For their establishment, two factors appear to be necessary— neurasthenia and neuropathy. Persons otherwise normal who acquire neurasthenia do not acquire the special fears (see also pp. 18 and 19).

A similar explanation applies also to the origin of *folie du doute*. The madness of doubt is in reality an insanity of indecision, and I believe it to be a neuropathic exaggeration, so to speak, of the indecision which is commonly seen in ordinary neurasthenics. That profound neuropathic elements, hereditary or acquired, are necessary for its formation there can, I think, be no doubt. To me, the term insanity of indecision appears to be better than *"folie du doute"* or "obsession of indecision," and it is the one which I am in the habit of employing.

A somewhat similar explanation may be applied to so-called "insanity with irresistible impulse." That the inhibition of the neurasthenic is deficient, we have already seen, and that this defect should manifest itself in various bizarre and erratic forms in persons who are also of neuropathic organization, is not surprising. The normal brain is constantly eliminating impulses which are as constantly restrained or diverted into special channels. In the neuropathic neurasthenic, these impulses not only cease to be restrained, but manifest themselves as pathologic associations of movement in relation to the environment. To my mind, the term insanity from deficient inhibition is better than "*Zwangs-irresein*," "compulsion neurosis," or "insanity with irresistible impulse." The pathologic association that gives birth to the impulse is formed in the same manner as are numerous other, often irrelevant, associations in the normal mind; but in the latter such associations are repressed or inhibited and give no outward manifestation of their existence, while in the neurasthenic-neuropathic subject, they are given motor expression as rapidly as they are formed.

The psychic symptoms observed in the simple neurasthenia of non-neuropathic individuals, suggest also an explanation of so-called "aboulic insanity," or, as I prefer to call it, insanity from deficient will. The condition is closely allied to the insanity of indecision and is characterized by the inability of the patient to perform some special act or acts which are, as a rule, simple in themselves, and which are habitually performed by normal persons without hesitation and even subconsciously. Thus, there may be a psychic inability to rise from a chair, to walk forward, to walk in a given direction, to ascend a certain stairway, or to perform

some other act, equally simple, but concerning which some pathologic association has been formed.

The foregoing considerations, while they give a full value to the
factor of neuropathy, furnish us an important indication of treatment, because of the underlying neurasthenia. Cases of neurasthenic insanity are to be treated vigorously by physiologic methods.
In given cases, full rest treatment is to be employed, and everything possible is to be done to force up the nutrition and the general
health of the patient. While this is being done, it is necessary,
of course, that the patient should have assigned to him a nurse
who is not only experienced in rest methods, but is possessed of
intelligence and of sufficient force to be able to influence the
patient. The nurse should tactfully endeavor to break up the
absurd associations upon which special fears or other obsessions
depend; thus, she should combat, when present, the tendency of
the patient to count or to be dominated by certain numbers; she
should oppose indecision by a persistent method of retraining; and
in cases of deficient will, the will of the patient should be reinforced by that of the nurse.

It is almost unnecessary to add that after a course of treatment by rest, an elaborate method of physical exercise and mental
training should be instituted, which should extend over many
months. In young persons and in comparatively recent cases,
such a course of treatment is often followed by gratifying results.
In older patients, in whom the fears or obsessions have been long
established and in whom the neuropathic factor is dominant,
treatment is of little avail, even when carried out elaborately.
This fact should not, however, discourage us from making the
attempt, especially in young individuals and in whom there is
marked impairment of the general health.

Psychotherapeutic methods are especially applicable here.
These together with psychoanalysis, so much advocated by the
Freudians, are discussed in Part III.

DEMENTIA

A detailed discussion of the treatment of simple demented
states is unnecessary. In the management of dementia, as it

presents itself in the simple and uncomplicated senile form, simple hygienic measures alone are applicable. These should include especially rest and full feeding. A systematic treatment by rest in bed is, however, not practicable, nor can massage, so valuable in asthenic states, be employed save exceptionally and in a limited degree. Full feeding, careful attention to the digestive tract, tonic medication, occasional medicines to induce sleep, cleanliness of the person, and general supervision and care are the measures to be followed. So far as possible open air occupation should be instituted and the general interest of the patient should be aroused. The nature of the affection sets a narrow limit to our efforts.

PARESIS

In regard to paresis, as in all else, clear conceptions are absolutely necessary to any rational attempts at treatment. The recent developments in our knowledge of the relation of the Treponema pallidum to so-called parasyphilis have greatly influenced our conceptions of syphilis of the nervous system. The discovery of the spirochetes in the brain of the paretic by Noguchi, was soon confirmed by Marinesco, Marie, Levaditi and Bankowski, Foerster and Tomasczewski and others. The demonstration of the presence of living spirochetes in material obtained from paretics by brain puncture and the successful inoculation of rabbits with the substance of paretic brains, have permanently placed the earlier belief as to the syphilitic nature of paresis upon the permanent basis of fact. These great discoveries did not, however, lead to the erroneous conclusion that all syphilis of the nervous system is the same; indeed, the old clinical distinctions between syphilis of the vessels and membranes, on the one hand, and paresis and tabes, on the other, were emphasized. It came to be recognized that, in a sense, we have in the former affection an interstitial syphilis and in the latter a syphilis of the nerve substance, a parenchymatous syphilis. Further, the difference in the course and symptoms of the two groups of affections suggests a possible difference in the character of the infection; as though paresis and tabes were caused by a special strain of the spirochete. Many clinical observations point to such a fact; such, for instance, as cases in which husband and wife both suffer from paresis or both from tabes. It is a significant fact that one of them does not suffer from syphilis of the membranes and vessels and the other from parasyphilis. Equally convincing are the instances in which a number of men all acquire syphilis from the same woman and all subsequently develop paresis. It would seem that either at times the germs of syphilis undergo some change, acquire some quality which especially favors the development of paresis or it may be that, as Mott has expressed it, there are varieties of spirochetes as there are different varieties of the trypanosomes, the morphological character of which would not permit of differentiation. However, whatever the fact may be, for us the truth remains of the great clinical difference between the two groups of syphilis of the nervous system; a truth which is in keeping, further, with the vastly different results of treatment.

Let us briefly review the methods of treatment at the present time in vogue in paresis and tabes. A new impetus to our efforts for the cure or arrest of these affections was, of course, given by the introduction of salvarsan. It was given a most extensive trial, while the old remedies, the mercurials and the iodids, were for a time set aside. It was soon found, however, that the intravenous injections of salvarsan *alone* achieved comparatively meager results. Perhaps cessation of pains in tabes with some general improvement, and little or no definite gain in paresis were the results. It was found that the salvarsan diffused with great difficulty into the intradural space, if at all, and a decided advance in method was made when direct intradural injections were devised. Various procedures were tried by Marinesco, Robertson, Sicard and Lapointe, Forrester and others but that which first achieved a definite character was that devised by Swift and Ellis. According to this method, the patient is first given an intravenous injection of salvarsan or neosalvarsan. After an interval of an hour—though some physicians prefer to wait only twenty minutes —blood is again drawn from the vein. The blood, thirty to forty cubic centimeters in amount, is allowed to stand over night; the supernatant serum is pipetted off and then thoroughly centrifuged;

later, it is inactivated at a temperature of 56°C. Ten to twenty cubic centimeters, diluted according to judgment with the addition of twice or an equal amount of salt solution, is then injected intraspinously. As a rule, the intraspinous injection is given about twenty-four hours after the intravenous. The patient either lies upon his side or sits upon the edge of the bed with his back to the operator. A lumbar puncture is then made with a Quincke needle, and the spinal fluid allowed to run off to the amount of forty cubic centimeters or more. In some cases, it is wise and expedient to thoroughly drain the dural sac. The serum, which has been warmed to the body temperature, is then introduced by means of the Luer syringe and allowed to flow in by gravity, reenforced if necessary by the piston. The patient is then placed upon his back upon the bed without any pillow under his head, while the foot of the bed is slightly elevated. He is allowed to remain in this position for about three hours, when the foot of the bed is lowered and the patient permitted to assume a more comfortable position. I have been in the habit of repeating this procedure about once in two weeks, rarely once in ten days, until three, four or more treatments have been given.

Ogilvie has devised a method in which the salvarsan is directly added to blood serum outside of the body, thus avoiding the twenty-four hours' delay of the Swift-Ellis method. Forty or fifty cubic centimeters of blood are obtained in the usual manner, are allowed to stand for three or four hours, the supernatant fluid pipetted off and centrifuged. Salvarsan, one-fourth milligram, which has been dissolved and neutralized in the usual way, is then added to the serum; the mixture is incubated for an hour at body temperature, and then inactivated for half an hour at 56°C. The amount injected into the dural sac is about ten cubic centimeters. Another method, which has not been much followed, is that of injecting a salvarsanized serum obtained after an intravenous injection and prepared as in the Swift-Ellis method, directly beneath the intracranial dura. Previous to the injection the intracranial pressure is first reduced by making a lumbar puncture. The objection to this ingenious method, which is to be credited to Wardner, is the operative procedure; namely, the giving of an anesthetic and the trephining. **Byrnes** has devised a bichlorid of mercury method. The blood—about six ounces—is allowed to stand, the serum collected, centrifuged and inactivated. One-fiftieth of a grain of bichlorid is then added, precipitation being prevented by shaking and by the addition of more serum. Several manufacturing chemists have marketed bichlorid serum. Cotton has used both the Ogilvie and bichlorid serums intracranially and intraventricularly.

Cotton who has made perhaps the most elaborate study of the various methods, expresses himself as to their relative value as follows:* "We are still undecided as to the best method to be adopted and, consequently, are using all the methods in order to ascertain which is preferable. Given an early case of paresis, from our experience we would say that the Swift-Ellis method was as efficacious as any. In other words, if the Swift-Ellis treatment fails to arrest the process, we have not been able to produce better results in these cases by the other methods." He does not, however, claim that it is the exclusive method.

As to the efficacy of the treatment, Cotton draws very positive conclusions. He claims, among other things, that in the use of salvarsanized serum we have an agent which causes definite arrest in paresis. He also points out that the case must be treated in the early stages, as advanced stages show no favorable reaction to the treatment; that the majority of cases cannot be helped after two or three years have elapsed. Further, treatment must be persistent and uninterrupted, and also that the efficacy of the treatment depends not upon the type of method as upon the stage of the disease. Of great significance is his statement that remissions occur in 35.5 per cent. of cases treated by salvarsanized serum, while only 4 per cent. of remissions occur spontaneously. The latter figure is much lower, however, than the experience of others would indicate.

Personally, I have used the Swift-Ellis method in a large number of patients, many of them relatively early cases; at times with a favorable result as to both symptoms and progress. In some

---

* "American Journal of Insanity," 1916 vol. lxxii, p. 548.

cases, a remission of longer or shorter duration was established and in a few instances remissions or improvements of such long duration that, perhaps, they can be regarded as arrested cases. I am not, however, by any means so sanguine as are others as to the efficacy of this treatment in paresis. On the other hand, in locomotor ataxia, it has in my experience led to results often surprising in the degree of the improvement, in the disappearance of the pains and in the lessening of the ataxia. Some of these doubtless deserve to be regarded as arrested cases; but the future only will tell.

Improvement is indicated not only by a favorable change in the symptoms, but in due course by a change in the serological reactions and, especially, by a fall in the lymphocyte count of the cerebrospinal fluid. The latter is sometimes a very striking feature of the treatment and is looked upon as a very encouraging sign.

A simple expedient and one that is remarkably productive of good results is that of **simple drainage** as carried out by **Gilpin and Earley** in my own clinic. They began by instituting spinal drainage in every case of tabes and paresis *before giving the intravenous* injection in the hope of influencing the diffusion of salvarsan into the dural cavity. The improvement, especially in tabes, was so striking that very soon they began to study the effects of spinal drainage alone, and to their surprise found that without salvarsan or other treatment, marked signs of improvement made their appearance. The patients are put to bed and drained of every possible drop of fluid about once a week or once in two weeks. The pains immediately become less, the ataxia diminishes and even the lymphocyte count in the spinal fluid falls.

I believe it to be of the utmost importance not to lay aside the mercurials in patients in whom treatment by salvarsanized serum is adopted. It has been my custom, after having submitted a patient to a course of Swift-Ellis treatments, to give the patient a series of hypodermatic injections of some soluble salt of mercury or, better still, a course of mercurial inunctions. It is important, however, to note that the patient is not as tolerant to mercury as before the salvarsan treatment and that the physiologic effects

16

of the mercurial may become rapidly pronounced. It should, therefore, be given with care. Conversely, salvarsan seems to be more effective when the patient has been previously treated with mercurials. The iodides, now so much neglected, are also still of value. They probably do good by stimulating absorption and, indirectly, making the treponema more accessible to the mercurial or salvarsan as the case may be.

Finally, we should employ, in addition, whenever possible, physiologic methods of treatment. Whenever circumstances permit, I institute both in tabes and paresis full rest methods—continuous rest in bed, massive feeding, massage, gentle bathing, etc. (see pp. 40 et seq.). This merely means that in addition to the parasiticide we are using, we are stimulating the defensive resources of the organism to the uttermost. Such results as I personally have had both in tabes and paresis—especially in tabes —have been due to a combination of all the therapeutic measures, and of these the physiologic have not been the least important. In tabes, I need hardly add, I have also made persistent use of the Frænkel method of exercises (see p. 169).

The care which paretics require after they have passed the stage of possible treatment is, of course, very general and largely protective in its nature. Adequate institutional care must sooner or later be established in the average case.

THE INSANITIES OF INTOXICATION AND THE DRUG HABITS

A discussion of the treatment of mental diseases would be incomplete without a consideration of the treatment of the conditions resulting from the abuse of stimulants and drugs. Manifold disturbances of function are met with, varying greatly in degree. Frequently, there is mere general nervous weakness and relatively slight functional impairment; at other times actual insanity is present. The first group of cases presents symptoms resembling neurasthenia, but which are properly termed neurasthenoid. The second group of cases presents symptoms of mental derangement more or less clearly expressed. Numerous instances are, of course, found, presenting intermediate conditions between these two extremes.

Drug habits have their origin in a large number of cases in an underlying neuropathic constitution. Persons do not ordinarily acquire alcoholism, for instance, from the use to which alcohol is put for social or medical purposes. This may be the apparent origin of some cases, while in many patients a drug habit can be traced to the first administration of a drug by a physician; but it is nevertheless true that in a far greater number of instances, the drug habit exists not because of these incidental factors, but because the nervous system of the patient is of itself pathologic. The close relation, observed in so many family histories, of alcoholism, tuberculosis, and insanity can have but one significance; namely, an enfeebled organization with diminished powers of resistance. Frequently, the neuropathic condition does not assume a definite clinical form, the patient merely presenting a tendency to neurasthenic breakdown, to general nervousness or hypochondria. In other cases, the history suggests very strongly recurring waves of depression, analogous to those which are observed in a frankly developed melancholia.

A brief consideration of the subject will convince us that the various stimulants and drugs have an effect upon the nervous system which is intrinsically the same. The clinical picture presented, of course, varies in its details according to the special poison which has been at work. Many poisons—for in the sense in which we are discussing them all of the stimulants and drugs are poisons —act upon the nervous system primarily as stimulants and secondarily as depressants; while others act as depressants and destroyers of function from the very beginning. Alcohol may in a sense be taken as the type of the poisons under consideration, and it will serve our purpose best to consider its action briefly.

In an ordinary attack of alcoholic intoxication, there is, at first, an increase in the ease with which ideas are eliminated; speech and memory are stimulated; the individual is talkative; there is a tendency to reminiscences, to jests, to rhymes, to puns. At the same time there is noticeable an increased difficulty of apprehension and comprehension and an undoubted diminution of inhibition or self-control. There is an increased evolution of impulses of various kinds, sudden and unrestrained. Later, there is a slowing of mental action and the difficulty of apprehension is increased. After a while, the individual is no longer able to understand what is said; judgment is gone, language becomes exaggerated, boastful, profane, or maudlin, and finally ends in a mere jargon. The attack terminates in unconsciousness and stupor. While alcohol apparently acts as a stimulant in the beginning, it is doubtful whether it does not from the very first retard rather than facilitate intellectual functions. Every brain-worker will, I believe, admit that even small doses of alcohol increase decidedly the difficulty of intellectual labor.

The picture presented is confirmed when we turn our attention to the symptoms presented by **chronic alcoholism.** Here the individual presents undoubted, continued, and persistent diminution of the ability to work. Especially is it noticeable that he has difficulty in taking up new subjects. His intellectual life is contracted. It is difficult to deflect his mental processes from their accustomed channels into new ones. He apprehends and he acquires with difficulty, and he forgets with great readiness. Judgment is dulled and impaired. If the condition progresses, the mental impairment becomes more pronounced and tends to permanence. Symptoms of well-marked dementia make their appearance. There is loss of the sense of the proprieties; parental and filial love and the sense of shame become obtunded. It need not be pointed out that such a patient fails to realize his own condition, that he resents the accusation that he is drinking to excess, and, indeed, may sooner or later develop the idea that he is being injured and oppressed by those about him. Emotionally he is irritable, he is restless and he is unreliable in statement. In addition to these nervous phenomena, he presents various physical signs; among them are chronic gastric catarrh, morning nausea, headache, dizziness, tremor of the tongue and hands, and weakness of the extremities. Depending upon personal peculiarities or upon the long continuance of the alcoholic abuse, changes may become evident in the peripheral nerves; indeed, these may become pronounced before dementia is decided, and the patient then presents the all too common picture of alcoholic multiple neuritis. That epilepsy may develop, that optic atrophy may occur, is also well known and need not be here dwelt upon. The foregoing picture is not invariable. In many cases of chronic alcoholism, there is present merely a mild obtusion of the mental faculties; the patients have not actually crossed the borderline into insanity. While any case may eventuate in insanity, there is nevertheless a broad line of distinction between chronic alcoholism, as it is ordinarily met with, and alcoholic dementia. Nevertheless, that the action of alcohol is throughout that of a destructive agent must, I think, be admitted.

When we analyze the mental affections that result from the abuse of alcohol, we find that they readily separate themselves into, first, alcoholic **delirium,** so-called delirium tremens; second, alcoholic **confusion,** so-called alcoholic confusional insanity; and, third, alcoholic **stuporous insanity** or alcoholic dementia. Clearness of conception necessitates a word as to the nature of the intoxication present in these affections. In alcoholic confusional insanity, for instance, the symptoms persist for many months after the patient has ceased to take alcohol. The persistence of the symptoms cannot, therefore, be due to the alcohol, but is due to the presence of autogenous poisons themselves the result of disturbances of function in various organs, e.g., in the liver, the thyroid, the kidneys, adrenals and other glands and tissues.

Alcoholic delirium closely resembles delirium from other causes. It is characterized by active and numerous fantastic hallucinations, among which visual hallucinations predominate. Illusions are present; consciousness is obscured; the patient is no longer in touch with his surroundings; mental confusion, pronounced and active, completes the picture. As in delirium from other causes, the patient sleeps little or none; the nutrition fails rapidly; the temperature is generally normal, though at times there is fever. As in other deliria, the reflex excitability is increased. Tremor of the tongue and fingers is present; epileptiform convulsions may occur. The duration is usually short, the delirium continuing from one or two days to one or two weeks. In favorable cases, the symptoms gradually subside. Recovery may ensue after a sound sleep, after

the taking of food, or after general quiet has been brought about.
On the other hand, the patient's mental faculties may become more
and more impaired, he may gradually become profoundly unconscious and may die of exhaustion, of renal complications, of enfeebled or fatty heart, or, it may be, of pneumonia.

Instead of an acute alcoholic delirium supervening in a patient,
there may develop a condition of more or less persistent **confusion**.
Especially is this result apt to ensue when a chronic alcoholic increases his potations beyond their usual amount.   Alcoholic confusion is characterized by the same symptoms as characterize
confusion dependent upon other causes.   Hallucinations and
delusions, unsystematized in character, are again present.   Sleep
also is disturbed.   Auditory hallucinations are numerous and pronounced.   Visual hallucinations, on the other hand, are not so
prominent in alcoholic confusion as in alcoholic delirium.   Alcoholic confusion, like confusion due to other causes, runs, as a rule,
a prolonged course—many weeks or months.

Lastly, the patient may develop **alcoholic dementia.   In this**
dementia the patient may become stuporous or he may present
symptoms vaguely suggesting paresis, such cases being sometimes
spoken of as alcoholic paresis.   Other cases, again, present systematized delusions and very closely resemble paranoia.   It is
highly probable, when the picture of paranoia is closely simulated,
that we have to deal with a patient who is a paranoiac at the same
time that he is a sufferer from alcoholism.   It is very probable also
that alcohol may in a neuropathic subject of bad heredity be an
exciting factor in the development of paranoia.   It is a remarkable fact, further, that "alcoholic paranoia" so-called is frequently
characterized by a special delusion, namely, that of marital infidelity.

From the foregoing brief summary of facts, we are to draw the
conclusion not only that alcohol acts as a poison to the nervous
system, but also that in its action it resembles in a general way
other poisons and toxins.   The delirium, the confusion, and the
stuporous insanity resulting from alcohol differ in no essential particular from the deliria, confusions, and stupors due to other
poisons or due to the various infectious diseases.   Intrinsically the
phenomena are the same.

DETAILS OF TREATMENT OF DRUG HABITS AND INSANITIES OF INTOXICATION

The outline given of the action of alcohol will serve as a text for general remarks upon the treatment of the drug habits and toxic insanities as a whole. Three important facts should be prominently borne in mind: first, the **underlying neuropathic constitution**; secondly, the **damage** done to the nervous system and other organs by the poison; and lastly and especially, the **secondary autointoxications**. These considerations at once indicate that treatment must consist in something far more radical than the mere withdrawal of the stimulant—that a plan of procedure must be instituted which will favor as large a degree of recovery in the nervous system as possible, and which at the same time will take cognizance of the various visceral disturbances that have been induced. With these preliminary considerations, let us turn our attention to the treatment of the various drug habits and insanities of intoxication in detail.

Alcoholic Delirium (Delirium Tremens)

The treatment of delirium tremens is to be conducted upon the same principles as the treatment of delirium due to other causes. The underlying **asthenic state** is, however, so pronounced that our efforts to support the strength of the patient must, if possible, be redoubled. Food should be given in as large quantities as possible and at short intervals, say of one or two hours. At the same time, strychnin and digitalis should be administered freely. Strychnin especially is indicated, and is most efficacious when used hypodermically. The use of the hypodermic syringe, however, may for the time being exaggerate the terror and enhance the delusions from which the patient is suffering, so that if nervous collapse does not seem imminent, it may be well to give the strychnin by the mouth. Digitalis can be used freely in doses of from fifteen to twenty drops of the tincture at intervals of four hours, or of half an ounce or more of the infusion at like intervals. We must remember that in alcoholism the patient is far less susceptible to the action of digitalis than under other circumstances. The moment, of course that an impression is made upon the pulse, the drug should either be stopped altogether or the dose much diminished.

The delirium is dependent not so much upon the presence of alcohol in the tissues, as upon the damage that the poison has already produced; it is best, nevertheless, in the majority of cases, to withdraw the alcohol. It is desirable, of course, to withdraw it altogether if possible; however, if the alcohol be withdrawn suddenly, it occasionally happens that the heart fails, that nervous collapse follows, or that the delirium itself assumes for the time being a more ominous character. Whether or not alcohol is to be administered in a given case, therefore, must depend largely upon the individual judgment of the physician, and also upon the effect which is obtained from the use of strychnin and digitalis. When in spite of other measures the pulse fails, and becomes frequent and weak, and the skin becomes cold and clammy, it is quite obvious that alcohol must be given in full doses. Indeed, such a condition of affairs should be anticipated. Frequently, solution of ammonium acetate, a half-ounce every hour or two, proves very serviceable in permitting a more rapid or earlier withdrawal of the alcohol, keeping up elimination and stimulating the heart. At times it is well to combine with it ammonium carbonate. As in other forms of delirium, it is also necessary to administer remedies to produce sleep. If the delirium be very active, medinal and sulphonal, so efficacious in ordinary forms of delirium, may be insufficient. Here full doses of paraldehyd will in the majority of cases prove effectual and will greatly enhance the action of medinal and sulphonal. Now and then, though not often, the physician may be compelled to fall back upon other narcotics. In this connection, the depressing action of large doses of bromid should not be forgotten, nor should the untoward cardiac effect of chloral be lost sight of. We should remember, in regard to morphin, that alcoholics are sometimes dangerously tolerant to the drug. Failing to induce quiet, a second dose may be resorted to after too short an interval. The fact, also, of the frequency of renal involvement in alcoholism, should make us additionally careful with regard to the use of this drug. Under certain conditions, however, when other narcotics fail, it is perfectly proper to use a combination of bromin, chloral and morphin. Such a combination is, as a rule, very efficacious. It should contain a maximum amount of bromid and but moderate doses of chloral and morphin. The bromid should preferably be in the form of the ammonium salt. Hyoscin hydrobromate or scopolamin may also be employed, especially in association with other remedies, e.g., morphin. We should be satisfied if only a moderate degree of sleep is obtained, for as time passes and the symptoms subside, sleep comes on spontaneously. If the case be complicated by pneumonia or other visceral disease, this, of course, will demand especial attention. Supporting measures are then doubly indicated. If there be suppression of urine or serious renal involvement, intravenous saline transfusion or hypodermoclysis, with or without venesection, should, among other measures, be held in mind.

Two facts of great importance have, of late, given rise to a method of treatment of alcoholic delirium that is remarkably efficacious. The first fact is that of the edema of the brain and the second that of acidosis. The latter is incident to the alcoholic poisoning and it is a result of the starvation of the brain substance. A hypertonic injection, intended both to dehydrate the tissues and to neutralize the acidosis and containing sodium bicarbonate, sodium chlorid and sodium bromid is injected intravenously and followed immediately by a solution of glucose. The latter is given because of the energy which it furnishes. Hogan[1] of Vallejo, California, whose experience embraced sixty-five cases with a mortality of but 9.3 per cent., has published the following details of the method as employed by him.

"In the preparation of the solution 5.8 gm. of chemically pure sodium chlorid and 8.4 gm. of chemically pure sodium bicarbonate are boiled in 120 c.c. of distilled water and filtered through paper, then placed in a flask and reboiled. In addition 10.2 gm. of chemically pure sodium bromid is boiled in 30 c.c. distilled water, filtered and reboiled. These may be kept ready for use, and when needed are added to 850 c.c. of either freshly distilled water or tap water that has been filtered and boiled. Under no circum-

---

[1] Hogan, James J., M. D., "Treatment of Acute Alcoholic Delirium," The Jour. of the Amer. Med. Ass'n, Dec. 16, 1916, p. 1826.

stances should old distilled water be used, as I have found that it produces severe chills. This mixture is heated to about 110° F. and is ready for use.

"The glucose used in the early cases was the anhydrous variety, but on account of the price and our inability to procure it in sufficient quantity, I found that I could prepare the glucose crystals found in the market and that the results w re satisfactory. In a flask with 250 c.c. distilled water 80 gm. e placed and boiled. To this is added 0.25 gm. of blood charco. . This is allowed to stand for twenty-four hours, is then filter d into a clean flask, reboiled, and is ready for use. This solu'.'on may be made up and kept ready for use.

"Both of these solution must be given ve y slowly, from twenty to thirty minutes being taken for the 1,250 c.c.

"A small percolator, such as is used in giving salvarsan, with rubber tubing and needle attached, is all the apparatus that is needed.

"The after-treatment followed in these cases consisted of active elimination, produced by 0.3 gm. calomel followed by 30 gm. magnesium sulphate."

The blood pressure, instead of being raised, was reduced proving that the injections were unattended by any danger on this score. Both the edema of the tissues and the acidosis were remarkably influenced. The delirium and struggling rapidly subsided and the patients recovered in between two and three days. This method may, of course, be combined, when necessary, with the supporting and sedative measures previously detailed.

Chronic Alcoholism

In the management of chronic alcoholism, we are especially to consider the underlying neurasthenic or neuropathic factors, and whatever plan of treatment we institute must take these factors into account. Secondly, and of equal importance, is the detailed study of the patient's symptoms. There is almost invariably present a marked chronic gastritis. The liver also should be carefully examined, bearing in mind, of course, the relation of alcoholism to cirrhosis. The heart and blood-vessels and the urine should be similarly studied. It is unnecessary to point out here possible changes in the lungs, save to mention the not infrequent coexistence of tuberculosis and alcoholism, and the further fact that many confirmed alcoholics suffer from chronic bronchitis. The practical point for the physician to remember, is the fact that the alcoholic is a man who is ill; that he is suffering not so much from the presence of the poison, as from a diseased nervous system and from various visceral complications, slight or pronounced, as the case may be.

We are confronted at the outset of the treatment by the problem of the withdrawal of the stimulant. I believe that it is always best to attempt rapid or immediate withdrawal. If no recent alcoholic excesses have been committed, this can, as a rule, be accomplished without much difficulty. When, however, the patient is just passing through an exacerbation of his alcoholism, withdrawal will have to be more gradual. It is to be remembered, however, that the moral effect of a too gradual or too prolonged withdrawal is bad. As the stimulant is withdrawn, food, tonics, and supporting measures must be substituted, and the treatment thenceforward does not differ from that adopted in other asthenic states. Special symptoms and special visceral complications, as already indicated, must be treated appropriately.

Unfortunately, the management of chronic alcoholism is not so simple as the foregoing paragraphs might seem to indicate. The patient is but rarely a willing subject of treatment. He is quite commonly impatient of restraint or control of any kind. It is true that men sometimes voluntarily enter institutions for inebriety, but, as a rule, they do so with the understanding that they are to have as much stimulant as they think they need. In the United States—speaking generally—and in many other countries, inebriates cannot be restrained unless they have crossed the borderline into actual insanity. Forcible restraint of inebriates can be carried out in America, however, in a few States. In Massachusetts, for example, by special provision of law it is possible to subject confirmed topers to the same dicipline as applies to the insane elsewhere; and a somewhat less satisfactory law has also been passed in Pennsylvania. Drunkards really need the same degree of care as the insane, and special institutions for their control should be provided everywhere. In Austria a procedure, known as the "Curatel," has been established. This consists in the local appointment of a curator or administrator who acts in the capacity of a guardian to the patient, and, under the same provision, the patient may be placed in an asylum. In more conservative countries, physicians are restricted to less effectual means.

If the patient's circumstances permit, the best plan of treatment consists in withdrawing him from his ordinary surroundings, instituting a system of **absolute isolation,** and at the same time placing him under the care of a **trained nurse.** Such a plan as this is, in suitable cases, almost invariably followed by the most gratifying results, results which are also far-reaching and frequently permanent; the isolation of the patient gives the physician the best opportunity for the study of the morbid conditions underlying the disease, and for their appropriate treatment.

Whenever practicable, it is wisest to institute a form of **rest treatment.** The isolation of the patient in a room with a special nurse of the same sex, constitutes the most effective means of restraint that can be devised, while the moral effect is of the very best. Under these conditions the stimulant can be withdrawn as rapidly as the symptoms of the patient justify. The patient should be kept in bed for a number of weeks in succession, and during this time massage, baths, Swedish movements, electricity, and such other expedients as suggest themselves should be employed from time to time. Under rest, full feeding, and full physiologic measures, it is found that the craving for the stimulant rapidly grows less.

It is a good plan at the beginning of the treatment to administer small doses of calomel and to follow this after a time by a saline cathartic. A diet should then be instituted, adapted to the digestive tract and the needs of the patient. In many cases it is necessary to begin with a liquid diet—beef-tea, broths, soups, and meat preparations generally. If the stomach tolerates it, however, some solid or semi-solid food should be given at the outset, or at least should be begun as early as possible. The weakness of the alcoholic is, as a rule, very pronounced, and is not relieved by mere beef preparations. Milk also should be added to the diet at as early a date as possible. A great many alcoholics have an aversion to milk, but, as a rule, they can readily be brought to take it if a small dose of alcohol be added. As the treatment progresses, the alcohol can, of course, be withdrawn. Frequently, instead of adding alcohol to the milk, our purpose is answered equally well by diluting the milk with some carbonated water, such as soda water or Apollinaris. In other cases, again, it is a good plan to peptonize the milk, the cold process being generally preferable. At times, some other expedient may be better, *e.g.*, giving instead of whole milk, skimmed milk or buttermilk. The patient should be fed at frequent intervals; that is, about six times daily, as in ordinary rest treatment. The solid food, which is given in small quantity at first, should gradually be increased until it is brought up to a normal amount. When the patient is **obese,** the diet is modified accordingly. Starches are excluded in all cases because of the gastric catarrh so commonly met with, but here, other fattening foods also should be avoided. Lean meats, fish, green vegetables, may be given; in general, we should follow the ordinary diet adapted to obesity.

The general principles which obtain in ordinary rest treatment for neurasthenia are fully applicable here. **Massage** should at first be given somewhat gently, as patients not infrequently present some soreness of the limbs, suggestive of neuritis. In many cases undoubted neuritis is present, and in these cases massage can only be employed partially. **Baths, electricity, passive movements, and Swedish movements** with resistance are to be employed as indicated. After a while a marked improvement is noted in the patient's general condition, and soon it becomes necessary to permit him to leave his bed for brief periods of time, and increased daily, so that at the end of six or more weeks he is up the greater part of the day. As soon as this is the case, some form of **active room exercise** should be instituted. The exercise should, of course, be gentle at first and only very gradually enlarged in amount. Subsequently, according to the progress of the case, these exercises should be followed by **exercise in the open air,** always, of course, in the company of the nurse.

In mild cases, it is possible to conduct the entire treatment without the use of medicines, but usually the latter are indicated, and may be employed with great advantage. They are roughly grouped into three categories: first, those indicated by the symptoms arising from the withdrawal of the alcohol; second, those indicated by the deranged visceral functions; and, third, those which are stimulating, or antagonistic to the action of the alcohol.

The symptoms which arise during the withdrawal of the alcohol consist generally in marked increase of nervousness, of insomnia, and sometimes of headache. As a rule, these indications can be readily met by the administration of the milder sedatives and hypnotics—the bromids, medinal, or sulphonal given alone or in association with hyoscin hydrobromate, scopolamin, or occasionally, chloral. Morphin and chloral are best avoided or their use limited to occasional administration only. The use of hypnotics should as far as possible be conjoined with the administration of some form of bathing. In most cases a warm sponge-bath between blankets or a warm tub-bath of short duration greatly enhances the action of the sedatives.

In the second category of drugs, we have those whose action is directed to the condition of the digestive tract, of the kidneys, or of the heart and general circulation. As already stated, there is almost always present a gastric catarrh, and this must be taken into consideration not only in the diet, but also in the medicines prescribed. Silver nitrate, one-fourth grain, in pill, with one-fourth grain extract of hyoscyamus, administered three times daily, half an hour or twenty minutes before meals, has, as a rule, a very happy action. At times lavage is necessary, though except in severe cases, this need not be continued very long. Sometimes the morning nausea and vomiting of chronic alcoholism are troublesome, but usually they readily subside. Occasionally, a course of divided doses of calomel, at other times of sodium phosphate, is of value. Small doses of other saline laxatives may likewise be employed. A little later the fluid extract of cascara can be given, just as in the rest treatment of neurasthenia.

In the third category of drugs we have, as already stated, those which are tonic and stimulating, or possibly antagonistic to the action of the alcohol. They are, however, to be regarded merely as adjuvants in the treatment, and should not be relied upon to any great extent. Strychnin generally proves very valuable. Usually moderate doses, say one-fortieth grain (1.5 milligrams), answer every purpose, though if there be marked cardiac weakness, much larger doses—for instance, one-twentieth grain (3 milligrams)—should be given. It is not improbable that strychnin, so employed, decidedly diminishes the appetite for alcohol. When used in large doses, however, it may at first increase the nervousness from which the patient suffers. It is wisest for a time to begin with moderate doses. Atropin is another highly useful drug. Like strychnin, it appears to lessen the depression caused by the withdrawal of the alcohol. It appears not only to act as a stimulant, but also to diminish somewhat the epigastric sinking sensation from which alcoholics suffer. It should be administered in moderate doses, say one one-hundredth of a grain (0.6 milligram) twice daily, and if it is found that the patient is tolerant of the drug—that it does not produce dryness of the mucous membranes or other unpleasant symptom—the frequency of the dose may be increased to three times daily. Now and then cases are met with in which larger doses, say one-sixtieth or one-fiftieth of a grain (1 to 1.2 milligrams), are well tolerated. It proves especially valuable in cases in which there is marked depression with coldness and clamminess of the extremities. Like strychnin, atropin may be given hypodermically, and when the depression caused by the withdrawal of the alcohol is very marked, this method of administration should be resorted to. In other cases, it is most conveniently given by the mouth. Coffee should, of course, also be used; occasionally caffein proves most valuable. Digitalis, strophanthus, or other cardiac tonics may be given with good result. These drugs are of as much service as the strychnin and the atropin, if not of greater value than either. They should be given in sufficient dose to produce a full physiologic effect upon the pulse. Later in the treatment, other drugs, such as arsenic, iron, and the bitter tonics, may be administered as indicated. We should, of course, never prescribe the bitter tonics in the form of tinctures. As a rule, their exhibition in pill form, with or without a small quantity of capsicum, answers every purpose. Gold and sodium chlorid, which, under the name of bichlorid of gold, was much vaunted by advertising pretenders some years ago, as a specific for alcoholism, is almost inert, its action being that of a very feeble tonic and alterative. The use of apomorphin or of other nauseant drugs in the treatment of alcoholism is unscientific and is to be strongly deprecated. The plan also of substituting some other drug, such as morphin, cocain, or chloral, as the alcohol is withdrawn, cannot be too strongly condemned.

The patient should be kept under treatment for as long a period as possible. After he leaves the immediate care of the physician, he should be under the supervision of a well-instructed professional nurse. As a rule, when a subject of alcoholism has been properly treated and for a sufficiently long period, the tendency to relapse is comparatively slight. It is exceedingly important, however, in the after-treatment to guard the patient against nervous or physical strains of any kind. Relapses are not infrequently to be traced to indiscretion in overwork or to taking part in social functions with the attending loss of sleep and the temptation to the convivial use of wines and liquors. The danger of the depression caused by the excessive use of tobacco, and the consequent craving for stimulants, should be especially pointed out. The greatest difficulty is, of course, experienced in the treatment of those cases in which there is a marked neuropathy. Especially is this the case with patients in whom the drunkenness comes on in spells or well-defined attacks, attacks which probably correspond to waves of emotional depression, hypomelancholia. As far as possible, the life of the patient who has been treated for alcoholism should be based upon physiologic principles. Everything should be done to keep the organism at as high a physiologic level as possible. The importance of physical exercise, especially out-of-door exercise, in this connection is obvious.

Hypnotism was some years ago suggested as a mode of treatment of alcoholism, especially by Forel. Of its efficiency I have no personal knowledge. It is very doubtful, however, whether any method of treatment which fails to recognize fully the pathologic groundwork underlying the alcoholic habit, can be successful. Certainly, in all but very slight cases, hypnotism can be no more efficient than it is in actual organic disease. We should remember also, as has been pointed out by Crothers, that alcoholics are generally very poor subjects for hypnotism. Finally, we should remember that the state of hypnosis is merely a state of hysteria artificially induced (see p. 90; also p. 301).

Alcoholic Confusional Insanity, Alcoholic Dementia, and Alcoholic Paranoia

The treatment and management of the insanities resulting from alcohol are to be based upon the general principles elucidated in the foregoing discussions. The management of alcoholic confusional insanity does not differ from that of confusional insanity from other causes. Rest methods and general physiologic measures must again be applied. It is remarkable in how great a degree alcoholic insanities yield to treatment, provided they have not advanced too far or continued too long. Even in cases of alcoholic dementia so profound as to simulate paresis, most remarkable improvement is observed. Alcoholic paranoia alone offers an exception. In alcoholic paranoia we have to deal with a patient who has, so to speak, the paranoiac constitution; the alcohol has merely been the exciting cause of the development of the disease, the patient being already predisposed by his organization to that form of nervous degeneration which manifests itself as delusional insanity. When improvement or recovery follows in alcoholic confusional insanity, or alcoholic dementia, it usually does so only after many months of treatment; but the degree of improvement is at times remarkable, the patient becoming apparently normal, save for some persistence of nervous weakness or a degree of inability for sustained intellectual effort.

The expedient of a hypertonic, alkaline and sedative intravenous injection, such as has been described in considering the treatment of alcoholic delirium, might be tried in these cases. While the results would probably not be as prompt and as satisfactory as in delirium, it could do no harm and might possibly lessen the duration, especially of alcoholic confusion.

Morphinism

Much of what has been said in regard to the treatment of alcoholism is applicable to the treatment of morphinism. The same general principles are applicable. The treatment resolves itself into the treatment of the **habitual** and of the **occasional** users. There are some patients who, like the periodic alcoholic, make use of morphin or of opium at certain periods only, and then again voluntarily abandon the drug. It is a common thing to find persons who suffer from recurrent attacks of headache or neuralgia, or from menstrual troubles, using morphin periodically. Women especially are prone to form such a habit—a very dangerous one, for sooner or later the periodic users of morphin become slaves to the medicine. It is obvious that if patients come under our care for such a use of morphin, the pathologic condition which necessitates this use—the headache, the neuralgia, or the menstrual pain —should be the first object of our attack.

The treatment of the periodic users of morphin is far more difficult than that of those who use the narcotic continuously. It is also a remarkable fact that it is, as a rule, less difficult to treat successfully a patient who has used rather large doses of the drug, but who has done so for a short time only, than it is to treat one who has used only small quantities, but has used them for many years. Physicians cannot rid themselves of the great responsibility involved in the abuse of morphin; for it must be admitted that it is too frequently prescribed for comparatively trivial affections, and that some physicians are altogether too ready with the use of the hypodermic syringe. Prescriptions for the relief of pain should be for a few doses only, and the patient himself should be warned against the unnecessary repetition of the dose. Happily, the "Harrison Act" in this country now effectually forbids the renewal of prescriptions save by the explicit order of the physician, while the illegitimate sale of the drug is also stringently controlled.

Unlike the abuse of alcohol, the long continued use of morphin is but rarely followed by frank and outspoken insanity. There is, however, a marked diminution in the capacity of the patient for work or for sustained effort of any kind. The mental faculties are usually somewhat obtunded, though not always to a marked degree. The moral sense, however, always suffers severely. Generally, the statements of the patient are absolutely unreliable in regard to everything that pertains to his use of the drug. A patient whose pupils are profoundly contracted and who presents the brilliant countenance and the evident signs of well-being following a recent dose of morphin, may assure the physician in the suavest manner possible that he has not had a dose for many days or weeks. Sleep is always greatly disturbed. Not infrequently, diurnal somnolence alternates with nocturnal insomnia. Now and then, hallucinations and mental confusion make their appearance, especially during periods of the withdrawal of the drug. The hallucinations are mainly auditory and are painful in character. The delusions are persecutory and terrifying.

If the morphin has been used for a long period, more or less decided and persistent mental impairment follows; this condition is analogous to alcoholic dementia but less marked. The patient frequently presents, besides, hyperesthesias and paresthesias of the extremities. His nutrition is poor, the skin is yellow, relaxed, and dry, while the superficial fat largely disappears. The appetite is diminished, cardiac palpitation is of frequent occurrence, while asthmatic symptoms, more or less marked in character, make their appearance, especially in the intervals of the taking of the drug. Sexual power and desire, as in alcoholism, are much diminished.

As in the case of alcoholics, we are confronted with the difficulty of controlling the patient. Only in exceptional cases can success attend the physician's efforts when continual supervision is not possible. No treatment is so efficacious as that by full rest methods, largely because of the complete control which is gained over the patient. Partial rest methods fail. Full rest methods on the other hand, are very frequently crowned with success. As in the case of alcoholism, the patient should be placed in bed, should be carefully isolated, and should be placed upon a diet especially adapted to the case—one which contains large amounts of milk, fruit, and vegetables, and a relatively small amount of beef and lamb. Morphinists, as a rule, have a diminished appetite, especially for meats. The remarks already made in regard to the diet in alcoholism apply with but slight modifications here. As a rule, the white meats (fish, oysters, breast of fowl, etc.) are well digested, and are found more beneficial than the red meats (beef, lamb, etc.). In addition to the rest and the special feeding, bathing, massage, and electricity should be employed systematically. Isolation is absolutely imperative. No one should have access to the room save the nurse and the physician. No letters, packages, or newspapers should be admitted to the room under any pretext. Patients practise all sorts of devices to secure possession of the coveted stimulant. Bribery of servants is attempted, or an order may be written on a piece of paper, the paper wrapped about a coin, and the missive thrown out of a window; in my own observation this method upon one occasion actually enabled the patient to procure the drug. It is remarkable also to what extent friends and relatives will enter into collusion with the patient to supply him with the stimulant, all fearing that the doctor is practising great cruelty and is withdrawing the drug too rapidly. Vigilance in such cases cannot be too great.

The question of the rate of withdrawal is not susceptible of a routine answer, but must be decided with special reference to all the circumstances in each individual case. Some writers advise immediate withdrawal, others rapid withdrawal, and others again very gradual withdrawal. Thus, Gilles de la Tourette advises sudden withdrawal if the patient has been taking large doses, say, five to six grains daily, and gradual withdrawal if the patient has been taking less than five grains; while Comby advises sudden withdrawal invariably. It is my own practice not to begin withdrawal until rest treatment is fully under way. We must remember that the morphin habitué labors under an excessive fear lest the drug be withdrawn too soon. Besides, sudden withdrawal always implies a period of frightful physical and mental suffering. Further, the patient is, as a rule, intensely distrustful. I know of no class of patients with whom it is more difficult to establish friendly relations, or in whom it is more difficult to inspire confidence. However, if the patient learns after his first days of rest and isolation that he is still receiving his hypodermic injections, or that he is still being allowed his usual quantity of laudanum or opium, confidence sooner or later asserts itself, especially as the physical comfort resulting from the bathing, massage, and proper diet soon becomes pronounced. Withdrawal may then be commenced, and it is almost always best conducted very gradually. At first, the diminution of the dose is practically imperceptible; later on the reduction may be more rapid. If the patient has been in the habit of receiving hypodermic injections, it is my practice not only to reduce the dose gradually in the manner indicated, but also to begin adding to the injection small doses of strychnin nitrate, say one-fiftieth of a grain (1.2 milligrams), and if the skin be very moist, small doses of atropin sulphate, say one two-hundredth of a grain (0.3 milligram). Hyoscin or scopolamin may also be employed in doses of one one-hundredth or one two-hundredth of a grain (0.6 to 0.3 milligram). These drugs markedly allay the nervousness and suffering of the patient. It is needless to say that after the morphin has been discontinued entirely, hypodermic injections of strychnin or of strychnin and atropin may be kept up for some time without informing the patient of the change. Cocain should never be used; a large number of patients that come under our care for the morphin habit have already acquired the cocain habit. The same remarks apply to the use of alcohol. Many of our cases, indeed, are instances of the "triple" habit, namely, morphin, cocain, and alcohol.

The reason for withdrawing the drug in the gradual manner I have described, is not only to diminish the sufferings of the patient, but also to prevent the onset of serious symptoms. Every now and then, if the drug be abruptly withdrawn, signs of collapse—diarrhea, sweating, cardiac weakness, and dyspnea, with excessive prostration—may set in. In other cases, again, mental symptoms resembling those of confusional insanity make their appearance, the patient becoming hallucinatory, delusional, and finally delirious. Such symptoms are not likely to make their appearance if the drug be withdrawn in the manner indicated and under fully established rest conditions. When drugs are used habitually, tolerance to their use is sooner or later established and an increasing dose is required to produce an effect. The establishment of this tolerance doubtless depends on the formation of antibodies; in the case of morphin the formation of an antitoxin has been definitely proved. Hirschlaff some years; ago demonstrated this fact experimentally in animals. It would seem that the symptoms arising during the withdrawal of the drug are largely due to the unantagonized action of the accumulated antitoxin; the vomiting, the diarrhea, the sweating are the efforts on the part of nature to eliminate this substance itself now acting as a poison. Similarly, it is extremely probable that the nervous disturbances, delirium and confusion, are the result of its unopposed action upon the nerve-centers. Stimulation of the emúnctories, especially brisk purgation, is indicated provided the general condition of the patient justifies such a course.

Because morphin patients are so untrustworthy, and because the means of obtaining the medicine save under rigid isolation are so many, the physician should carefully watch the patient in order to learn whether withdrawal is actually taking place. Absolute supervision is possible only under absolute isolation, and even then, by the most unexpected means, the patient may be placed in possession of the stimulant. However, if the quantity administered is really being diminished, certain symptoms inevitably make their appearance. They are, first, restlessness, which may become very marked, and is accompanied by more or less insomnia. The patient also yawns a great deal or sneezes, complains perhaps of having caught a slight cold, or perhaps has an attack of difficult respiration, simulating asthma. In addition to restlessness, he manifests signs of fear, complains of a sense of oppression, declares himself dissatisfied with the treatment, and insists upon going home. Involuntary movements of the legs and arms also make their appearance, the limbs being thrown about the bed. At times this is merely due to restlessness; at other times distinct involuntary jerkings are observed. Intention tremor also becomes evident. When, for instance, the patient attempts to pick up a glass of water, it is noticed that he trembles decidedly. Sometimes, instead of an asthmatic attack, all the symptoms referable to a cold in the head or a spasmodic cough may be noted. Sometimes vesical tenesmus is present. Palpitation of the heart may also be evident, or the patient may complain of fluttering sensations in the precordia.

Obviously, if none of these disturbances be observed, and if the patient continues comfortable and in good spirits, sleeps well, and is contented with his surroundings, he is obtaining the drug surreptitiously. It should be remembered that even under very gradual withdrawal some of the symptoms described make their appearance, and may, indeed, become so marked as to necessitate for a time a return to a larger quantity. No picture is more alarming than that often presented by morphin patients in the stage of withdrawal, especially if the depression produced by the vomiting and diarrhea be accompanied by mental confusion and delirium. These symptoms cannot be relieved by other remedies, and a recourse to morphin for a time is not only indicated, but is really the only course to pursue. The history of the withdrawal in a confirmed case of morphinism is, in my experience, not a steady and unbroken decrease in the quantity of the drug, but embraces a series of diminutions, the progressive decrease being every now and then broken by a return to a slightly larger quantity.

The detailed method of diminution depends largely upon the individual case. As a rule, I continue for a number of days the quantity of morphin that the patient is habitually taking; I then begin to diminish the doses given in the early part of the day; those given at night are continued in full quantity for a somewhat longer period. This is contrary to the practice of others, who begin by diminishing the evening doses. I have observed, however, that cutting off the evening doses makes the patient restless and sleepless; while the reduction of the morning doses, though producing restlessness, is not attended by the great disadvantage resulting from insomnia and its attendant evils. No hard-and-fast rule can, however, be said to apply. The patient should be given the drug when he needs it most, and it should be first diminished or withdrawn at those periods when he needs it least. Inasmuch as morphin injected hypodermically is eliminated by the stomach and is subsequently reabsorbed by the intestines, Hitzig has suggested that in treating morphinism we should systematically wash out the stomach. This seems to me an unnecessary precaution. The procedure adds greatly to the distress from which the patient is already suffering, and it is doubtful whether the quantity of morphin thus gotten rid of is really large.

Auxiliary Drugs.—As already stated, during withdrawal, we should, according to judgment, use hypodermic injections of strychnin and atropin. As in the management of alcoholism, the dose must be adapted to the case. In morphinism relatively larger doses of these drugs are tolerated. However, in many cases it is possible to bring about withdrawal without their use. Occasionally it is a good plan to use digitalis or strophanthus. As the treatment progresses, and during the convalescent period, bitter tonics, mineral acids, iron, arsenic, or malt and other nutrients may be added, as seems expedient.

Among drugs to which especial virtue in the treatment of morphinism has been ascribed, we should mention sodium phosphate. It has been especially advocated by Luys. He believes that it has a supporting action on the nervous system and should be given hypodermically. Beyond purely theoretic considerations, the practice has nothing to recommend it. Dr. W. W. Winthrop, of Fort Worth, Texas, has recently called attention to the employment of "husa" as a remedy for the cure of the opium habit. Husa is an unclassified, or at least unidentified, plant found in the Everglades of Florida. According to Winthrop, it is a diffusible stimulant, causing gentle excitement, followed later on by sedation and sleep. From three to four months are necessary to effect a cure. It appears, also, that precaution must be taken to prevent the formation of a husa habit. The treatment of the opium habit by this means is, therefore, open to the same objection as any other method depending upon the substitution of one drug for another. Cocain, which has been recommended by Skene, Mattison, and later by Keugla, is merely a makeshift substitute, and should not be resorted to. Caffein, also recommended by some writers, may occasionally be used in cases in which withdrawal is followed by great depression, or in cases in which the early morning depression is very marked. It should not be given toward evening for fear of adding to the insomnia.

Insomnia and restlessness not infrequently demand the use of the bromids. Ammonium bromid may be given in doses of thirty to forty grains (2 to 2.5 grams) at intervals of four hours. Better still, hyoscin or scopolamin may be given in small doses twice or three times daily. At times, medinal may be given; if possible, sulphonal should be avoided, as should also chloral, both of these drugs favoring the confusion and delirium occasionally met with in severe morphinism. The hot bath offers a harmless, and often a very efficient, method of combating the insomnia.

Suggestion, advocated by some writers, with or without hypnotism, is of little or no value in the treatment. Hirt, for instance, treats cases outside of institutions, if the daily dose be not greater than 0.25, 0.50, or at most 0.75 gram (4 to 12 grains), with the aid of hypnotism. He places a reliable female nurse in charge of the patient. The morphin is then suddenly withdrawn. Sleep is produced by chloral or trional or by warm baths. In four or five days the treatment by hypnotism is begun. Hirt states that only a slight degree of hypnosis is required. The treatment extends over a period varying from twenty-one days to eight months, but recovery can be regarded as established only in one and a half to two years after the last hypodermic injection has been given. Certainly, the method has nothing to recommend it on the ground of economy of time. Besides, success seems to be very doubtful. It cannot but be greatly inferior to treatment directed primarily to the reëstablishment of the general health, such as is embodied in the application of rest methods.

Duration of Treatment.—The treatment of the morphin habit by rest methods should be continued for a very long period; that which is sufficient for ordinary cases of neurasthenia or hysteria being totally insufficient for cases of morphinism. A course of three months of treatment is, as a rule, absolutely demanded, and, for many patients, the treatment should embrace five, six, or even seven months. I do not mean to imply that the patient should be kept in bed during all of this period, but that full rest methods should be kept up for from three to four months, and after this a partial rest treatment should be instituted, the patient being up and out of bed, and exercising out of doors, daily for some three or four hours. In cases so treated I have met with most gratifying results. Success, it need hardly be stated, is still further assured if the patient's nurse accompany her to her home or elsewhere and remain with her for a period of several months longer. If practicable, the entire length of treatment under the supervision of the nurse should extend over a year. In no class of patients is relapse so apt to occur as in morphin users, and it is for this reason that every possible precaution should be taken, provided the patient's means permit it.

After-treatment.—With regard to the management of morphin cases subsequent to the rest treatment, the general principles already indicated in the section on Alcoholism are applicable here. Everything should be done in the way of proper diet and exercise to keep the patient's health at as high a level as possible. Here also it is important to avoid fatigue, and especially strain, excitement, and worry. Cases presenting special difficulties, are those in which the habit has been acquired in the attempt to relieve a painful affection which still continues, as, for example, a persistent neuralgia, frequently recurring headache, or painful menstruation. It is needless to point out that every effort should be made to discover and, if possible, eradicate the cause of the painful affection, whatever it may be, treating the headache or neuralgia upon such principles as are indicated; or if functional or organic disease of special structures be present—*e.g.*, pelvic disorders, in women—instituting such means, medicinal or surgical, as are necessary.

Cocainism

In the treatment of cocainism, we have again to apply the principles already detailed in the consideration of the treatment of alcoholism and morphinism. Cocainism arises usually in one of two ways. It may be acquired as a concomitant of the morphin habit, the patient having learned to take cocain in order to diminish the amount of morphin, or perhaps it has arisen in the unscientific treatment of morphinism by cocain substitution. The second and far more frequent cause of the cocain habit is the use of the drug in the treatment of affections of the nose. Not only is cocain applied by the surgeon preparatory to the performance of operations, but it not infrequently happens that the patient secures a solution containing the drug and makes his own applications. Within my own knowledge, not a few cases of cocainism can be traced to some such misapplication of the drug, the victim not infrequently being himself a physician. In prescribing cocain for purely local affections, we incur a responsibility not less than that which we incur in prescribing morphin. We should never lose sight of the fact that every local application is accompanied by a certain amount of general action. After the use of cocain over a mucous surface, such as the nasal chambers, the patient experiences not only local anesthesia, but also a comfortable sense of warmth and well-being diffused over the body. Further, the nerve-centers are stimulated, especially if the doses have been large, very much as they are stimulated with alcohol, save that the stimulation is far more marked and sudden.

There is intense excitement with increased pulse-rate, accompanied by a sense of intoxication. There is a marked increase of the nervous irritability and the ideas flow much more rapidly than normally.

A form of cocain inebriety is also now and then met with, which is due to the abuse of various coca-containing medicines. The continued use of the so-called "tonics," "restoratives," "elixirs," and "wines," which, in addition to alcohol, contain coca, cocain, kola, and like drugs, is much to be deprecated. These preparations are not tonic but merely stimulating, and they cannot fail to prove injurious. Occasionally, they give rise to drug habits and to alcoholism as well. In many cases a fancy name, in others an incomplete chemical or pharmaceutical name, disguises, or at least fails to reveal to the careless user or prescriber, the true nature of the harmful compound.

The cocain habit is frequently established with rapidity. If the drug be withdrawn for a time or if the patient fail of access to it, he is seized with a feeling of great discomfort, of marked oppression, of faintness, palpitation, and general nervousness. The cocain user becomes excessively irritable, sharp and short in his speech, jerky in his manner, and exceedingly restless. Inability to work and ready fatigue are prominent symptoms. There is more or less impairment of will-power and loss of memory, and the patient grows as unreliable in his statements and as reckless of the truth as the morphinist. He is pale and haggard; his general nutrition is much impaired, and his weight is below normal. Often he presents a picture of premature senility. His reflexes are exaggerated. His movements are those of unrest and constant change of position. At times his muscles are the seat of spasmodic twitchings. His pupils are dilated. Frequently, there is a tremor of the tongue and sometimes of the hands. His pulse is rapid and he frequently suffers from palpitation. His skin is likely to be cold and moist. He sleeps but little—often, indeed, insomnia persists for days. Later, he may, as in the case of alcoholism, develop a true confusional insanity. In this state he may be the victim of delusions of persecution. At other times he may, as in alcoholism, entertain the delusion of marital infidelity. Not infrequently hallucinations, visual and auditory, and especially hallucinations referred to the cutaneous surface, develop. The patient frequently believes that there are vermin or fleas upon his person, or in his bed or about his room; and he often spends a large part of his time in bathing, rubbing, scratching, or in making efforts to rid himself of the imaginary pest. So striking is this hallucination of cutaneous sensibility in cocainic insanity, that a patient presenting it is said to suffer from the "cocain bug."

Withdrawal.—During the withdrawal of the drug, the symptoms just detailed become much exaggerated. If no exaggeration is noted, it is very probable that withdrawal is not actually taking place, or that some other drug is being substituted. Usually this substitute is morphin. Contrary to what one might expect, it is generally practicable to withdraw cocain far more rapidly than either morphin or alcohol. Curiously enough, after the cocain has been withdrawn for a period, the patient sleeps without the administration of drugs; frequently, indeed, he cannot keep awake. At times, however, it is necessary to give moderate doses of hyoscin or scopolamin, the bromids, or medinal or sulphonal, for some time. It is proper, in order to relieve the depression from which the patient suffers, to allow a cup of strong coffee in the early part of the day.

As already stated, the cocain habit may have been acquired in the attempt to cure the morphin habit, and cocainism and morphinism may exist together. In such cases, the cocain may be entirely withdrawn at once. The morphin, however, should be withdrawn in the gradual manner already described. Similarly, the patient may be the victim of the so-called "triple habit;" that is, he may use not only morphin and cocain, but also alcohol. Here the problem presented often taxes our ingenuity. As a general rule, however, it may be stated that it is expedient to withdraw the cocain at once, the alcohol rapidly, and the morphin gradually. Morphin distinctly overshadows the other drugs, and, as a rule, it is best to continue this agent in full doses for a number of days. In other words, the treatment of the "triple habit" resolves itself sooner or later into that of simple morphinism.

It cannot be too strongly insisted upon that rest and isolation, as detailed in the sections on Alcoholism and Morphinism, apply equally to the treatment of cocainism. Cocain users are even less to be trusted than are morphinists. They are, when the habit is confirmed, tricky, treacherous, and utterly untrustworthy. I know of no cases more difficult to control. They betray a degree of shrewdness and cunning in circumventing the physician and deceiving the nurse that is almost incredible. They are, on the whole, far more difficult to treat by rest methods because of their extreme restlessness. The inclination to move and to be about is so great as to make restraint doubly difficult. So well known is this fact that hospitals which receive alcoholics or morphinists for treatment will very frequently decline cocainists. The latter will often, in spite of the utmost vigilance, smuggle into their rooms, or conceal about their persons and belongings, quantities of cocain, or will succeed, if the nurse be not careful, in stealing or otherwise obtaining a supply. A hypodermic syringe is often a coveted object, and one of my patients upon one occasion stole a hypodermic syringe, the whereabouts of which the closest search failed to reveal, until finally a digital examination was made of the rectum. Here the syringe was concealed. No expedient is too disgusting, no conduct too objectionable, so long as the coveted stimulant is obtained. Noise, threats of legal prosecution, and defiance of nurse and physician are the order of the day. The term "cocain fiend" has not been applied to these patients without cause.

Confinement, under the supervision of a trained nurse, in a room to which no other person but the physician has access, presents practically the only favorable prospect. As in the case of morphinism, this isolation should be practised for from two to three months or longer. The general principles already indicated with regard to the use of tonics in the convalescent period of morphinism, apply equally here. We should remember that our patient is below weight, and that he presents the symptoms of nervous exhaustion to a profound degree.

The prolonged abuse of cocain more frequently than morphin gives rise to insanity. Like alcohol, it may give rise to a dementia resembling paresis—a pseudo-paresis, which is in reality a profound confusional insanity with expansive or persecutory delusions as the case may be. It may become more pronounced and finally terminate in a more or less prolonged stupor or dementia, a so-called cocain-paresis. When cocain-poisoning has attained so severe a degree as this, the prognosis is, as a rule, unfavorable as regards recovery.

Chloralism, Trionalism, and Other Forms of Chronic Intoxication

It is not necessary to consider in detail the other forms of drug intoxication with which the physician has to deal. Enough has been said in the foregoing pages to indicate the general plan of treatment which is to be followed in given cases. The temptation is always to replace the drug that is withdrawn by another, and indeed, in practice, especially in the treatment of chloralism, such a procedure is for a time necessary, but it should be discontinued as early as possible.

Chloral is a poison depressant to the heart and vasomotor apparatus. Dyspnea, vertigo, and general sense of weakness are among the symptoms likely to be present. In well-established cases there are marked nervousness, marked insomnia, and a certain degree of mental weakness, as manifested by loss of will-power and failure of memory. In some cases an emotional depression is present which may simulate melancholia. The patient is weak, his movements are tremulous, and he frequently complains of palpitation of the heart. These symptoms must be combated by food, by rest and by other physiologic measures, and by tonics, such as digitalis, strophanthus, and strychnin. When the habit has been long continued and the doses large, the patient occasionally suffers from attacks of delirium closely resembling delirium tremens. Chloral, it should be added, has been so largely displaced by other hypnotics that chloralism is at present a very infrequent condition.

It not infrequently happens that patients become the victims of narcotic habits other than those already discussed—*e.g.*, veronalism or sulphonalism. Sometimes, also, one of the less commonly used narcotics, such as **paraldehyd, somnal,** or **chloralamid,** is the intoxicant to which the patient becomes addicted. One of the worst and most horrible cases of drug inebriety that I have been called upon to treat, was a case of paraldehyd habit in which a woman took enormous doses of this disgusting narcotic daily. She constantly reeked with the unpleasant odor of the drug, while her mucous membranes were ulcerated and her form much emaciated. Occasionally ether and chloroform are used by inebriates. Among the rarer forms of drug addiction met with at the present day are the **phenacetin** habit and the **antipyrin** habit. These habits, however, are less harmful than those already mentioned, and can, as a rule, be treated more readily.

General principles, of course, are to be applied in the treatment of a drug habit no matter what its cause. Among these, let me repeat, are, first, the isolation of the patient in such a manner that his access to the drug, save as administered by the physician, is absolutely cut off; second, the employment of such therapeutic measures as will raise the general health of the patient to the normal level. The permanence of the result obtained, depends in a large degree upon the influence of friends and relatives.

Insanities from Lead Intoxication

Lead intoxication, so far as the cerebral symptoms are concerned, may manifest itself either in an acute or a chronic form. In the acute form the patient presents headache, insomnia, frightening dreams, tinnitus, flashes of light, mental slowness, and depression. Soon delirium ensues, which is often very violent. Hallucinations of sight especially are prominent. The delirium may become more and more pronounced, and may pass on to coma, or the patient may survive and there may be remissions with occasional recurrences of the delirium. Epileptiform convulsions also may make their appearance. In the chronic form, a dementia is observed which, like alcoholic dementia, bears some crude resemblance to paresis, and is sometimes spoken of as lead-paresis. At other times, the patient manifests delusions which are more or less systematized in character and generally persecutory in type. In other words, there is present a paranoia which resembles the paranoia of alcoholism. This form of mental affection is very rare.

The treatment of the insanities of lead intoxication is to be based, as before, upon general principles. Every effort is, of course, to be made, as soon as the diagnosis is established, to bring about the elimination of the lead. The iodids should be cautiously administered, while the bowels should be kept freely open by salines, more particularly the sulphates. General physiologic measures, with tonic medication and liberal feeding, are, of course, to be employed as in the other forms of mental disease. The prognosis, on the whole, is not favorable.

Part III
SUGGESTION

PART III.—SUGGESTION

CHAPTER I

NORMAL SUGGESTION

Legitimate Field of Suggestion; Direct and Indirect, General and Special Suggestion. Suggestion in Hysteria, Hypochondria, and Neurasthenia. Suggestion in Other Forms of Functional and Organic Disease.

A discussion of physiologic methods of treatment would not be complete without some consideration of **suggestion.** Whatever view one may hold as to the therapeutic efficacy of this measure, its study will prove not only interesting, but also of practical value.

Much unnecessary mystery attaches to the term. Unfortunately it has been associated very closely with hypnotism, and has acquired an almost specific meaning. To make a suggestion, however, does not mean to impose a hallucination or a delusion upon a person in the condition of hypnotic sleep, but merely to convey to, or arouse in the mind of another, some thought or idea, in an unobtrusive manner. It is a process that is always taking place, usually unconsciously, among the various individuals of the social body, and is in itself the outcome of perfectly normal mental functions.

Physicians employ suggestion habitually, though most frequently they do so unintentionally and unconsciously. That it often powerfully affects the progress of a case, for good or for ill, every experienced practitioner will admit. Mental factors influence more or less the physical condition of every patient, and this fact is true whether the patient be suffering from an acute or a chronic, a general or a local affection; from disease of the nervous system or of other structures; from organic lesions or from a purely functional disorder.   Suggestion as an adjuvant to treatment may, in skilful hands, aid in the most unmistakable manner in bringing about recovery.   Even in incurable cases it may assist materially in keeping the patient comfortable.   It may diminish the necessity for the administration of drugs, or it may enable us to give placebos in place of the latter.   Without stooping to any dishonest procedure, or imitating the methods of the various mind-curists, faith-curists, faddists or other unqualified practitioners, striking results can frequently be achieved by simple and perfectly proper means.   It is rarely, of course, that we can rely upon suggestion alone; it is commonly as an adjuvant to a treatment by physiologic methods and medicines that suggestion proves of value.

It is hardly necessary to point out how the belief in eventual recovery affects the patient's general condition and nutrition. Other things being equal, the man who feels sure of getting well eats better and sleeps better.   The very action of the heart is promoted by this hopeful and contented attitude of mind.   Compare such a condition with that of a patient who is tormented by doubt and fear, or in whose mind the conviction has become settled that he is stricken with a serious, or possibly fatal, malady. Instead of coöperating with the physician in a whole-hearted manner, he looks upon the treatment and its various details with doubt and suspicion.   That he takes less food, that he digests it less well, that his sleep is more disturbed, that he feels his pains more acutely, that his various symptoms present themselves to him in a grossly exaggerated and distorted form, need hardly be pointed out.

Every physician knows how smoothly the ordinary self-limited and curable affections progress when the patient has confidence in his medical adviser; every physician knows not only this fact, but is even aware of the effect of each separate visit upon his patient. Irrespective of the instructions given to the nurse, or of the modifications in the details of treatment resulting from the observation of conditions present, each visit has a distinctly tonic and bracing effect upon the patient.   The nurse, too, acts no inconsiderable part.   By the way in which she attends to her duties, by her general demeanor and conduct, even by such trivialities as the raising or lowering of the curtains, will she convey indirectly to the patient suggestions for good or for ill. Many nervous patients are intensely susceptible to such indirect suggestion. Indeed, this is true of many persons who are apparently well. In a previous chapter allusion was made to the case of a sufferer from hypochondria, who upon hearing of an attack of appendicitis in an intimate personal friend, was himself almost immediately seized with diarrhea and abdominal pain, and going at once to bed, sent for his physician under the belief that he too had appendicitis. Such instances are by no means rare. I need only instance how in the contagion of hysteria, the symptoms may spread from patient to patient until large numbers of persons are affected.

The manner in which suggestion acts offers an interesting problem. The rôle which the nervous system plays in the function and nutrition of every structure of the body is well known. It is probable that every tissue has a nerve-supply that directly dominates its nutrition, though the assumption of special trophic nerves is not necessary to explain this relationship. In the case of the circulatory apparatus, of the glands, of the muscles, and of the bones and joints, physiologic, clinical, and pathologic evidence of direct nervous control is incontrovertible. In the case of other structures, such as the blood-making organs and the ductless glands, this control is a matter of legitimate and logical inference. A moment's reflection calls to mind the relations existing between the cells of the anterior cornua of the spinal cord and the muscles, between the lesion of tabes and the nutrition of the bones and joints, between syringomyelia and painless ulcers, and between lesions of nerve-trunks and changes in the muscles and skin. Fixed relationships such as these, however, are but little influenced by mental and emotional conditions; at least, not demonstrably so. Different, however, is it in the part taken by the nervous system in such functions as circulation, digestion, and secretion. It is in this field that we touch upon facts, elementary in character, but which when considered in their possible relation to suggestion become of the very greatest importance. The intimate union between the sympathetic nervous system and the cerebrospinal nervous system is such that it is readily conceivable that the functions of the former should be influenced by the latter. The cerebrospinal nerves, which execute the mandates of the will, that is, carry out voluntary movements, terminate only in striated muscle fiber. The sympathetic nerves, on the other hand, terminate in smooth muscle fiber and in glandular tissue; in other words, the sympathetic fibers include all efferent nerve-fibers except those which go to the voluntary muscles. The first or proximal neuron of the sympathetic nervous system is always situated in the gray matter of the cerebrospinal axis, that is, in the cord or in the brain stem. This proximal neuron gives off an axon which, passing out by way of the rami communicates, terminates in an arborization about the distal neuron situated in the sympathetic ganglion. Thence fibers pass to smooth muscle or gland. The sympathetic nervous system thus has an origin which is primarily cerebrospinal, and, in a sense, it is really an integral portion of the cerebrospinal apparatus. It is only in a limited measure independent or "autonomic."

Mode of Action of Suggestion

Suggestion—and we are still speaking of suggestion without hypnotism—may act in two ways. It may expend itself upon the mind of the patient alone. Thus, it may affect the emotions and the general mental state of the patient; or it may affect one or more of the special functions of the nervous system. That the functions of the nervous system are greatly influenced by the mental condition is evidenced not only by numerous physiologic facts, but by a still greater number of clinical facts. That the mental state may be a preponderating factor in an attack of vomiting, of diarrhea, of cardiac palpitation, in changes of the temperature of the extremities, or even in such phenomena as the degree of the patellar reflex, is well known. The common functional nervous diseases, notably hysteria, furnish a still more remarkable series of facts.

Illustrations from the domain of hysteria are especially significant because in this affection, as I have shown in the preceding pages, psychic factors are dominant. All of the symptoms bear the impress of their psychic origin and, notwithstanding, there are present the most remarkable physical and visceral manifestations. Among the more frequent are vasomotor disturbances, such as pallor, flushing, erythema, mottling of the skin. In rapid pulse, rapid respiration, hysteric cough, and vomiting, in hysteric yawning and hysteric aphonia, in hysteric anuria and polyuria, we again have incontrovertible evidence of profound somatic disturbances.

How the various portions of the nervous system itself yield to the dominant psychic factor is evidenced by the existence of the numerous hysteric motor and sensory palsies—hysteric hemiplegia, paraplegia and monoplegia, stocking-like or glove-like anesthesia, segmental anesthesia, geometric anesthesia, hemianesthesia and the various forms of hyperesthesia. Diminution in the size of the muscles may follow persistent hysteric palsy. However, it is in the more readily disturbed functions alone that the influence of psychic factors becomes evident. Gross organic changes, such as brittleness of bone, arthropathies, and reaction of degeneration in nerves and muscles, do not follow from mere perversions of psychic action.

Methods of Suggestion.—In a book devoted to purely practical questions, psychologic and metaphysical theories as to the action of suggestion would be out of place. They would yield little of practical value, and, after all, it is the facts of suggestion that interest us as physicians, and with which alone we are concerned. In a study of suggestion, the subject naturally separates itself into a consideration of suggestion without hypnotism and of suggestion with hypnotism.

Suggestion without hypnotism is susceptible of scientific application and is often profound and far-reaching in its effects. It may be employed either in the form of indirect or of direct suggestion, and it may be general in its character or it may be special. **Indirect and general suggestion** is the form which is habitually employed by physicians, though, as has been pointed out, such employment is usually unintentional and even unconscious. In it the patient is always unaware that suggestion in any form is being made, but it is none the less potent. **Direct suggestion,** on the other hand, consists in the frank statement to the patient that he is improving or that he will get well. The manner in which the direct suggestion is to be made will depend largely upon the mental make-up of the patient. To patients who are educated, if the facts permit, it is a good plan for the physician to give a brief explanation of the symptoms present, couching his language in the simplest and most elementary terms. Many patients are in such cases completely satisfied. With other persons, the explanation must of necessity be avoided—first, because of the nature of the symptoms, and, secondly, because a discussion of the viscera or of other structures of the body arouses mental pictures that are at once disagreeable and alarming. Direct suggestion is, in my experience, most efficacious when the statement is made moderately. The patient readily builds upon and adds to the suggestion thus thrown out. An overstatement or one made with unnecessary emphasis or exaggeration may fail of effect, while a moderate statement may prove of enormous and convincing force. Care, tact, and judgment must be used in the employment of direct suggestion, for it is not without its dangers. The patient may, for instance, be led to expect a change of symptoms before a sufficient time has elapsed for a change to ensue. Under these circumstances the influence of the physician and the confidence reposed in him by the patient may be seriously shaken. Again, if the suggestion be made in so blatant and unreserved a manner as to excite the suspicion of the patient, the result may be equally disastrous. Notwithstanding these obvious dangers, there can be no doubt that, when properly employed, direct suggestion is of the utmost value, especially if the physician be one whose personality is forceful and impressive.

Therapeutic Suggestion in the Neuroses

Direct suggestion, as can readily be understood, is most valuable in hysteria, less valuable in neurasthenia, and least valuable in hypochondria. In hysteria both direct and indirect suggestion should be employed. Its detailed application depends upon numerous factors, such as the sex, the age, the education, the emotional and mental peculiarities of the patient, and his social state. Details can hardly be entered into for individual cases. When and how, or when not, to employ suggestion in hysteria must depend entirely upon the personal tact and judgment of the physician. It is remarkable how greatly not only the general condition, but various special symptoms, can be influenced. In discussing the treatment of hysteria (see p. 122) I pointed out many of the methods by which special suggestion is to be employed. Suffice it here to say that, other things being equal, special suggestion, *i.e.*, suggestion for the relief of individual symptoms, had best be made indirectly. Owing to the peculiar mental condition of the patient, direct suggestion sometimes produces the very opposite result from that intended.

In neurasthenia indirect and general suggestion is of undoubted value. Direct and special suggestion has, on the other hand, a limited application. A placebo that will induce sleep in hysteria will frequently fail in neurasthenia. A placebo that will cause the disappearance of a headache or neuralgia in hysteria, is not unlikely to fail when prescribed for similar symptoms in neurasthenia. As a rule, general suggestion only should be employed in neurasthenia; special suggestions may, however, be made, when the physician can safely predict the change of symptoms.

In hypochondria we have to deal with a condition in which suggestion has, because of the persistent nature of the affection, a very secondary value. Suggestion does, however, influence the progress of a case for the time being. Not infrequently an individual symptom may be suppressed. We are apt, however, soon to be confronted by a recurrence of the general sense of ill-being or by an onset of new symptoms that take the place of those which have disappeared.

Suggestion as an Adjuvant

In the employment of suggestion, even in those cases in which it is most effective, that is to say, in the great or cardinal neuroses, as they may be termed—hysteria, neurasthenia, and hypochondria—we should bear in mind that it is never to be relied upon of itself, but that it should be employed only as an adjuvant to physiologic and medicinal methods of treatment. In other functional nervous diseases, as chorea and epilepsy, suggestion is of little or no value, while in others still, as **paralysis agitans,** it is of value only in contributing to the general comfort of the patient. In paralysis agitans the physician often pursues a wise course in frankly saying to the patient that the symptoms will not disappear, but that the disease is not immediately dangerous to life, that the patient is in no danger of a "stroke," or palsy, and that he will continue to be quite comfortable for a long time to come. This also is the rôle of suggestion in **organic nervous** diseases. Limited though its function may be, it is not to be despised or thoughtlessly thrown aside. Many a tabetic patient is benefited by a full and frank statement as to the nature of the affection from which he suffers, especially if the statement be coupled with the further declaration that the disease is often self-limited, that the pathologic process frequently becomes arrested or that its progress is exceedingly slow. There is a remarkable quality entering into the psychic make-up of every human being, which enables him to become accustomed to some fact in regard to his life, disease or death, no matter how unpleasant this fact may be. There is a veritable psychic compensation that to a large degree eliminates such a fact from his daily thoughts, his daily consciousness; and he learns to put it aside, as it were, and to make the most of the life that is his. To favor and to bring about such a mental attitude, is the only, but very important and legitimate, function of suggestion in cases of organic disease. How powerful suggestion is, even in face of a certain and impending death, to enable the individual to maintain a nervous equilibrium, and even a relative degree of psychic well-being, is seen in the influence of the religious preparation for death in the case of criminals sentenced to the scaffold. The eagerness with which a commutation of a death sentence—a commutation which usually means imprisonment for life—is accepted by prisoners, is another instance of the same thing. It is this factor in the psychic make-up of man that the physician should bear in mind even in dealing with cases of hopeless disease.

Occupation and Amusement in Conjunction with Suggestion

One application of suggestion it is necessary to mention, especially, because of its importance. There is a group of cases in which the influence of suggestion is marked, provided the patient can at the same time be kept actively employed or mentally diverted. We have seen in the preceding pages how marked is the tendency in the various great neuroses to introspection—to analysis of symptoms, to self-examination. This condition is manifested in a typical degree in hypochondria, on the one hand, and in melancholia, on the other, while it is present to a less pronounced extent in neurasthenia and in hysteria. In all of these affections, as I have pointed out, suggestion should be employed habitually as an adjuvant to the ordinary physiologic methods of treatment. There is, however, a special field for its application in connection with occupation, amusement, and change of scene. So employed, it proves useful in a large number of cases of mild neurasthenia and hysteria, some cases of hypochondria, and a small number of cases of mild melancholia. Everybody knows the benefit that ensues from travel, ocean voyages, moderate social relaxation, play or amusement. Especially valuable is such diversion if it be coupled with the direct suggestion that the patient's symptoms are of little consequence and that he will soon be well. Again, in discussing the management of hypochondria, I pointed out how important it is to keep the patient occupied. Other things equal, the hypochondriac is better when he is under the pressure of work. Work is a physiologic stimulant to both mind and body. The mere maintenance and stimulation of function will not only in certain cases of hypochondria, but also occasionally in mild cases of nervous or mental depression of various kinds, serve to tide a patient over his period of ill health. It is of the utmost benefit in certain cases to minimize the symptoms and to make powerful and repeated suggestions to the patient that he is not ill, or, at least, not sufficiently so to justify him in giving up his work. Of course, at the same time that work is urged upon the patient, his personal hygiene, his habits, his exercise, bathing, food, and sleep, should be carefully regulated; that is, in addition to suggestion and occupation, he should receive the benefit of various physiologic procedures.

The number of cases of melancholia permitting of such a method of treatment is, of course, small. Furthermore, it is necessary that the cases should be carefully selected, lest harm be done.

A patient passing through the early stage of melancholia might, by the injudicious application of this method, be made very much worse. It every now and then happens, however, that, owing to the position which a patient occupies, either in public life or by reason of his responsibilities, it is of the utmost importance to keep him in a measure discharging his duties. In such a case, provided it is merely one of simple mental depression—and not, of course, one of frankly developed melancholia with its hallucinations and delusion of the unpardonable sin—much success may attend the application of the method. Occasionally the patient can be taken away from his routine work and interested in some other form of occupation or some sport or amusement. The latter is best if it take the patient out-of-doors. Skilful individualization must, of course, come into play in the prescription of the daily life, the occupation, amusement and entertainment of the patient, and the choice of surroundings, including in the latter the personality of the associates or of the trained attendant. It is obviously impossible to enter further into details.

CHAPTER II

SUGGESTION BY MYSTIC AND RELIGIOUS METHODS; SUGGESTION UNDER ARTIFICIALLY INDUCED HYSTERIA—HYPNOTISM; PSYCHANALYSIS

Pythonism, Shamanism, Magnetism, Mesmerism, Hypnotism Psychanalysis, Metallotherapy, Perkins's Tractors, Mind Cure Faith Cure, Eddyism

In a book like the present, a discussion of the subjects of this chapter is—so far as its direct teaching is concerned—somewhat out of place. The procedures employed certainly do not constitute physiologic methods of treatment. On the contrary, they usually call into being, as there will be no difficulty in pointing out, nervous states that are both abnormal and pathologic. However, because of the necessity of placing in bold contrast mystic and religious methods of treatment with physiologic procedures, the following sections have been appended.

For public reasons, too as well as for personal fulness of knowledge, physicians should understand the various methods of so-called "mental healing," etc., that from time to time find vogue among large sections of the community. Thus, they will be able to recognize and to point out both the positive and the negative dangers that these methods involve; as well as to differentiate clearly in their own minds between such practices and the legitimate employment of psychic influences to promote the recovery of the sick. The subject of hypnotism again, has attained a certain importance in medical jurisprudence that must be alluded to.

Superstition and Magic

Since the dawn of history, superstition and magic have played a large part in the treatment of disease. That they have continued to do so, even down to our own times, no one will deny. Large numbers of lay persons are at this very day earnest advocates of religious and superstitious methods, while the medical profession itself is not free from the charge of having at various, and indeed quite recent times countenanced procedures whose sole recommendation has been the mysticism involved. Four thousand years ago, religious and mystic rites were practised in the treatment of disease in Egypt. Prosper Alpinus informs us that the Egyptian healers subjected their patients to mysterious manual operations, that they enveloped them in the skins of sacred animals and conveyed them into holy places, to be visited by dreams and inspirations. Similar practices were in vogue in ancient Greece and Rome, while among the Hebrews, the prophets practised the healing power of bodily contact—often by the laying on of hands. The Psylli, a people of Lybia, were famed for their magic cures; these they performed by stretching their bodies on the bodies of the sick and by making the latter swallow water impregnated with their saliva.

Among the ancient Greeks, a practice called **pythonism** also prevailed. From a cave sacred to Apollo, a stupefying vapor issued, which had so powerful an effect as to throw men into convulsions. These phenomena were ascribed to a supernatural agency, while the incoherent ravings of those who inhaled the toxic vapor were regarded as prophecies uttered under the inspiration of the deity. A priestess, called a pythoness, was appointed to inhale the prophetic fumes. In order to enable her to perform the duty assigned to her, a seat, called a tripod, was constructed over the mouth of the cave. Thus, the pythoness, inspired by the fumes, made known the will of Apollo to the attendant priests, who communicated the revelations to the inquirer. The disconnected words and cries uttered by the pythoness in her ravings, were carefully framed into sentences. The priests filled up the breaks with such words and in such construction, as to give coherent meaning to the whole, and it is not strange, perhaps, that the content of the revelation expressed whatever was most essential to the interests of the shrine. The pythoness was supposed to give advice in regard to private enterprises, public affairs, and, also, the healing of disease. Crude survivals of similar practices, in which hysteria and deception are commingled, are still found among the north Asiatic races, and, for that matter, among all the savage races of the world. Shamanism, as practised among the Ural-Attaic people, is a good illustration. The Shamanic priests know the secret of the coming and departing of evil spirits. Their offices are generally called in requisition in cases of sickness or death, which are ascribed to the presence or ill-will of demons. By shouts, incantations, by the beating of drums and blowing of horns, the demon is supposed to be driven out. Quite frequently the priest will work himself into a condition of hysteria and even of trance. In Siberia, the priest usually sucks the part of the body of the patient which aches the most, and finally takes out of his mouth a thorn, a bug, a stone, or some other object, which he then asserts to have been the cause of the pain.

More rational and less crude were some of the other methods pursued in ancient times. Thus Asclepiades, it is said, quieted by manipulations the mild insane, and when the manipulation was carried to excess, the patient fell into a lethargic sleep. Cœlius Aurelianus prescribed friction by the hand for the cure of pleurisy and also gave instructions for the manipulation of epileptics. Practices similar to these prevailed at various times in other countries. In the fifteenth century, Pomponatius, in the sixteenth century Agrippa, the famous Paracelsus and later Bacon, Cardanus, and Van Helmont, were advocates of the doctrine that the body possesses an influence of magnetism—that there is a certain energy which acts beyond the body, that this action is in accordance with the will of the possessor, and that, by this means, various qualities can be imparted and results brought about.

Mesmerism

The greatest magnetizer that the world has ever produced was Mesmer, who appeared in the latter part of the eighteenth century. In 1774, Hell, professor of astronomy in Vienna, informed Mesmer that he had cured rheumatism in himself by a magnetic process. In consequence of this, Mesmer immediately entered upon a career of treating by magnets every one who applied to him. He distributed magnets in every direction, and in his memoir, published in 1779, he maintained that the heavenly spheres possess a direct power or influence over animal bodies, particularly over the nervous system, and that in this way arises animal magnetism. Being persecuted for his doctrine, he removed to Switzerland, and later, in 1778, to Paris. There he announced that he could operate powerfully upon the nervous system, and he established himself in a magnificent house in the fashionable quarter of the French capital. His patients were seated around and were in contact, directly or indirectly, with a wooden vessel or "*baquet*" which contained the magnetic fluid. He was regarded as a great magician, and received big fees, while his artful and occult procedures produced astonishing effects. In response to a request from the government, the medical faculty of Paris appointed a commission in 1784 to investigate his claims. This commission consisted of prominent physicians and physicists. Among its members were such men as Franklin, Bailly, Lavoisier, Guillotin, and Poissonier. Mesmer, however, declined to submit his practice and theories to this body, and the commission were forced to undertake their investigations with the aid of d'Eslon, the ardent pupil and disciple of Mesmer. The commission freely acknowledged the facts disclosed by their investigations, but denied the connection of these facts with animal magnetism. Mesmer vigorously protested against this adverse report, but he could not withstand the reaction which it caused. The magic of his spell was broken, and in the following year he left Paris.

Notwithstanding the decision of the Paris commission, adherents made their appearance abroad. Physicians in Bremen, Karlsruhe, Heilbronn, Strassburg, and Berlin followed Mesmer's practices, and during the latter part of the eighteenth and the beginning of the nineteenth century, his teachings were actively studied in Germany. Among others, Wolfahrt, who was sent in 1812 by the Prussian Government to Mesmer at Frauenfeld for the purpose of studying animal magnetism, returned an enthusiastic advocate of Mesmer's doctrines. In France, on the other hand, the Abbe de Faria in 1814 strongly opposed the existence of a magnetic fluid and declared that the phenomena observed in the so-called magnetized subjects were not due to a fluid emanating from the magnetizer, but had their origin in the imagination of the subject, and that the causes of all the phenomena were to be sought for in the subject himself. Faria fully recognized the importance of his views, but he was unable, in spite of the clearness and logic of his position, to make converts of the believers in mesmerism. In 1821, Dupotet actually introduced the practice of mesmerism into the Paris hospitals. The learned bodies of France, however, consistently maintained their unfavorable attitude toward the subject. In 1826 a second commission, in which Laennec and Majendie took part, again rendered an adverse decision, and although in 1831 Husson made a report to the Academy favorable to mesmerism, it made but a slight impression upon the members. In 1837 a final commission was appointed to investigate the subject; the report was again unfavorable, and the Academy finally decided to concern itself no longer with the subject. Interest in animal magnetism, however, did not entirely die out. In 1842, Gauthier published his "History of Somnambulism," which contributed numerous additional facts to our knowledge of this and related conditions.

While mesmerism was at its height, **three schools** of animal magnetism were developed:

First, the school to which Mesmer himself belonged, and which asserted that the effects obtained were due to physical agency alone. The means employed were friction, touches, passes, and grasping. The resulting phenomena were explained on the theory that a fluid or ether passed from the magnetizer to the magnetized, or *vice versa*. The adherents of this school were the original advocates of "animal magnetism."

Second, the school of Barbarin, the adherents of which maintained that faith was the principal factor required, in consequence whereof, they were known as "spiritualists." In their minds all physical means were merely accessories. They asserted that the effects attributed to animal magnetism were the products of the resolution or will of the operator, and that the latter could produce identical effects, whether he were in contact with, or at a distance from, the patient.

The third school, that of the Marquis de Puysegur, occupied a position midway between the others; explaining the results obtained, by physical or psychologic means, as the case required.

The term "mesmerism," while still used popularly and in general literature, has in medicine, to-day, historic interest only; the practice it denoted, however, persists in a modified form under another name, and to this we shall now give attention.

HYPNOTISM

In England, the subject of animal magnetism was taken up in 1841 by James Braid, who had witnessed the public demonstration of Lafontaine in Manchester. The circumstance that Lafontaine used, besides passes, the expedient of fixing the eyes of his subjects upon a bright object, led Braid to study especially the effects of this fixation, and he concluded that the ocular fatigue thus caused, sufficed to bring about the magnetic sleep; he held the object immediately before and somewhat above the eyes of the subject. In his work upon "Neurypnology," published in 1843, he, like Faria, opposed the theory that any force passed from the magnetizer to the subject. Thus, he showed that the experimenter could induce the sleep in himself without the assistance of any other person. Braid also showed how dependent upon suggestion were many of the phenomena observed. He reported the employment of hypnosis in numerous diseases with success. Many of his assertions were corroborated by the distinguished physiologist Carpenter and others of high standing, for example, Bennet, Simpson and Laycock; notwithstanding these facts, mesmerism or braidism made but little impression upon England.

Grimes, in America, obtained independently results similar to those of Braid, as did also Liébeault in France. In 1866, Liébeault published a work on artificial sleep and related conditions. Like Faria, he recognized the subjective nature of the hypnotic phenomena. Bernheim, who attended in 1882 Liébeault's Policlinic at Nancy, became an enthusiastic disciple and an active advocate of the therapeutic application of hypnotism. In 1875, Charles Richet published in detail an essay on artificial somnambulism which led Charcot to study extensively the phenomena of hypnotism as induced in the hysteric cases of the Salpêtrière. The results were embodied in a large volume by Paul Richer, under the title "Clinical Studies in Grand Hysteria or Hystero-Epilepsy." Charcot, further, in 1882 made an extensive report to the Academy of Sciences in which he analyzed the various phenomena observed and separated them into three fundamental groups, namely, those of the cataleptic state, those of the lethargic state, and lastly those of somnambulism.

There were, for the time being, two schools of hypnotism—that of Nancy, founded by Liébeault and Bernheim; and that of the Salpêtrière, founded by Charcot and his pupils. Charcot regarded the symptoms of hypnotism as those of a neurosis and as belonging to the domain of hysteria. This also is the attitude of his followers to-day. Thus, Babinski says that *grande hysterie* is a sine qua non of *grande hypnotisme*, while Gilles de la Tourette declares that hypnotism is nothing else than a paroxysm of hysteria which is provoked instead of being spontaneous. Bernheim, on the other hand, insisted on the essentially psychic character of hypnosis; he denied that it was a neurosis, and found only a superficial resemblance between it and hysteria, asserting, moreover, that Charcot's three stages were artificial products. The uniform results obtained by Charcot, he maintained, were due to the fact that his observations were made on hysteric subjects, who were unusually susceptible, and who were, besides, unconsciously "trained" by the experiments and by the surrounding patients.

Without pausing at this point to discuss these divergent views, let us turn our attention to the manner in which the hypnotic state may be induced.

Methods of Inducing the Hypnotic State

Hypnosis may be induced in a variety of ways. All of the methods, however, can be grouped under the following heads: first, those depending upon sensory impressions; secondly, those depending upon sensory impressions plus fatigue; and, thirdly, those depending upon conceptions or hallucinations of sleep aroused in the subject by suggestion.

In the methods of the first group—sensory impressions—

monotonous or sudden impressions may be made upon various organs; as the eye, the ear, the cutaneous surface. For instance, the subject may gaze steadily at an object which may or may not be bright, or he may gaze at a part of his own person. Again, he may listen to some monotonous sound, as the ticking of a watch or clock, to monotonous musical sounds, or to gentle rustling or rushing sounds like that of running or falling water. Lastly, a part of the cutaneous surface may be gently stroked, always in the same direction. All of these methods have this in common —they bring about a concentration of the attention upon a single impression. The impression being monotonous and continuing uniform, arouses sensations of fatigue; these are in turn followed by the mental attitude of sleep. The attention, being arrested by the continuous or constantly recurring impression, becomes fixed; trains of thought are not produced—the function of association is more or less in abeyance; sooner or later the fatigue sensations are attended by sleep hallucinations and hypnosis is established. Sudden or violent impressions may act in a similar way; thus Charcot and his pupils made use of the sudden flare of a calcium light, an electric spark, or—to affect hearing instead of vision—blows upon a tomtom, or other loud and sudden noises. The hypnosis so produced has been spoken of as "fright hypnosis;" the sudden emotion of fright appearing to be the immediate cause. In this respect it resembles a form of hypnosis induced in animals.

Methods belonging to the second group, namely, those embodying a sensory impression plus a fatigue effort, have been practised since time immemorial. The Indian fakirs fixed the eyes thousands of years ago, as they do to-day, upon the point of the nose, while the monks of Mount Athos fixed their eyes upon the navel. Other races and other times made use of magic mirrors, of crystal globes, or of vessels containing water. The monotonous chanting of incantations, again, embodies the principle of the continuous sensory impression and the fatigue effort. Braid, as is well known, made use of fixation of the eyes in such a way as to involve early fatigue of convergence and accommodation. Mesmer, on the other hand, made use of "passes." These, when made in contact with the body, acted by monotonous cutaneous impression; or, if at a distance from the body, acted by monotonous visual impression, but more especially by suggestion. Lafontaine, again, practised the combined method of fixation and of passes. Braid's method was gradually used less and less frequently; in later years it was employed in conjunction with the verbal suggestion of sleep. Various objects may be used for fixation of the eyes, especially glass balls, metallic buttons, or other small bright or shining objects. Luys made use of a rotating mirror; Preyer employed a candle-flame, the latter being somewhat raised above the level of vision and close enough to cause marked convergence. Hansen placed large false diamonds upon a dark background. The eyes or the finger of the operator have often been used; small magnets also. An objection to fixation has been advanced in the fact that the method is frequently not successful, and that if long persisted in, it leads to nervous disturbances of various kinds, more especially fatigue and headache.

In regard to passes or stroking, most operators agree that complex movements are unnecessary; it suffices to stroke gently with the palm of the hand—always in the same direction—some one part of the surface of the body, more especially the face, the brow, and the eyelids; or, the hands having been raised, the hands, arms, and body are gently stroked downward toward the hips. According to Löwenfeld, passes made over the face and in direct contact with the latter, are the most effective. In many subjects, however, the stroking really prevents sleep instead of furthering it.

In the form of monotonous verbal suggestions, auditory stimuli have proved most effective. The method is essentially one of suggestion. It is the object of the operator to induce in the subject, as gently and yet as persistently as possible, the conceptions and sensations that obtain in a person about to go to sleep. This is the method that was introduced by Liébeault and was later practised by Bernheim. An explanation should first be given to the subject regarding the nature and action of hypnotism and regarding the nature of the procedure. This is done to obtain his confidence, to allay nervousness, to obtain his entire acquiescence and willingness. It is of the very greatest importance also to have present one or more individuals of the same sex as the patient. The presence of such persons reassures the patient and is a protection, it need not be added, to the operator. The procedure should take place in a quiet room, moderately lighted. The subject, clad in loose and comfortable clothing, should be seated in an armchair, or should recline upon a sofa or lie upon a bed. The operator should then speak to the patient somewhat as follows, in a voice gentle, steady, and rather low: "Look at me and think of going to sleep. You are resting; you have a feeling of restfulness in your entire body; you are becoming more and more sleepy; your arms, legs, your whole body, feel tired. In a little while your eyelids will grow heavy; your eyes will fall asleep; your eyes are closing; you are unable to keep them open; you cannot see with them any more; your eyes are closed; you are sleeping." In some persons sleep follows almost immediately. In others the procedure must be repeated many times with gentle and drawling, but recurring emphasis. Should the suggestion of going to sleep fail of itself, the procedure may be repeated combined with fixation—any small bright object or the finger of the operator sufficing. Thus, while holding before the subject's eyes the bulb of a thermometer, or, it may be, for the sake of the added mental impression, a magnet, the operator may say: "Look steadily, now, at the object which I hold in my hand and think only of going to sleep." Then he should say, as before, in a monotonous and rather subdued voice: "Your eyes are heavy, they are beginning to close, your eyes are growing moist, you are not seeing clearly, they are closing, you are very sleepy, you are becoming more and more sleepy; your head and body, your arms and legs are tired; you are sleepy; so sleepy, you feel nothing; everything sounds far away, you see nothing, you are very sleepy, your eyes are very heavy, you are asleep." Only exceptionally is the procedure entirely successful at the first attempt. Löwenfeld employed a method somewhat as follows: The subject is comfortably placed in an armchair or a sofa. His eyes are closed and he is told to count for a number of minutes quietly to himself from one to one hundred, the counting being continuously repeated. After a while, the operator begins to suggest sleep in the manner already described. Löwenfeld used the method of fixation in a majority of cases, but only for a very brief time.

The subject presenting now the appearance of sleep, the presence of "suggestibility" can be tested by raising the arm of the patient; the arm is gently stroked, while the operator says that the arm is stiff, that he (the subject) will not move it, that the arm is becoming more and more rigid all the time, and finally that he cannot move it. If a fair degree of hypnosis has been induced, the arm remains fixed in a cataleptoid position. The establishment of cataleptoid rigidity is, however, not necessary to demonstrate the existence of the hypnotic state. As a rule, hypnosis is induced more and more readily upon each successive attempt, and, instead of making the test by catalepsy, the patient can be awakened during the procedure a number of times; at each time, he can be questioned directly as to whether he has been asleep, and if so, to what extent. Each time the hypnotic procedure is repeated, the suggestion of sleep is aroused more strongly than before. This method is known as the "fractional method."

With refractory subjects, hypnotizers have not hesitated to call to their aid drugs and anesthetics. The patient has, previous to the séance, been given a dose of bromid, chloral, paraldehyd, or an inhalation of chloroform or ether has been given during the procedure. The mere act of holding a chloroform or ether funnel before the face is itself suggestive of sleep, and both Bernheim and Wetterstrand believed that they noted the existence of hypnosis before the subjects were actually anesthetized by the drug. As might be supposed, the use of drugs and anesthetics as adjuvants to hypnotism has not been followed by uniform results.

Autohypnosis.—As was proved long ago by Braid, it is perfectly possible for an individual to hypnotize himself. Especially is this the case in persons who have been previously repeatedly hypnotized; either the autosuggestion of sleep or fixation of the eyes suffices. Indeed, a "subject" sometimes passes spontaneously and involuntarily into a condition of hypnosis, when looking at bright objects. This is one of the dangers to be guarded against by appropriate countersuggestion in the hypnotic state. There is reason to believe, however, that this countersuggestion is not always effective.

Awakening of the Subject.—It is usually much easier to awaken the subject than to induce hypnosis. The mere command to the patient to awake is, as a rule, sufficient. At other times, along with the verbal command, the operator may blow into the subject's face, slightly smack his cheek, shake him by the shoulder, call him by name—in other words, he is to imitate the procedures that would be used to awaken a person from normal sleep. Most subjects awaken spontaneously from hypnosis in a few minutes— say in about a quarter of an hour, if undisturbed; quite commonly they awaken almost immediately after the operator has withdrawn from the room. The sleep may, however, exceptionally persist for a much longer period; from one to two hours or even longer. Other things equal, the deeper the hypnosis, the longer the sleep. When the hypnosis is extremely profound, the patient is sometimes awakened with great difficulty. Sudden awakening is, as a rule, unpleasant to the subject; indeed, it is occasionally followed by a period of depression, or the subject is for a time dazed or confused and sometimes complains of headache or sensations of fatigue. It is always wiser to suggest in the course of the hypnosis that the subject will awaken after a stated interval, say five minutes, or that she will awaken when a certain signal—for example, a knock upon the floor—is given.

Phenomena of the Hypnotic State

The phenomena of hypnotism, like those presented by hysteria, are classifiable into psychic, sensory, motor, and somatic. Among the **psychic phenomena** is especially to be noted an *increased susceptibility of the subject to suggestion.* Ideas verbally or otherwise suggested by the operator are, in the absence of contrary influences, readily accepted by the patient. No matter how absurd intrinsically or how completely out of keeping with the actual facts or surroundings, the suggestion is, as we shall see, received and treated as true. It is clear that the mental processes that would normally correct such a suggestion are in abeyance—

that evidence, intrinsic to the falsity of the suggestion or derived from the senses, does not find its way to the field of cortical activity. In other words, the function of association is in abeyance or impaired, and with this change, the faculty of judgment falls wholly to the ground. Again, the suggestion may be one that under normal conditions would be resisted strenuously, but in hypnosis it is accepted tamely, or at most after ineffectual resistance. Certainly, the next inference that is justifiable is that the *function of the will is in abeyance* or greatly weakened. Memory also is seriously influenced, both according to the degree of the hypnosis and according to the suggestions offered; but more of this later.

Among the **sensory phenomena,** there may be anesthesia, local or general, blindness or deafness, suggested or spontaneous, or, other modifications of the special senses. Among the **motor phenomena** are palsies, tonic spasm, contractures or even convulsions. Among the **visceral phenomena,** modifications of the pulse and of the heart's action, vasomotor disturbances, and even modifications of the secretions have been observed. The resemblance or rather the identity of these phenomena with those manifested in hysteria will presently become more apparent.

The **sequence of phenomena** observed in a person undergoing hypnosis is somewhat as follows. Let us assume that the person experimented upon has already been hypnotized a number of times and is, therefore, what is known as a "good subject;" and that the operator is using suggestion, together with fixation of vision. The subject, we will say, is comfortably seated in a chair. The operator holds a bright object, *e.g.*, the bulb of a thermometer, a few inches in front of the eyes and a little above their level. At the same time, he makes the verbal suggestion to sleep in the manner already described. Gradually the eyelids grow heavy, droop by degrees, and finally close. Just before this happens, it is observed that the eyes cease to converge upon the object, that the pupils become dilated, and that the subject makes one or two movements as of swallowing. As hypnosis becomes established, the entire body becomes relaxed, the patient lolls in his chair, and now presents the outward appearance of sleep.

If the sleep has been produced by verbal suggestion alone, without fixation of the eyes, failure of convergence and dilatation of the pupils, are, of course, absent and swallowing movements may not occur.

Various **degrees of the hypnotic sleep** are recognized; thus, Bernheim speaks of nine stages, Liébeault of six, Fontan, Ségard, and Forel of three, while Gurney, Delboeuf, and others speak of two. Forel classifies the stages as follows: (1) somnolence, (2) light sleep, and (3) somnambulism. In the first stage, that of somnolence, the subject is still able to resist the suggestions of the operator, to open his eyes, and to perform other volitional acts; in the second stage, that of light sleep, the subject can no longer open his eyes, and accepts more or less readily the suggestions that are offered to him, but he subsequently remembers the events of the hypnotic séance; in the third stage, that of deep sleep or somnambulism, the subject, in addition to a ready acceptance of suggestions, subsequently betrays a loss of memory with regard to the events of the hypnosis and also manifests post-hypnotic phenomena.

As already stated, **cataleptoid** phenomena may be induced in hypnosis, and, indeed, the possibility of inducing this condition has frequently been used to test the degree or the reality of the hypnotic sleep. By Charcot and his disciples, who studied hypnotism in the hysteric patients of the Salpêtrière, catalepsy was induced in a different way. The subject was asked to look attentively at a bright object held at a distance of some centimeters before his eyes; after the lapse of a few moments, the object was suddenly withdrawn. When the experiment is successful, the patient becomes immobile; his eyes are fixed and open and staring directly in front of him. His eyes are also moist, or tears may make their appearance. There is anesthesia of the cornea, and indeed of the entire body. At the same time, catalepsy is marked and typical. The limbs retain whatever positions they may be placed in; if the subject is stood upon his feet, he remains in the position which has been given him. He presents the symptom which has been termed "flexibilitas cerea." If the condition persist for any length of time, it may eventuate in an attack of "grand hysteria." During its continuance, marked suggestibility is noted. Subsequently, no recollection of the events of the hypnosis is retained. There is also marked fatigue.

When the bright object, instead of being suddenly withdrawn, is held persistently before the subject, a different set of phenomena are observed. The eyes gradually become closed and the subject falls asleep. He now presents, instead of rigidity, complete muscular relaxation. Anesthesia is present, as in catalepsy, while mental obscuration is more profound. To this form Charcot applied the term **lethargy**. It can be produced notably by persistent fixation of a bright object, but a catalepsy can be converted into a lethargy by merely closing the eyes of the subject. Indeed, by opening one eye and closing the other, the same subject becomes hemi-cataleptic or hemi-lethargic.

In lethargy, the knee-jerks are said to be exaggerated and there is also present a condition of hyperexcitability of the nerves and muscles. The latter phenomena have, however, been much disputed.

The term **somnambulism**, Charcot applied to a state which he induced in subjects already lethargic or cataleptic, by slightly rubbing the top of the head with the tips of the fingers or the palm of the hand. The subject passed into a condition in which his senses seemed more acute and it became possible to provoke very complicated automatic actions. Neither Charcot nor his followers believed that his three forms really represented three different conditions. Various transitional stages were observed, and, not infrequently, instances occurred in which the symptoms of the various stages were present at the same time and commingled.

The truth of such essential and elementary facts as the artificial induction of catalepsy, and the opposite condition of muscular relaxation or lethargy, together with anesthesia, has been abundantly demonstrated not only upon human beings, but also upon animals. It is hardly necessary to refer to the well-known fact that many birds and small animals become motionless when in the presence of danger, and this, too, when escape would seem possible; e.g., the catalepsy of the bird fascinated by the serpent, the lethargy of the opossum in the extremity of its peril. Experimentally a condition of absolute immobility can readily be induced in chickens, ducks, geese, turkeys, canary birds, rabbits, guinea-pigs, and other animals, simply by firmly holding them and gently pressing the extended head and neck upon the surface of the ground or table. The animal then allows itself to be manipulated in various ways. Its muscles are flexible or catatonic, as the case may be, and it can be made to assume the most grotesque positions. Generalized catalepsy can be induced very readily in the rabbit, for instance, by holding the animal in the manner just described; a line is then gently traced with a piece of chalk down the nose, and when the chalk reaches the table, a white streak is suddenly drawn along the surface of the latter. Every muscle of the rabbit instantly springs into contraction and it sprawls with limbs and head extended at full length. A similar method may be adopted with other animals; the chalk is not always necessary, the mere finger of the experimenter sufficing. Not only are lethargy and catalepsy readily induced in animals, but anesthesia also is present; this is readily demonstrable, and lasts, as Danilewsky has shown, for from ten to thirty minutes. It is needless to point out that experimental catalepsy in animals is identical with catalepsy in the hypnotized human being. It is interesting to note, also, that Charcot induced catalepsy in his human subjects by the sudden drawing away of the object of fixation.

Nature and Pathology of Hypnotism

The phenomena of hypnotism are beyond all doubt **pathologic.** So evidently is this the case that it is difficult to conceive that physicians can be found who entertain the opposite view. On the other hand, it is perhaps not surprising that in that hotbed of hypnotism, the Nancy school, and by some of its advocates elsewhere, this rational view was indignantly rejected, for example, by Liébeault, Bernheim, Liégois, Baunis, Forel, Löwenfeld, and Wetterstrand. The Paris school, on the other hand, promptly recognized the identity of the symptoms presented by hypnotism with those of hysteria. It does not weaken this position, to reproach the Paris school, as did Bernheim, Wetterstrand, and others, with studying hypnotism in cases already hysteric.

The identity of the catalepsy and lethargy induced in animals, with the catalepsy and lethargy induced in the patients of the Saltpêtrière, is a sufficient answer. To say that many human beings are susceptible to hypnotism, is to say that many human beings under given conditions become hysterical, a truth which our ever-increasing experience with the "traumatic neuroses"— *i.e.*, traumatic hysteria—most clearly shows. Again, the contagiousness of hysteria—so old a story as not to bear extended repetition—is abundantly demonstrated as to hypnotism by Bernheim's own clinic. Here the patients fell asleep with surprising ease. They saw daily large numbers of hypnotizations. Each awaited his turn with the expectation of falling asleep. Each was impressed with the wonderful and mysterious power of the operator, his faculty of imitation was unconsciously stimulated, and when his turn finally came, he was so well prepared that the slightest verbal suggestion sufficed.

As has already been pointed out, the phenomena of hypnotism are classifiable into sensory, motor, psychic, and somatic. The sensory phenomena are always those of impairment or loss. In light hypnosis, there is merely diminution of sensation; in more marked hypnosis, abolition of sensation. This abolition of sensation is indistinguishable from the anesthesia of hysteria. As in hysteria, it may be general or limited in distribution; as in hysteria, it may involve the special senses. The motor phenomena consist of paralysis, tonic spasm, contractures, or convulsions, as the case may be. The suggested palsies of hypnotism are indistinguishable from those of hysteria, as are, indeed, the other motor disturbances. Convulsions may be induced with the greatest ease, as was demonstrated many years ago by A. J. Parker and myself.

If, in consequence of a suggestion, a palsy occur in an hypnotic subject, it is interesting to note that, just as in ordinary hysteria, the paralyzed limb also becomes anesthetic; in other words, a true segmental anesthesia is spontaneously established. A more convincing or significant fact it would be difficult to imagine.

As in hysteria, the palsies and anesthesias of hypnotism are to be referred to a contraction of the field of cortical activity; a similar explanation holds good for the psychic phenomena. This contraction or reduction is seen typically in the impairment or abolition of the function of association and of the function of the will. Thus, the subject is unable, because of impaired association, to correct the erroneous conceptions that the suggestions of the operator arouse in his mind; for instance, when he accepts the suggestion that he is in the midst of a garden of flowers when in reality he is in a room, it is because impressions made upon his senses do not reach the field of cortical activity; or when he accepts a suggestion that is intrinsically absurd and out of keeping with his past experience, it is because the memory of these experiences and of the actual facts of his existence are not aroused and do not enter his field of consciousness. Owing to great depression of cortical function, association is for the time being lessened or even destroyed. It is not surprising, finally, that in hypnosis there is a lessening in that summation of cortical activities which we term the will; the latter is at first impaired and finally abolished. Intrinsically, the state of hysteria and the state of hypnosis are the same. Not even with regard to the phenomena of suggestibility does hypnosis differ from hysteria, for hysterical patients are notoriously open to suggestion (see Part I, Chapter IV).

The fact that in decided hypnosis there is an abolition of memory for the events of the séance, is in keeping with the fact of the general reduction in the field of consciousness. In addition, memory presents other phenomena liable to misinterpretation. Thus, during the hypnotic state memory may, as a result of suggestion, be stimulated, so that the subject is able to recall events and circumstances which he is apparently unable to remember in his normal condition. The cortical activity, being stimulated, may flow along old and long-neglected channels. A memory thus brought to light *may be* accurate, but this is never certain; unfortunately, it is possible to suggest to a subject that he has participated in or been present at events that have never occurred, and if asked to give an account of them, he may recite in great detail and with the appearance of truth a long train of fictitious happenings.

It is but a step from this to the phenomena presented by the clairvoyant or the spiritualistic medium. Autohypnosis, like the ordinary form of hypnotism, relieves the cortex of the corrective restraint imposed in the waking condition by the contact of the senses with the outer world. Under these circumstances, the hallucinations pursue an untrammeled course; nor is it strange that they should follow the trend indirectly suggested by the questions of the anxious and too willing listener. Instead of dealing with a fictitious past or an unreal present, the hallucinations may project themselves into the future, and thus assume the form of prophecies. Of similar value are other phenomena, such as telepathy; seeing and hearing at a distance; transposition of the senses, during which the medium may hear with her stomach or read books through her back; also conversations in foreign, and to the subject totally unknown tongues; and, lastly, even the invention of entirely new and unheard-of languages!

It is certainly not in my province to discuss these various manifestations, except in the way of warning. To practical physicians they have but the significance of abnormal mental states, and when so analyzed and stripped of the unconscious exaggeration and overstatement of the believers, and of the admixture of fraud and legerdemain of the medium and her friends, they cease to be mysterious. It does not serve to point out that there are specific instances which are unexplained—it does not serve to call attention to special cases of the accuracy of this or that prophecy or of this or that telepathic or mystic communication. The sources of error, the possibilities of self-deception or of gross fraud are always so numerous as to be beyond control; they cannot be eliminated. In every instance, personally known to myself, scientific evidence—evidence such as is demanded by scientific investigations in other fields—has not been present. On the other hand, the facts of the mental state of hypnosis, of autosuggestion and of the unconscious suggestion of the environment, afford an abundant explanation for so much as has been plainly genuine. For the rest, let him believe who will. Many years ago, I attended a séance at which the medium during her autohypnosis became possessed of the spirit of a departed Persian princess. During this condition she wrote many pages of Persian manuscript, which she subsequently read aloud. The manuscript consisted of cursive and connected loops and strokes, with here and there well-formed letters in English script. I did not think it necessary to pursue the investigation further; and I need hardly add that a savant who was present, failed to detect the remotest resemblance between the curious sounds made by the medium and any Persian dialect known to students. Need I refer to the case of the young lady who, knowing only English and French, conversed in modern Greek? Again, I say, let him believe who will. Or shall allusion be made to the medium who became possessed of the spirit of a young and departed Swedish preacher, and who began preaching in the Swedish language? Unfortunately, among the observers present was one who had the right to marvel at the completeness with which the young Swede had forgotten his native tongue. Probably no more thorough or sincere study was ever made of an autohypnotic subject than was made of Hélène Smith by Flournoy, and so interestingly told by him in the volume "From India to the Planet Mars." The visions of this medium are interesting and the invention of the two Martian languages wonderful, and yet, as Flournoy points out, the conclusion is inevitable that all these Martian communications had their origin exclusively in Hélène's own brain.

In addition to the impairment of the function of association, of the will, and of the modifications of memory, the subject also presents, as we have just seen, hallucinations and illusions. In ordinary hypnosis these hallucinations and illusions are suggested by the operator and are readily accepted by the subject. That the subject may also suffer from spontaneous hallucinations, just as do cases of hysteria, we have also seen. Sometimes the state of hallucination is a negative one; thus, it may be suggested to the subject that a certain person or object present in the room is absent, and the subject accepts the suggestion, notwithstanding all ocular or tactual demonstration to the contrary. This condition has been termed **negative hallucination.** It may likewise be induced in regard to pain and other subjective symptoms of disease, as we shall see when we come to study certain mystic methods of "healing." Lesions are, of course, uninfluenced.

Post-hypnotic Suggestion.—A suggestion may manifest itself in various ways in relation to the hypnotic state. Thus, first, it may manifest itself only during the hypnosis; secondly, it may persist after the patient has been awakened; thirdly, it may reveal itself only after the hypnosis has been concluded; lastly, it may become active only after a specified interval of time, the so-called "*suggestion à échéance.*"

Usually, but not invariably, suggestions show no tendency to persist after the hypnotic séance has terminated; such persistence can, however, be secured by suggesting it to the subject. The term post-hypnotic suggestion is, however, properly applied to the suggestions which become manifest only after the subject has been awakened. A common instance is one in which the operator suggests to the subject that after he awakens he will perform some definite act—for example, rise and bow to a stranger, to a piece of furniture, or to an imaginary person. The suggestion may, of course, be made very complex, and yet it may be followed quite closely. Experience shows that in most subjects, post-hypnotic suggestions have their limitations, both as regards their complexity and as regards their nature; in others they are very closely followed, even when they are intricate, or are unpleasant or repellant to the individual. The hallucinations that accompany the post-hypnotic suggestion are apparently very vivid and often very persistent. Thus, Bernheim suggested to a lady that on awakening she would see the portrait of her husband; she saw the portrait immediately, and the vision persisted for twenty-four hours. Londe suggested a portrait, the hallucination of which persisted, it was said, for two years. How vivid and intense a post-hypnotic hallucination may become, is instanced by an experiment of Forel. He said to a young woman during hypnosis: "You will see on awakening three real, dark, sweet-smelling violets with leaves and stems which you will feel." He handed her, however, only one violet. After being awakened, the subject could not tell whether one or two or all three of the violets she seemed to perceive were real or suggested. She thought all three were real; one hand held empty air, the other the real violet.

The post-hypnotic suggestion which makes its appearance only after a fixed interval of time (*suggestion à échéance*) is very interesting. A definite act is suggested, to be performed at a definite time; it may be after a given number of minutes, days, months, or even, it is said, a year or more. The subject is apparently in her normal condition on awakening and does not perform the act until the precise time has arrived. If minutes be suggested, the accuracy of the subject is often remarkable. Without a watch or other guide, the suggested act is either performed at the exact time suggested or nearly so.

The post-hypnotic suggestion is not, however, so wonderful as it seems; the suggestion made during hypnosis is received, retained, and perhaps relegated to the field of subliminal consciousness. In other words, the paradox exists that it is forgotten after the hypnosis, but still remembered and recalled into the field of consciousness at the exact time. After all, everything depends upon the reality of the absence of memory of the events of the hypnosis; that some kind of memory does persist—call it subconscious memory, if we must—is self-evident. Besides, if it be suggested to the subject that on awakening all recollection of the séance will disappear, she will, as a matter of course, when questioned, say that she remembers nothing. I am of the opinion that in many cases conscious memory persists, and that the subject is self-deceived. In a successful case, the instructions are carried out at the exact time and to the exact letter, even when the period which intervenes presupposes a complex mental calculation and the act itself is difficult of performance. Sometimes the patient will say that she does not know why she performs a certain act at a certain date; as often, however, if questioned by the operator as to her reason, she will say, "Why, you wanted me to do it," or "Did you not tell me to do it while I was asleep?" The performance of an act after an interval during which the patient is apparently unmindful of the suggestion finds its counterpart, perhaps, in the power which many persons have, of awakening at a predetermined and unaccustomed hour, after having gone to sleep at night as usual.

The somatic phenomena of hypnotism are those of hysteria. Thus, we have the same vasomotor disturbances; e.g., local flushings, pallor and the like. As in hysteria, the pulse-rate is not especially changed. This is true also of the digestive functions; hunger and thirst can, of course, within limits, be suggested or dispersed by suggestion. The secretions also are not especially altered. The urine, however, may be greatly increased in amount and may show a relative diminution in solids.

Krafft-Ebing and a few other experimenters have maintained that they could produce organic changes in the skin by suggestion. Thus, during hypnosis, a key at ordinary temperature was held before the subject, who was told that the key was red-hot. It was then firmly pressed against the surface of the body; after a number of hours, a blister appeared having the shape of the key. Rybalkin, it is said, obtained similar results at the Salpêtrière, while Focachon states that he has produced blisters by means of postage stamps. These experiments are all of them open to serious objection, for it appears that in no instance was possible deception guarded against. This view is shared by Schrenk-Notzing, who does not regard the evidence as either conclusive or satisfactory. Vesication by suggestion does not, up to the present time, rest upon a scientific foundation.

Krafft-Ebing has further maintained that the temperature of the body can be influenced by suggestion. Thus, he suggested to a patient, whose temperature in the morning was 36.8°C. and in the evening 37.4°C., that the temperature should for three days be 37°C. On the first day it was 37.1°C., and on the two following days 37°C. He suggested to the same patient a few days later that the temperature on the day following would be 36°C. It should be added that at the time the suggestion was made, the temperature was 40°C. from emotional excitement (?). As suggested, the temperature ranged on the following day from 36° to 36.1°C.! No credence can, in my judgment, be attached to these observations, considering the vagaries and untrustworthiness of hysteric subjects.

Claims as to the Therapeutic Value of Hypnotism

If, as I believe, the phenomena of hypnotism belong unequivocally to the domain of hysteria, the question as to the propriety and the wisdom of employing it as a method of treatment assumes a very serious aspect. To induce hypnosis in a patient is to induce hysteria. To answer, as do Wetterstrand and others, that the larger number of persons who are capable of being hypnotized are not hysteric, is merely to say that a large number of persons not previously hysteric, manifest hysteria under given conditions. If a patient be already hysteric, the process of hypnosis merely deepens the hysteria into somnambulism.

The state of hypnosis is beyond all doubt pathologic. Have we the right to superimpose upon the disease from which a patient suffers, another morbid condition—especially, when the result, so far as the original disease is concerned, is, to say the least, doubtful and the expedient is itself attended by a danger more or less grave? The evidence goes to show that the effect of an hypnotic séance is not limited to the actual period of the hypnosis, but endures for some time thereafter; permanently, I believe, in some cases. The very existence of post-hypnotic phenomena proves this proposition. Some change in the psychic make-up must obtain to make the post-hypnotic suggestion (á échéance) possible, and the more remote in point of time is the completion of the suggestion, the more profound must this change be. Further, such a serious psychic disintegration as is implied by the persistence of hallucinations, can only be viewed with alarm. How profound must be the disturbance which permits a woman in her waking state to see upon a blank wall the portrait of her husband—a hallucination that is accepted as true by the subject and which persists for days and even years! How grave must be the derangement of function of senses and cortex implied by Forel's experiment with the violet; the subject, let us remember, could not when awake tell the real violet in the one hand from the two imaginary violets apparently in the other. In the normal or waking state, impressions made upon the senses find their way to the cortex and there give rise to images which become associated with the previous experiences of the individual. In other words, they are normal phenomena, normally correlated. Vastly different is it, however, in hypnosis or post-hypnotic suggestion. Here the patient becomes the victim of hallucinations which bear no relation whatever to his environment or to the impressions upon his senses, and, what is worse, he accepts these hallucinations as real; in other words, he has lost the faculty of distinguishing between normal mental images or concepts, and hallucinations. To maintain that such conditions are normal, or that such perversions of function are without danger to psychic integrity, is to fly in the face of truth; but more of the dangers of hypnotism later. Let us now turn our attention to the assertions that have been made of its therapeutic utility.

Hypnotism is believed by its advocates to be of value in the various functional nervous diseases and in some that are organic or possess a fixed pathology. Thus, Forel asserts that hypnotism is efficacious in pains of all kinds—headache, neuralgia, sciatica, toothache that does not depend upon abscess, insomnia, functional palsies and contractures; that it is palliative in organic palsies and contractures; that it acts very favorably in chlorosis, menstrual disturbances (both metrorrhagia and amenorrhea), loss of appetite and all nervous disturbances of digestion, constipation and diarrhea (when the latter does not depend upon fermentation), psychic impotence, pollutions, masturbation, sexual perversion, alcoholism, morphinism, muscular and articular rheumatism, neurasthenic complaints, stammering, nervous disturbances of vision, blepharospasm, pavor nocturnus of children, nausea, seasickness, vomiting of pregnancy, enuresis nocturna, chorea, nervous coughing, hysteric disturbances of all kinds inclusive of hystero-epileptic attacks, anesthesia, bad habits of all kinds, and epilepsy. Wetterstrand, Bernheim, Berillon, Barwise, Herman, Drayton, and Rose also speak of treating epilepsy successfully. Van Renterghem and van Eeden, who enumerate in addition among affections benefited by hypnotism, anemia and psychic depression, were less fortunate in chronic alcoholism, stammering, chorea, hypochondria, nervous asthma, habitual constipation and masturbation, and obtained no result or no noteworthy result in epilepsy, in chronic articular rheumatism, tabes, writer's and piano-player's cramp, organic diseases of the nervous system, and internal diseases. Hilger failed in epilepsy; in Löwenfeld's experience, also, little is to be gained in this disease. Wetterstrand, Bernheim, van Renterghem, van Eeden, Dumontpallier, and others report satisfactory results in chorea. Löwenfeld affirms success in nervous coughs, asthma, and affections of the heart—including even dilatation of the heart. He, also, together with Schrenk-Notzing, Bernheim, Fuchs, Wilkin and others, reports favorable results in sexual perversions.

Certainly, organic nervous diseases would seem to offer a most unfavorable field for hypnotism. Notwithstanding this, Bernheim, Fontan, Grossmann, Lloyd Tuckey, and others assert the achievement of very noteworthy results in both organic brain diseases (focal lesions) and organic cord diseases (tabes, myelitis, etc.).

As further instances of the character of the assertions concerning affections more or less successfully treated by hypnotism, we may mention brain abscess (Starck), hemorrhoids (Brown), arthritis (Desplats), albuminuria (Desplats), scurvy (Bertschinger), periostitis (Ringier), chronic articular rheumatism (Ringier, Behring, Delius), carcinoma of the kidney (Ringier), post-diphtheritic palsy (Luys), sycosis (Berillon), paralysis agitans (Osgood), paranoia (Bauer, Ringier), trichinosis (van Renterghem), and osteomyelitis (van Renterghem). This list, it need not be added, could be still further and greatly extended, were it to serve any rational purpose.

Regarding the efficiency of hypnotism in **hysteria**, Löwenfeld says that the results are not always what one would expect à priori; opposed to the large number of successful results, there is a large number in which but temporary improvement or complete failure obtains, and in which suggestion during the waking state and other therapeutic measures achieve more than hypnotic suggestion. Curiously enough, Forel also declares that in his experience more can be accomplished in hysteria by skilful suggestion during the normal or waking state than by formal hypnosis, and this is fully in accord with my own observations made many years ago. Do not such admissions as this knock the very keystone out of the arch of therapeutic hypnotism? If there is one disease in which the patient is susceptible to suggestion, it is hysteria, and to admit that normal suggestion equals, if it does not surpass, in efficacy, suggestion under hypnotism, is to admit the needlessness, if not the uselessness, of hypnosis as a method of treatment.

When we turn our attention to another field in which hypnotism should be useful, if ever, namely that of mental diseases, we meet with a like disappointing result. To begin with, only a small percentage of the insane can be hypnotized, and even here the effects are unimportant. Most of the advocates of hypnotism lay claim to success in "mild melancholia," whatever that may mean—probably hysteria—but when any real affection exists, outspoken failure is the result; or if not failure, a result that is, to say the least, questionable. Not even in the neurasthenic-neuropathic psychoses—the psychasthenias—the insanities of the special fears, of indecision, deficient will, or deficient inhibition, is a result achieved. In the first place, in genuine cases of these affections, the patient can rarely be hypnotized; secondly, when the patient is hypnotizable, the benefit is very doubtful, while there is grave danger of injury. A new neurosis, hysteria, with its manifold possibilities for harm, is imposed upon a nervous system already the seat of grave degenerative changes. The same truth obtains with even greater force in diseases in which the neuropathic degeneration is more pronounced; to wit, paranoia, mania and melancholia, hebephrenia, catatonia, dementia paranoides—in short, the whole group of the neuropathic insanities. How helpless, again, is hypnosis in delirium, confusion, or stupor!

Surgical Anesthesia by Hypnotism

A limited number of surgical operations have been performed under hypnosis. In 1821, Recamier in Paris performed painlessly minor surgical and dental operations. Cloquet in 1826 removed a cancerous breast under hypnotism; the patient manifested no pain during the operation and subsequently had no recollection of what had transpired. Esdaile and Loysel had similar success in the performance of operations. In 1859, Guerineau amputated the thigh of a man under hypnotism; during this operation the consciousness of the patient was fully preserved and he had complete recollection of the operation afterward. Broca, Pozzi, Fort, Tillaux, Johnson, Clark, MacDonald, and others have likewise performed operations on persons under hypnotic anesthesia. It would appear that it is usually extremely difficult to hypnotize patients about to be operated upon; the nervousness and fear are generally so pronounced that hypnosis cannot be induced, and even when induced, we are confronted by the danger that it is neither so deep nor so persistent that the surgeon can count upon an undisturbed opportunity for the performance of a long operation; further, the necessary absolute quiet is not always secured by hypnosis. At most it can be said that only under very exceptional circumstances can hypnotism be employed for the purpose of surgical anesthesia. Löwenfeld, with Wetterstrand and Davis, believes that the quantity of an anesthetic necessary can be diminished by the simultaneous use of hypnotism, and that complete narcosis can be obtained in a much shorter time than by the ordinary method. Liébeault, Messnet, Dumontpallier, Wetterstrand, Journée, Schrenk-Notzing, and Lugeol assert that the pangs of labor can be relieved by hypnosis. Fontan, Fraipont, and Delboeuf believe that hypnosis can hasten or prolong the act, and also that the occurrence of pains at regular intervals can be successfully suggested. Liébault states that a number of times he was able to prevent threatened abortion.

Bernheim believes that hypnosis may be of value for diagnostic purposes, particularly that it may help us to distinguish between organic and functional disturbances; that it may also be of use in setting aside hysteric symptoms which now and then are associated with organic diseases; further, that hypnotic anesthesia may be employed in diagnosticating local affections; similarly, Löwenfeld is of the opinion that hypnotic anesthesia is of special value in gynecologic investigations, and that anesthetization of the patient by chloroform or ether may be avoided by this means. Messnet and others have affirmed that the suggested anesthesia of hypnotism may involve the genital apparatus, and that under this condition various gynecologic manipulations may be performed, the subject being entirely unconscious of them.

Conclusions

In reviewing the assertions quoted as to the value of hypnotism, it is difficult to draw intelligent conclusions. That many of the statements are out of harmony with accepted facts of pathology and out of all keeping with common experience cannot be denied. One cannot but suspect errors of diagnosis, enthusiastic over-statement, and gross self-deception. In what other light, for instance, can we regard the cases of organic hemiplegia recorded as cured by Bernheim?* What view shall we take of the cases of myelitis cured by suggestion? What of lead-poisoning successfully treated by the same method? Bernheim, for instance, records a case of lead-poisoning with paralysis of the extensors of *one* hand and with analgesia and anesthesia in the forearm *at different times*, in which amelioration of the paralysis followed the first séance, and gradually total cure was brought about. Can one be censured for doubting the correctness of the diagnosis? Is not the suspicion, to say the least, justified that such cases are proved to have been hysteric by the very fact of their amenability to suggestion? That improvement—not cure—may now and then occur in an organic case is not strange when we remember how frequently actual organic disease is complicated by hysteria. Again, when we review in our minds the various functional nervous affections enumerated by the various authors, suspicion as to the hysteric character of the greater number cannot be suppressed; indeed, it seems to be well grounded. What shall we say as to the menstrual disorders, the amenorrhea, metrorrhagia, metritis, chlorosis, anemia, and epilepsy successfully treated by hypnotism? For one, I can but repeat, let him believe who will. As to the cases of epilepsy reported to have been cured by hypnotism, I prefer to believe either that hystero-epilepsy was mistaken for epilepsy or that the cases were incompletely observed; and as regards the diseases of the blood, I cannot exclude from my mind the suspicion that if such disease were really present, other factors were at work to which the recovery was due. Does it seem worth while to discuss the efficiency of hypnotism in chronic

* "Treatise on Suggestive Therapeutics," translated by Herter, New York, 1900; and elsewhere.

articular rheumatism? Here again I must be pardoned if I question the diagnosis and think of hysteric arthralgia. There is hardly an affection which hysteria does not simulate, and it is often extremely difficult to obtain a correct history from a hysteric patient. The latter is often unable by reason of her condition to give an accurate account of herself, but relates to the physician such a history as his questions suggest to her mind, or such history as she involuntarily and unconsciously infers that he desires.

Another question that arises is, whether the relief or cure afforded by hypnotism—say in a favorable case, as hysteria—is permanent, or do the symptoms tend to recur? A fact which does not appear in the reports of published cases, is that the **tendency to recurrence** is very great. True, it is unusual for exactly the same symptom to repeat itself, but commonly *entirely new symptoms* of the *same underlying morbid condition* make their appearance. Some years ago a young woman presented herself at my clinic; she complained of a severe pain in the right shoulder, and the case was regarded as rheumatic. Antirheumatic remedies, however, failed to produce relief, and this was also the case with massage and the local application of electricity. A hysteric joint was finally diagnosticated, especially as several other surface stigmata of hysteria—for example, inframammary tenderness and inguinal tenderness—were present. The patient further volunteered the information that she had been repeatedly hypnotized in Vienna with great success for a nervous affection. She was then promptly hypnotized, and in response to a suggestion the pain in the shoulder disappeared. Not many weeks elapsed before she came back with a severe globus hystericus; this being promptly relieved, she returned at a later period with severe neuralgia of both sides of the face. In other words, after one symptom disappeared, it was sooner or later succeeded by another —a not uncommon experience.

Unreality of Hypnotic "Cures."—The so-called cures of hypnotism cannot be cures at all. Let us take, for example, the case of a neuralgia in which, after a given number of hypnotic séances, the patient is said to be cured. The suggestion has not, of course, influenced the pathologic changes going on in the nerve. It has merely induced a **"negative hallucination"**—the fact of pain has been obliterated for the time being from the patient's consciousness. Morbid states themselves are never changed. It is the mind of the patient only that is acted upon; positive or negative hallucinations are induced, as the case may be; in other words, a pathologic mental state is superadded to the previous condition.

DANGERS OF HYPNOTISM

That the dangers of hypnotism are great and manifold is evident both from theoretic considerations and from demonstrable facts. In the first place, the very act of hypnosis implies a functional severance of the normal relations existing between the sense organs and the cortex, and between so much of the cortex as is active and that greater remaining portion in which are stored up the past experiences of the individual, his memory, personal and racial, his tendencies, inherited and acquired. How readily and how markedly this severance may persist in the waking period, we have already seen. Further, the hypnotic state is induced with increasing ease at each subsequent hypnosis: which merely means that this severance having once been brought about, recurs more and more readily. In short, a distinctly pathologic condition has become established, and this pathologic condition is, in many cases, persistent or even permanent. The person thus pathologically affected is now what is termed a "good subject!" He falls asleep at command, at a glance from the operator, at a knock on the door, or at such other signal as has been suggested under previous hypnosis. At times, indeed, a look, not intended as hypnotic, from a casual stranger, brings on the hypnosis; or it may come on spontaneously when the patient attempts to look fixedly at an object—an involuntary autohypnosis. We are told that autohypnosis and hypnosis by strangers can be prevented by precautionary suggestions to the patient in the hypnotic state —first, that no one but the operator will ever be able to hypnotize the patient, and secondly, that the latter will never be able to hypnotize himself. Unfortunately, these suggestions are not always efficacious. Like other post-hypnotic suggestions, they fade with time—just as the suggestion as to the disappearance of a headache or neuralgia may be efficacious at first, but gradually loses its effect.

Furthermore, spontaneous nocturnal somnambulism may be seen in subjects who have been repeatedly hypnotized. Dufay records an interesting example of such a case. A young woman, a servant, who had been many times hypnotized, was arrested, charged with theft. Her sister, however, testified that she arose every night, put on her clothing, and walked in her sleep. Dufay, on hearing this, hypnotized the young woman, and she then stated that one night during her sleep she conceived the idea that certain articles belonging to her mistress were not safe, that in consequence she had gotten up and removed the articles to a place of greater security. During her waking period she had remembered nothing of this. The articles were subsequently found in the place indicated by her to Dr. Dufay in the hypnotic séance.

The subject is also liable to certain dangers inherent in the act of hypnosis itself. Thus, patients who are hypnotized by the method of fixation may, as already stated, suffer subsequently from headache, depression, sleepiness, heaviness, fatigue, and disturbances of the general sense of well-being. It is therefore necessary, first, to make use of fixation as little as possible, and, secondly, to suggest during the hypnosis that there will be no headache, fatigue, or other unpleasant sensation afterward, but that the subject will feel bright and refreshed on awakening. We must remember, however, that while the sensations of fatigue may be suggested away, a certain amount of weakness or actual exhaustion may remain. Exhaustion is more likely to supervene when the hypnosis has been unduly prolonged, when catalepsy—especially general and long-continued catalepsy—has been induced, when painful and depressing suggestions have been made, when emotional crises—as paroxysms of weeping—have occurred, or when convulsions have supervened. Under these circumstances, the fatigue and exhaustion may be extreme, and it is needless to add that they cannot be removed by suggestion. In this connection, it is interesting to note that rabbits in whom catalepsy has been induced repeatedly, or maintained for long periods, may subsequently die of exhaustion. Such facts show that hypnotism is not to be undertaken lightly; nor is it to be regarded as a method of amusement or diversion. Again, the baneful effects of injudicious, reckless, and ill-considered suggestions, such as place the patient's health, happiness, circumstances, well-being of relatives, and the like, in an unpleasant light, need not be dwelt upon. Instead of being removed by countersuggestion, they may give rise to serious and persistent nervous symptoms—depression, hypochondriacal ideas and general sense of ill-being. Even death has been known to occur in hypnosis as a result of painful and horrible suggestions.* It is probable that in such instances the death is comparable to that which ensues upon great shock or fright.

Again, the fact must be borne in mind that in confirmed hysteric subjects, and also in others, in whom hysteria has not previously been manifested, severe convulsions may come on even before hypnosis is fully established. The hypnotherapeutists tell us that this tendency to convulsive attacks should be met by countersuggestions in the hypnotic stage, and especially by careful and repeated reassurances before the hypnosis is undertaken. Unfortunately, these precautions may prove unavailing.

Occasionally, patients return time and again for hypnotic treatment, establishing a kind of hypnotic habit. Janet especially has called attention to this fact. After a hypnosis, a patient who previously suffered from various pains and other distressing symptoms, experiences under the stimulating suggestions that her pains have disappeared and that she will feel well, bright, and refreshed on awakening, a grateful sense of elation, comfort, and well-being. Unfortunately, the suggestion persists for a limited time only—longer or shorter as the case may be—when a recurrence of the old symptoms takes place; and, now, with mental depression superadded. The patient again seeks the physician,

---

*Löwenfeld, "Der Hypnotismus," Weisbaden, 1901, p. 386.

experiences a like immediately pleasant result and subsequent sense of depression. The visit is repeated, a kind of craving ensues, and a hypnotic habit becomes established. Sometimes the recurring visit is interpreted by the patient or by her friends as an attachment, or a sympathy existing between the physician and herself. Cases are not unknown in which the patient has made the relations between herself and the operator the subject of mystic ideas, speaking ` of "influences," "spells," or "magic." Indeed, veritable psychoses have developed in this soil. The conversation of the physician with the patient and ofttimes the belief of the operator concerning "hypnotism at a distance," give further foundation for her delusions.

Advocates of hypnotism usually deny that any of the phenomena of the stage of hypnosis persist in the waking period. This is evidently an error, for, as we have seen, the very fact of the post-hypnotic suggestion evidences the persistence, or—in *suggestion à échéance*—the recurrence, after a stated interval, of hallucinations with their attendant gross modifications of will and judgment. Certainly, these phenomena are but the expression of the lasting impress made by the hypnosis, and if will and judgment can so readily be set aside, it is not going too far to assume that their integrity has suffered. A persistence of the increased suggestibility of the hypnotic stage is also usually denied, and yet the suspicion is more than justified that in a modified form this symptom does persist, and that in this respect the patient grows to resemble, more and more, the ordinary hysteric subject. Assuredly, the functional severance (see p. 308) of the integral parts of our psychic make-up necessary to hypnotic and post-hypnotic phenomena, cannot take place repeatedly without permanent danger to the psychic integrity. Indeed, I personally believe that hypnotism cannot with safety be practised at all, except perhaps within very narrow limits, and that a person repeatedly or frequently hypnotized is permanently damaged. Numerous instances could be selected from literature to prove this statement. A case, recorded by Bernheim, as an instance of the mixture of reality and imagination, of truth and falsehood, met with in a "normal" individual, will serve as an illustration.

The case is that of a young girl, and in abstract is briefly as follows: According to Bernheim, the subject was formerly hysteric but had for three years been cured by suggestion and no longer presented any nervous symptoms. She was a good-natured, respectable girl. In talking with her or questioning her, nothing unusual was noted in her conduct. A commission of alienists could find no trace of mental disease. "She is mentally sound. I know her to be," says Bernheim, "very susceptible to suggestion, to hypnosis, and to hallucinations in the waking state" (*sic*). He then undertakes an experiment with her which has not as yet been performed with her or in her presence. She enters the room and he says, "Henrietta, I met you yesterday on the street. You were in a remarkable situation, Henrietta! What were they doing with you when I saw you?" Bernheim repeats the question, and at the same time looks at her intently. Her facial expression changes and memory plays over her features. She blushes and says, "I do not like to tell you." Bernheim insists, "You must tell me." In a low voice she answers, "Some one struck me." "Who?" asks Bernheim. "A working-man." "Why?" She is silent, is evidently ashamed, and does not wish to tell. "Go on, tell me," says Bernheim. She whispers in Bernheim's ear, "Because I did not want to go with him." Bernheim looks at her severely. "Henrietta, you are lying, you are trying to deceive me. Why did he wish to strike you?" "I tried to steal his watch." "And then?" asks Bernheim. "He took me to the police." The poor girl was covered with shame. Bernheim declared that he then effaced this fictitious memory by saying, "You will remember nothing of this." Bernheim maintained that the case was one of a very suggestible person, whose imagination, trained by numerous hypnoses, converts her hallucinations rapidly into perceptions. It is both curious and interesting to note that Bernheim cites this case as that of a person in perfect mental health, and also as that of a patient cured by means of suggestion. It is, indeed, an overwhelming proof of the kind of cure brought about by hypnosis! Cured of hysteria, indeed! A remarkable cure, in which the patient has been so far damaged that she can no longer tell the difference between her hallucinations and actual occurrences! How baneful, how criminal, is this training in hypnosis! Instead of being cured, this poor girl was psychically ruined. The case further proves in the most striking manner that the increased suggestibility of hypnosis persists in the waking state; indeed, that the suggestibility of hysteria is enormously increased by hypnosis.

There is another danger to which the hypnotic subject is exposed, and that is from the **amateur hypnotist.** If hypnosis is attended by danger even in the hands of skilful and conscientious physicians, how much greater must be the danger in the hands of amateurs! All of the dangers of improper and unguarded suggestions become multiplied—of persistence of unpleaasnt symptoms, of convulsive seizures, or it may be of somnambulism so profound as to last unduly long or from which the subject can only be aroused with difficulty. How reprehensible are amateur hypnotic experiments, and, especially, the exhibitions of hypnotism by fakirs upon the public stage! That such exhibitions ought to be forbidden by law, should not need the saying. The harm is done not only to the silly dupes and confederates who occupy the stage, but to the young people of the audience, who become morbidly interested in the subject and essay experiments for themselves.

The danger to the subject from criminal suggestions will be discussed in a separate section. It is fitting here, however, to speak of another danger of hypnotism, and that is the danger not to the subject, but to the **hypnotic experimenter,** and this danger is not imaginary, but real.

I have already spoken of the **contagiousness** of hypnotism, how each patient is impressed by the hypnotic process in the others. Indeed, it is not unusual in a group of subjects for others than the one to whom the suggestion is addressed to fall asleep at the same time. It is true that the experimenter does not suffer from contagion in this form, but he suffers from contagion nevertheless. Sooner or later, if he but immerse himself in hypnotism long enough, he acquires the mental attitude of his subjects; namely, one of willing receptivity. He becomes possessed of an attitude of mind in which he accepts too readily as fact that which only seems to be fact—is too willing to believe that which he wishes to believe. In other words, he himself passes into a condition of abnormal susceptibility to suggestion; he becomes the victim of **autosuggestion**, and, in addition, reacts unconsciously to the communications of his subject. His attitude does not differ from that of the believer who sits in the spiritualistic circle, and who reacts alike to the suggestions of the medium and his own spontaneous mentation. That the faculty of critical judgment suffers in some experimenters, there is good reason to believe. In what other way are we to explain such statements as those affirming the successful treatment of genuine epilepsy and of organic diseases of the nervous system? How are we to explain the belief of otherwise reputable men in "hypnotism at a distance"—*i.e.*, hypnotism by mail, by telegraph, by telephone, and even by the simple act of will of the operator, the subject being at a distance and ignorant of the operator's intentions? Is it not probable that autosuggestion and contagion on the part of the experimenter offer a like explanation for such mysticisms as telepathy? In what other way are we to explain the "authenticated" instances of seeing and hearing at a distance, of conversations in unknown languages, or of such other absurdities as the "transposition of the senses" (see p. 303)? If the experimenter be not of good nervous fiber, and if he have the misfortune to hold mystic views and theories, his mental health may indeed be seriously endangered. At least two instances have come to my attention in which the mental integrity had suffered unmistakably through intense devotion to hypnotism. Hypnotism exerts upon some minds the charm of mystery, of a field as yet unexplored, of a means by which the intricacies of mind may be fathomed, the laws of "psychic force" determined, physics and chemistry set at naught—of souls communicating with souls distant alike in time and space, of fresh proof of the immateriality of the spirit—no wonder that under these circumstances some minds give way, sacrificed on the altar of hysteria!

Ethical Relations of Hypnotism.—The facts thus far considered certainly justify serious doubts first as to the propriety, and secondly as to the utility of hypnotism. However, if these doubts be waived and it be conceded that under certain conditions hypnotism is proper, it at once becomes evident that certain ethical relations must obtain. In the first place, the person to be hypnotized must be adequately informed as to the procedure and told exactly what the operator intends doing. The statement should be frank and full. Secondly, it is obviously improper to hypnotize a person against his will. At once we are met by the statement that a person cannot be hypnotized against his will. This is true in regard to a first hypnosis, but in persons who have been hypnotized many times, and who have been trained to go to sleep at command, or at a given signal, the hypnosis can probably be induced without any consent on the patient's part whatever. Again, it is obviously and necessarily an ethical part of the treatment that the suggestions be confined strictly to the purpose for which the hypnosis is induced. This is the only proper and legitimate course. The operator is not to allow himself to be tempted to use his patient for the purpose of experiment—not for the induction of catalepsy; not for the induction of somnambulistic phenomena; not for the performance or demonstration of post-hypnotic suggestions. Least of all is it right to induce in the patient grotesque, unpleasant, or painful hallucinations, the effect of which may persist in the waking state. Briefly summarized, the points which are to be borne in mind in a case in which hypnosis has actually been determined upon are as follows: First, the operator should make a preliminary statement to the patient as to the sleep about to be induced and as to the objects to be attained. Second, there should be present one or more witnesses, one of whom at least should be of the same sex as the patient. Third, the hypnosis should preferably be induced by verbal suggestion rather than by fixation—or, if fixation be used at all, it should be to as limited an extent as possible. Fourth, the fractional method should be employed, as by this means the degree of the hypnosis can be at any time determined, without the induction of an experimental catalepsy. Fifth, a moderate degree of sleep suffices to bring on typical suggestibility—very deep hypnosis lessens suggestibility. Sixth, the suggestion should be made gently, but firmly, persuasively, and with emphasis. It should be repeated eight, ten, or a dozen times. Some operators take hold of the right hand of the subject and accentuate their suggestion by pressure upon the hand. Grossmann has pointed out that the suggestion is more apt to be successful when it is made indirectly and embodies in itself some rational explanation; thus, in suggesting the disappearance of a pain, he thinks it best to suggest to the patient that the sleep is quieting the nerves, that by quieting the nerves it is greatly benefiting them, and that in consequence of this the pain will pass away. Seventh, the therapeutic suggestion having been made, it is now necessary to say to the patient that on awakening he will feel very well, bright and refreshed, and that he will experience no fatigue whatever. Eighth, the patient should now be awakened. This can be done in the manner already described (see p. 296), or it can be done by suggesting to the patient that in a given number of minutes, say two or three, he will gently awaken.

Criminal and Legal Relations of Hypnotism

When we turn our attention to the question as to whether it is possible successfully to suggest to a hypnotized person the commission of crime, we find that the evidence is altogether negative or nearly so. Taking, first, **crimes against the person,** assault and murder, we find no case upon record in which crime has been committed as a result of hypnotic or post-hypnotic suggestion. During hypnosis, suggestions contrary to the general habit or opposed to the moral make-up of the individual are successfully resisted. In other words, both the credulity and the obedience of the subject have their limits. Thus, Löwenfeld suggested to a young woman, whom, because of her pliancy, he frequently used for purposes of demonstration, that she was standing on the edge of a lake and was about to take a bath. This was said after the subject had already accepted and carried out a number of the most diverse suggestions. Notwithstanding this, she at once replied: "It is now April, and it is still too cold to bathe in the lake."

Lowenfeld insisted, "You are mistaken, it is July and a very hot day. You are very glad to be able to take a bath." However, the subject persisted, in spite of all the contrary efforts at suggestion made by Löwenfeld, that it was April and too cold to bathe in the open air. Löwenfeld is of the opinion that it was not her belief in the unfavorable season of the year, but the fact that bathing would necessitate the removal of her clothing, that prevented her compliance with the suggestion and served as the basis for her resistance. Another subject refused to enter into an imaginary conversation with a person with whom she was at enmity. One of Gilles de la Tourette's patients, to whom a bath was suggested, did strip herself, but here the personal equation doubtless enters, and perhaps the fact should be taken into account that in Continental clinics patients are accustomed to obey without question the instructions of physicians, whether these require exposure of the person or not. Another of Tourette's patients went so far as to open her corset, but instead of disrobing, passed into hysteric catalepsy. Cocke handed a card to a subject and commanded her to stab him, a suggestion which she tried to enact without hesitation. He then handed her an open pocket-knife and repeated the command. She raised her hand, but instead of stabbing Cocke, fell over in a hysteric paroxysm. Other "well-trained" subjects resist suggestions which merely offend the proprieties. Thus, a subject of Delboeuf refused to embrace a man, and another could not even be brought to embrace a clothes-pole. A patient of Pitres successfully resisted the post-hypnotic suggestion to embrace a young man; another when it was suggested to her that she must strike one of the bystanders and the enactment of the suggestion was insisted upon, passed into lethargy. A subject of Richet who impersonated various characters, resisted strenuously the suggestion that he was a priest. Another subject of Delboeuf, a young woman, refused to take a flower from an altar. A boy fifteen years old fled in terror at the suggestion that he should steal a watch. A patient of Pitres, as a result of post-hypnotic suggestion, took a coin from a table, but at once returned it to Pitres.

Abundant experimental evidence exists of the ability of the

subject to resist improper or criminal suggestions; on the other hand, as already stated, no evidence exists to prove the actual commission of crime as a result of hypnotic suggestion. In this connection, it is important to make broad distinctions between crime committed as the result of persuasion, argument, or inducement, and crime committed as a result of hypnotic suggestion. Every rational human being is influenced by argument, by the logical presentation of facts, by appeal to the emotions, by play upon the passions, fears, hopes, desires, and ambitions. It is in this way that leaders arise; it is in this way that strong minds dominate those that are weaker—it may be for good, it may be for evil; but surely the "influence" so gained is a very different thing from suggestion under hypnosis.

Several remarkable cases of crime, as a result of **personal domination** gained by means other than hypnotism, are upon record; but here the methods employed were those by means of which men in their normal condition influence each other. As to **murder**, it will serve to recall such cases as that of Gray and MacDonald, of Gabrielle Bompard, or that equally remarkable case in which a valet killed his employer at the instigation of another. The case of Gray and MacDonald is briefly as follows: MacDonald, recently married, was employed in Kansas by a farmer named Gray. It so happened that Gray had as neighbor a certain Thomas Patton, who was an important witness in a suit against Gray, and it was to Gray's interest that Patton should be gotten out of the way. Gray began in a systemic manner to arouse in MacDonald's mind the suspicion that Patton was saying things derogatory of MacDonald's wife, that he was ruining her reputation. Ere long MacDonald and Patton quarreled, whereupon Gray warned MacDonald that Patton intended to kill him at their next meeting, that Patton was a bad man who had already killed a number of people. Gray further advised MacDonald to be prepared and to anticipate Patton's designs; he gave to MacDonald, who had never before used firearms of any kind, regular instruction in their use, actually erecting a target and teaching the pupil how to aim. Finally, he gave gun and cartridges to MacDonald, led the latter to a place at which he knew Patton would pass, and again urged MacDonald to kill Patton, repeating and reiterating the assertion that otherwise Patton would murder MacDonald. Shortly after Gray left the scene, Patton appeared and was shot to death by MacDonald. Gray and MacDonald were both arrested and tried. Gray was convicted of murder in the first degree and hanged, while MacDonald was acquitted. It need hardly be pointed out that hypnotism played no rôle here whatever. As well might it be claimed that Othello was hypnotized by Iago. Murder was committed by a second person at the instigation of the real criminal, but the methods by which MacDonald was influenced were those of cogent argument and powerful persuasion. Again, Gabrielle Bompard was the willing *accomplice* of Eyrand in the murder of Huissier, not a hypnotic subject. That she was morally defective is a fact merely in keeping with her crime; that she was devoted to Eyrand and unhesitatingly coöperated with him, is no evidence of abnormal influence; other women have done the same. The manner in which she lured the victim to his death merely illustrates the extreme depth and degradation to which her moral nature had sunk. The murder of a millionaire, who was chloroformed to death by his valet, at the instigation of a third party, who did not even enter the house of his victim, is still fresh in the public mind. Here again there is no question of hypnotism, merely one of solicitation, argument, and promises of gain.

While the cases cited and others of a similar nature can be brought forward as instances of murder by **instigation,** I am aware of none that can be cited as an instance of murder as a result of hypnotic suggestion.

When we turn our attention to the question of **sexual assault** during hypnosis, or of **cohabitation** in consequence of a posthypnotic suggestion, the facts again yield a negative answer. We are told by Mesnet and others that anesthesia of the genitals may successfully be suggested to a subject and be so profound as to permit of various gynecologic procedures; if so, why may not sexual assault be committed? It is extremely probable that, in spite of the local anesthesia, the general reaction of the subject, physical and nervous, would be so great as to lead to immediate awakening.

Nor would suggestions by the operator that he is the lover or the husband of the subject, or that the latter ardently desires him, be of avail. The innate resistance of the woman of average moral make-up would here enable her to repel the suggestion. We have already seen that suggestions offensive to propriety and decency are spontaneously resisted. Again, one of Delboeuf's subjects denied the suggestion that she was engaged, another repelled the suggestion that she was married and fled at the approach of the supposed husband. Several cases of supposed sexual assault during hypnosis are, it is true, upon record; but they will not withstand investigation. One occurred admittedly in the person of a public woman, and her voluntary acquiescence is a matter of legitimate supposition. Another is stated to have occurred in the presence of the victim's mother, who noticed nothing of the assault! A third, the case of Castellan, did not occur either during the hypnotic state or as a result of hypnotic suggestion.

A very remarkable case of supposed hypnotic sexual assault— so believed by Grashey, von Schrenck Notzing, and Preyer— attracted considerable attention in Germany some twenty odd years ago. An Austrian lady of noble birth, the Baroness von Z., a spinster, thirty-eight years of age, rich and of a blameless religious life, not being well, and suffering from pain in the head and stomach, placed herself for treatment in the hands of a certain Polish hypnotizer and magnetizer, named Czynski, whose advertisement in the public press had attracted her attention. Czynski, as it subsequently transpired, was a man of unsavory record. He was thirty-five years of age, had taught French in Cracow, where, up to 1890, he had also advertised extensively that he had discovered a new method of cure by means of hypnotism and magnetism. About this time, he abandoned his wife and began living with a divorced woman, who subsequently bore him a child. Two years later he appeared with his mistress and child in Posen, where he gave public exhibitions in hypnotism, occultism, and allied subjects. Here and in the neighboring towns, which he visited, he met with extremely meager pecuniary success. He obtained some money by false pretense, and in consequence was driven out of Prussia. In April, 1893, he resumed his pursuits, with the addition of palmistry, in the city of Dresden. It was here that Baroness von Z. became his patient. Czyński treated the lady by laying on of hands, and, also, ordered various medicines. His relations with the patient gradually became more and more intimate, until in October or November, when the Baroness became his affianced. According to the Baroness's own account—given at the subsequent legal proceedings—Czynski some time in October declared his love for her, while she was asleep, *i.e.*, hypnotized. "I was surprised and frightened, but I felt great pity for him. He told me further that he was poor; that the woman who accompanied him was merely his medium; that his wife had been untrue to him and that he was very unhappy; that I alone could save his soul and make him happy; that he wished to procure a divorce, turn Protestant, and marry me. I wept, I deeply pitied him, and believed that I must do a good work. In reality, however, I felt no love for him." Czynski continued, thenceforth, to make declarations of love, both verbally and by letter. "He flooded me with letters, pressed me continually, and talked during my treatment only of love. He constantly besieged me. I did not want to agree to his proposition for a rendezvous, and yet I could not withstand him and had to go to him. We often spoke of religious matters, and then he would say to me that I could save his soul. This gave me a certain satisfaction and I consented. I no longer had any control over myself, I felt that I was entirely under his influence. Intercourse did not occur during the sleep-like condition, only I was influenced in such a way that I could not resist him. Even though I realized that what I was doing was wrong, I could not resist. I resisted sexual intercourse, but, in the end, I could not, and so it happened." In numerous letters written subsequently by her to Czynski, she evinced entire satisfaction with the relations existing between them, and further declared that she honestly loved him and would never part from him. The engagement was kept secret at Czynski's request for "political reasons." He told her that he was the last descendant of a princely house—Prince of Swiatopelk—also that he was a duke, and that a public engagement and marriage might result unpleasantly. He now parted company with his mistress, telling the latter that his wife was about to return to him; at the same time he took steps to secure a formal divorce from his wife, changing his religion from Catholic to Protestant, in order to facilitate his designs. Several months later, February, 1894, a secret pretended marriage took place between the Baroness and himself in Munich, a friend of Czynski's counterfeiting a Protestant clergyman.

The "marriage" proved Czynski's undoing. The father and brother of the Baroness, learning of the occurrence, notified the police, and Czynski was promptly arrested. Although the Baroness was made acquainted by her relatives with the fictitious character of the marriage, she declared, "I love Czynski! He is a man of honor; he has not deceived me; that is all wrong. Christ forgave the thief on the cross, why should not I forgive Czynski?" It was only later, when she learned through the court proceedings how Czynski had lied to her and deceived her, that she experienced a revulsion of feeling.

Czynski was indicted upon several points, only one of which concerns us; namely, that by means of hypnotism and suggestion he had reduced Baroness von Z. to a condition of loss of will—a condition in which, being without free will, she was subject to *his* will, and that while in this condition he had sexually assaulted her. This charge virtually represented the contention of the experts for the prosecution. However, the facts do not present the picture either of sexual assault during hypnosis or of sexual assault, the consequence of a post-hypnotic suggestion. What Czynski did was merely to use argument and persuasion and appeals to the emotions. Added to this, he was an unusually handsome man, with beautiful eyes and an attractive baritone voice. The Baroness, on the other hand, was no longer young; and here lay happiness clamoring at her feet! Further, we are informed that her family history presented both tuberculosis and repeated instances of insanity, that she herself had suffered from a series of nervous disorders in youth, that she showed undoubted signs of defective judgment, of lack of will-power, and, indeed, of actual mental feebleness. She was also exceedingly superstitious and believed the most absurd things. No wonder that she yielded to the handsome and youthful Czynski. Grashey, Preyer, and von Schrenck Notzing were opposed by Hirt and Fuchs, who maintained that the relations between the Baroness and Czynski had as their basis the natural emotions and needed no theory of hypnotism to explain them. The jury sensibly took the same view, and on this count of the indictment Czynski was acquitted, though on the others he was convicted.

Evidence with regard to the successful suggestion of other crimes by hypnotism is largely experimental. Thus, it has been proved experimentally that a hypnotized person may be induced to sign checks, papers, or legal documents. I do not know, however, of an actual instance in which this has been done for criminal purposes. Theft also has been suggested successfully in experiments upon hypnotized subjects, and in one case with disastrous results. Liébeault, at the instance of a colleague, made a post-hypnotic suggestion of theft to a young man of seventeen or eighteen years of age. As a result of this suggestion, the young man stole two small statuettes. These were subsequently returned by a messenger. Two months later, he stole an overcoat. He was discovered and arrested. Upon his person was found a notebook in which he had kept a record of a number of small thefts, and although his attorney maintained that he was a victim of hypnotic suggestion, he was sentenced to two months' imprisonment. Liébeault, who for a time was inclined to regard the subsequent thefts as indirect consequences of the original suggestion made by him, hypnotized the subject again, and now learned that the latter had, subsequently to Liébeault's hypnotism, been hypnotized again by Liébeault's colleague. It was the colleague who made the suggestion to steal the overcoat and other small articles of which the subject had kept a record. Liébeault considered that in this case the tendency to theft had been aroused by the experiments which he, together with his colleague, had performed. Whether the suggestion would have been successful if the subject had been a person of firmly established moral principles cannot, of course, be determined. In any event, the punishment of the thief is to be heartily applauded in view of what we know of the ability of the subject to resist, and, also, because a most dangerous precedent would otherwise have been established.

It is interesting to note that two of the most prominent apostles of hypnotism, Krafft-Ebing and Bernheim, held opposing views regarding the kind of individual who is most susceptible to hypnotism. Thus, Krafft-Ebing said that the susceptibility to hypnotism depends upon a special psychic and corporeal make-up. Indeed, he spoke of it as a "hypnotic gift," just as though it were some exalted quality with which special individuals are endowed. He stated further that it is found more frequently among persons who are nervously healthy than among those who are nervously ill, and especially did he maintain that the stronger willed a man is, and the more capable mentally, the more readily can he be hypnotized. Bernheim expressed himself in a diametrically opposite manner. Everything that lessens the power of reason, everything that depresses or weakens brain control, he said, increases susceptibility. Undoubtedly, Bernheim is right. It is the man who possesses less individuality, less personal force and less strength of will, who is the most pliable and the most receptive of suggestions; not the resolute, the strong-minded. Is it an evidence of exalted qualities of mind that one of Krafft-Ebing's patients, a woman of thirty-three years, under hypnosis and under the influence of the suggestion that she was a child of only seven years, at once assumed the manner, the conduct, and the characteristics of speech befitting the suggested age? Is this indicative of mental strength or stability? It seems unnecessary to carry the argument further. A typical "good subject" is Henrietta, the patient of Bernheim, whose case was quoted on page 319. Hysterical, neuropathic, defective in development—this is the kind of psychic make-up that becomes the sport of the hypnotist; not the healthy-minded man or woman.

Charcot and Gilles de la Tourette expressed themselves most emphatically on the general relation of hypnotism and crime. They pointed out that the subject is not always an entirely passive being, that he often examines the suggestions made to him, and that his credulity has its limits; that it seems proved by most careful observations that it is impossible, as a matter of fact, to make a somnambulist agree to commit an actual crime; and that, finally, while in the records of legal medicine, cases of violation are numerous enough, yet there does not exist a single case in which a somnambulist has acted criminally under hypnotic suggestion.

Legally, it is impossible to admit hypnotism as an excuse for crime. The standard by which a man is to be judged, in whose behalf absence of responsibility is alleged because of a hypnotic suggestion, is the same as that by which all other accused persons are to be judged. The *sanity of the accused* can furnish the only test. If a whilom hypnotic subject is sane, his responsibility is that of all other sane persons. It is too late, to-day, to accept the excuses of "witchcraft" and "possession."

A **legal danger** to which the **operator** may be exposed arises from the fact that hypnotic subjects may have **sexual hallucinations** or dreams, a memory of which may persist in the waking state. Charges of assault in hypnosis have actually been made in consequence of such hallucinations, as in the case cited by Löwenfeld of a physician who hypnotized a young girl alone; fortunately, the attendant circumstances were such as to clear the operator, but the case, notwithstanding, proves the reality of the danger. It is analogous to that arising from the erotic dreams of ether-narcosis and like conditions.

Hypnotism is now and then, upon theoretic grounds, looked upon as a possible means of obtaining **confessions** from criminals. In the first place, criminals are not very susceptible to hypnotism; and, secondly, Lombroso's experiments have shown that a criminal will lie as readily in hypnosis as in the waking state. Finally, that a fictitious memory may be developed under hypnosis, we have also seen (see p. 302). Almost any reply could be obtained under hypnosis by suggestive questions, and the statement of the average criminal under such a condition would have about as much value as the maunderings of the clairvoyant. Further, every one knows how, even in the waking state, suggestions with regard to past events are accepted by perfectly normal individuals. A familiar instance is seen in the unconscious training of witnesses previous to legal trials. A person whose memory of a given event is merely general, and often somewhat vague, may be led by suggestive questions to give his memory definite shape and form with regard to the most minute details. Opposing witnesses of apparently equal honesty and equal desire to tell the truth, often make very conflicting statements. If memory can be unconsciously so falsified in normal persons, how much more readily can it be falsified under hypnosis!

Summary

The foregoing considerations of hypnotism, to my mind, justify the following general conclusions. To begin, if hypnotism be at all applicable as a method of treatment, it is applicable to an exceedingly limited number of cases. Not even in hysteria is its use necessary or justifiable, save in rare instances. Experience shows (see p. 310) that suggestions in the normal condition are more potent in hysteria than suggestions under hypnosis; in addition to which, it must be remembered, that hypnotic suggestion enormously exaggerates the suggestibility of the patient during the waking state. I have no quarrel with him who tries to influence such affections as psychic impotence and sexual perversions, though the task is most frequently a thankless one. I can conceive, too, of surgical cases—rare to be sure—in which, for some reason, the ordinary anesthetics, ether or chloroform, cannot be used or in which cocainization is impracticable but in which hypnotic anesthesia may be tried and perhaps prove successful. On the whole, however, the field for hypnotism, under the best conditions, is practically *nil*. Of a truth, hypnotism never cures any affections except those which are readily curable by other and physiologic measures while it induces, let me repeat, a distinctly pathologic state. In spite of all that has been maintained to the contrary, proof is lacking that hypnotism possesses any genuine curative power. How "artificially induced hysteria" can cure, passeth human understanding. It ranks of necessity with "mind cure" and the imbecilities of Eddyism.

CATHARSIS

PSYCHANALYSIS

One of the most remarkable cults that has made its appearance in modern times, is that to which the name "psycho-analysis" has been given by Freud.   Just as mesmerism gave rise to animal magnetism and animal magnetism to hypnotism, so did hypnotism, in due course, give birth to "catharsis" and catharsis to psychanalysis.   In the early 80's Breuer of Vienna concerned himself with the study of hysteria by hypnotism and devised a method of treatment which he termed **"catharsis."**   This method was published some years later in a volume entitled "Studien ueber Hysterie," 1895, in which he had as collaborator Sigmund Freud.   These authors stated that they found, to their greatest astonishment, that the individual symptoms of hysteria immediately and permanently disappeared whenever they were successful in fully arousing in the patient the memory of the event which was causal to the development of the symptom, together with the accompanying emotion; if, added to this, the patient gave the fullest possible description of this event and gave verbal expression to the emotion. The symptom had existed as a substitute or in place of another past experience which had been suppressed, and the recollection of which had become subconscious—that is, it was a conversion of the original memory of an act and its associated emotion into a pathological symptom or obsession.   The therapeutic efficacy of their procedure Breuer and Freud explained as the catharsis of the repressed, "locked up," emotion, which had been attached to or associated with the suppressed psychic experience.   Withholding for the present our acceptance of this statement, let us examine the position of Breuer and Freud in detail.   They maintained that a hysteric symptom has its origin in a psychic trauma, which at the time of its incidence is accompanied by an emotion. The persistence or disappearance of the memory of such an event, depends upon several factors.   Above all, it is important whether the individual reacted energetically at the time or not.   Under a reaction are comprehended the entire series of voluntary and involuntary reflexes by which the emotions are commonly discharged, from weeping to an act of revenge. If such a reaction takes place in sufficient measure, the emotion in great part disappears. If the reaction be suppressed, the emotion remains attached to or associated with the memory. An insult for which apology is made is differently remembered from one that has to be pocketed. There is a hurt to the feelings which persists. Under these circumstances, the reaction of the injured person has only a full "cathartic" effect when it is an **adequate** reaction, as in revenge; but the human being finds a substitute for the deed in speech, with the help of which the emotion can be discharged—abreacted—almost as well. In other cases, speech is of itself the adequate reflex, as in the making of a complaint or a confession.

"**Abreaction**" or discharge is, however, not the only method by means of which the emotion may be disposed of. If not discharged, the emotion, in the normal individual, enters the great mass or complex of associations. It is ranged along with other, perhaps contradictory, conceptions and thus undergoes a kind of correction. For instance, after an accident, there becomes added to the memory of the danger and the lessening recollection of the fright, the memory of the subsequent rescue and the realization of the present safety. The memory of an insult is corrected by the realization of the actual facts, by the appeal to one's own sense of dignity and like procedures; and so the normal individual may, by the help of his associations, bring about the disappearance of the emotion.

Breuer and Freud declared that the memories which give rise to hysteric phenomena are preserved with remarkable freshness and with their full emotional tone for a long time. They added, however, that the patients are not in control of such memories as they are of others. On the contrary—and this is the weakness of their theory and subsequent procedure—they declared that these memories are completely absent in the usual psychic state of the patient or are at most only remembered in a "summary" (or condensed?) manner. Only when the patient is questioned under hypnosis do these memories reappear with the undiminished vitality of recent occurrences; they correspond to psychic traumas which were not sufficiently abreacted (*i.e.*, discharged). Such a discharge or abreaction is inhibited, repressed, at the time of the original occurrences, by various facts; for instance, the nature of the occurrence may make an adequate reaction impossible, *e.g.*, the loss of a beloved relative; or the social surroundings may make a reaction impossible; or the reaction may not take place because the occurrence deals with matters which the individual is anxious to forget, which he wishes intentionally to suppress, to crowd out of his conscious thinking. Again, as revealed by hypnosis, the occurrence may have had its incidence at the time of a seriously paralyzing emotion such as fright, or it may have had its incidence during an abnormal psychic state of the patient, as in the half-hypnotic twilight state of waking-dreaming, in autohypnosis and the like Here, it is the nature of the circumstances which makes a reaction to the occurrence impossible.

The method of **catharsis**—the method of Breuer and Freud—is operative as follows: It neutralizes the action of the originally unabreacted conception, by giving the associated imprisoned emotions discharge by means of speech, and brings them into corrective association, inasmuch as it brings them into the field of normal consciousness (in light hypnosis), or by means of medical suggestion, as is done in somnambulism with amnesia. To state it in other and less involved words, what Breuer did, was to hypnotize his patients and then endeavor to obtain from them memories of past occurrences, and in this procedure he does not seem to have relied solely upon the spontaneity of the patient but also to have made use of "medical suggestion" as is done "in somnambulism with amnesia."

We have just shown, in the preceding pages on hypnotism, how fictitious and utterly worthless a memory elicited under such circumstances may be. Indeed, the willing subject invents, fabricates the things for which—she cannot help but know—the physician is seeking. Again, we have already learned that hysteria and hypnosis are really identical states; namely, that hypnosis is merely an access of hysteria artificially induced, and, again, that the hysteric patient reacts to suggestion just as does the subject under hypnosis (see pp. 302, 94). Indeed, Breuer and Freud speak of the "hypnoid states" of their patients.

Further, such a modicum of truth as is embraced in the theory of emotional discharge, and for which Breuer and Freud have coined the entirely unnecessary word "abreaction," is not even new. It is a common experience with physicians, not only with neurologists but with practitioners in general, that if they can induce a patient to talk freely concerning his symptoms, especially dwelling upon the origin of the latter and the causes which led to them, the patient's mind is often relieved, the symptoms at once losing in importance and often fading away. There is an emotional relief akin to that which a child experiences when confessing to its mother some act of disobedience, some peccadillo or other trivial misconduct, the recollection of which is burdening its mind. So it is with the adult, as not only physicians but lay persons equally know. When a patient has unloaded his mind fully in regard to some real or fancied cause of worry, great relief is experienced. There is, as it were, a relief of tension, a reëstablishment of the emotional equilibrium, and a consequent sense of comfort and relief. Patients themselves know this, nervous patients in particular, and it is for this reason that they insist on describing their troubles in detail, often with such minuteness and with such wearisome repetition as to seriously tax not only the time but the endurance of the doctor. They want to tell their story, they want to tell it fully and completely without let or hindrance, and so anxious are they not to omit anything, that it is a common experience to have them come to our offices with long series of notes, mostly written upon small pieces of paper, in order that no point, no matter how minute, should be omitted.

The relief which patients experience by a full account of their symptoms, and the inevitable concomitant emotional discharge, is seen, in a more marked degree, of course, and yet typically, in the making of confessions; at times the demand for relief under these circumstances is so great and so insistent, that the sufferer voluntarily makes statements which he knows may lead to disgrace, imprisonment, and at times even to death.

Freud subsequently to his studies with Breuer, made what he

believed to be important modifications in the method, and renamed it "psycho-analysis." In the cathartic method the patient was hypnotized because of the "expansion of consciousness which ensues under hypnosis."* Freud dispensed, as he believed, with hypnotism; he made the following change in technique :† The patient lies upon her back upon a couch, while the physician sits upon a chair back of her and out of her line of vision. He no longer requests the patient to close her eyes as formerly, and avoids every touch or procedure such as would be in keeping with hypnosis. Such a séance has the character of a conversation between two persons equally awake (?), one of whom, the patient, is spared every possible muscular effort and every diverting sensory impression, such as might disturb her in her concentration on her internal psychic processes (sic). Freud believes that in this procedure there could not be any possibility of suggestion, and further that the method had an advantage in the involuntary (?) thoughts, to which under this method the patient gives expression—thoughts involuntary and almost always disturbing, which the patient under ordinary circumstances suppresses, and which usually interrupt a connected and designed account of the past history. In order to take advantage of these involuntary ideas or conceptions of the patient, Freud requests the latter to drift in her communication, just as one would drift in a conversation in which one passes in turn to the most varied subjects. He impresses the patient, before she enters into the detailed account of her history, to tell everything that comes into her head, whether she thinks it important or unimportant, whether it seems relevant or senseless. The patient is especially requested (sic) not to repress any thought or idea because this idea happens to be shameful or painful. This method later became known as that of "free association."

To begin, it is quite evident that Freud did not, in his modification, dispense with hypnosis. Have we not already learned that the hysteric patient reacts just as does the subject under hypnotism? Did not Breuer and Freud in their studies in hysteria

*See Freud's original communication in Löwenfeld's work on "Die Psychischen Zwangserscheinungen," 1904, p. 545, et seq.

†Loc. cit.

emphasize the hypnoid state of hysteric patients? How then can the element of hypnosis be eliminated? Finally, it is doubtful whether a method can be devised more favorable to the development of an autohypnoid state than that presented by Freud's technique. Again, in Breuer and Freud's "Studien," page 13, the employment of medical suggestion is freely admitted. Freud, however, in his psycho-analysis denies the possibility of suggestion. Let us see how much of truth there is in this claim.

Freud states that in the very beginning of the patient's account lapses of memory become apparent. These may have to do with everyday occurrences which have been forgotten, or with relations of time or of cause which have become disturbed, so that results are obtained which cannot be understood. Freud claims that no neurotic history can be elicited which does not reveal amnesias of some form or other. If the patient be urged (*sic*) to fill up these lapses of memory, it is noted that the ideas which now occur are repressed with every effort, until finally, if the memory really appears, the patient experiences a marked sense of discomfort. From this observation, Freud concluded that the lapses of memory are the result of repression and as the motive of this repression he recognized feelings of aversion or dislike. Thus arises a resistance to the reproduction of the memory.

As already pointed out, little credence can be given to memories evoked under hypnotism (see pp. 302, 319) and equally little credence can be given to the sayings of a case of hysteria under Freud's conditions. It is extremely probable, indeed, one may say certain, that, under such circumstances, the patient will respond with alertness to the slightest suggestions, inadvertent or unintentional though these may be on the part of the physician. Fictitious memories are thus doubtless elicited. Indeed, Löwenfeld who recognized the influence of suggestion in Freud's method, early gave an instance of a patient of Freud who subsequently came into his (Löwenfeld's) hands. The patient stated that the sexual events which she had related to Freud when under his treatment had really never occurred. She declared that the whole thing had

---

*Löwenfeld: "Sexualleben und Nervenleiden," 1899, p. 196.

been a piece of pure imagination.   As we will see later on, not only does suggestion occur in Freud's method, but owing to the peculiar nature of Freud's theories, suggestion occurs with especial force and directness.

Freud early arrived at the conclusion that the suppressed memories always have to do with sexual matters, and finally came to believe that every symptom—hysteric or otherwise—had its origin in some passionate sexual action or aggression of childhood! Others than myself have dwelt upon the glaring inconsistency of the sexual immaturity of children and the intrinsic biological improbability of this theory.   This inconsistency has been met by retreating to the age of puberty and attempting to save the situation by saying that the memory of these sexual events is projected from puberty into the period of childhood.

A special system was gradually evolved by Freud and by others who assumed the rôle of disciples.   Soon this acquired the character of a new cult with a new and strange vocabulary and strange symbolic interpretations.

Let us, without further delay, pass to the consideration of the mode of action of the psychic factors on which Freud and his disciples have laid so much stress, namely, psychic factors sexual in nature, sexual psychogenic factors as they might be called, or, to use the language of the Freudian sect, **sexual traumas**.   It is to these factors that this sect ascribes every known form of nervous and mental disease with the sole exception of those affections, the actual organic, infectious or toxic nature of which it is impossible to deny.   Further, these causes are said to be operative in intrauterine life as well as in childhood; and, from their very nature, are such that every human creature is or has been exposed to them.   At the very outset we are filled with astonishment at the fact that there are any normal boys and girls, any normal men and women, left in the world, and the inquiry naturally suggests itself, on what are these extraordinary claims based?   The Freudians assert that they derive their information from the unearthing —as they believe—of repressed memories of sexual occurrences— "traumas"—experienced in childhood.   Such memories being unpleasant or painful, are suppressed and not permitted to enter the field of consciousness, but commonly the attempt to suppress the memory is only partially successful. Though buried, it is supposed to be still active and manages to reach the field of consciousness by "displacement" and "conversion." The unpleasant feeling associated with the memory leaves the memory associated with the sexual trauma and joins itself to some other complex which has free access to the field of consciousness, and in so doing gives rise to fears, obsessions, delusions, tics, or other psychic phenomena; that is, a given symptom exists as a substitute of a past experience which has been repressed and the recollection of which has become subconscious. It is the conversion of the original memory of an act and its associated emotion into a pathologic symptom.

To the student familiar with the development of our knowledge of functional nervous disorders, the preceding interpretation at once recalls the writings of Janet. Janet, it will be remembered, showed that all of the various fears, phobias, obsessions, states of anxiety, indecisions and the like were really manifestations of but one disorder. He thus, by a brilliant generalization, brought them under one caption, for which he employed the term "psychasthenia." At the same time, he pointed out the fact that, in many of these cases, various acts of the patient in the past, breaches of conduct, of the proprieties, peccadilloes of various kinds, of which the patient was subsequently ashamed and which he tried to forget, played an important rôle in the evolution of the symptoms. Janet's observations were as important as they were satisfying. They really embody a kernel of truth, a modicum of actual scientific fact. Neither Freud nor his followers gave to Janet's discovery either recognition or attention, but restricting all causes to sexual transgressions, proceeded to erect a peculiar system of psychology; peculiar, first, in that it deals exclusively with sexual factors, and secondly, in that it constitutes a system of psychology of the unconscious mind. They formulated theories which deal with doubtful inferences and questionable hypotheses as though these were established facts, and this, too, in a field in which, from the very nature of the case, that which actually occurs is beyond the possibilities of human ken. A special terminology has arisen; for instance, "repression, displacement, condensation, transference, introjection, projection, introversion, conversion, sublimation, determinations, exteriorizations" and others still which might be added; all of these terms are used as though they dealt with actually observed concrete facts, and not with purely metaphysical abstractions.

The Freudians also lay a special stress on the study of the patient's dreams. Every dream is held to have a sexual content. It always deals with a subject of such a character that it cannot be entirely revealed without injury to the dreamer, without lesion of the proprieties. Lastly, the dream always deals with a desire. Sometimes the dream is a realization, unveiled and undisguised, of an unsuppressed desire; sometimes it is the realization of a desire veiled, latent and suppressed; sometimes it is the realization of a desire suppressed and little or but slightly veiled. The secret, non-communicable nature of the dream and the desire, veiled or outspoken, constitute, according to this theory, the important factors of the dream. In other words, in the dream suppressed sexual complexes are supposed to come to the surface and the desire, veiled or frankly expressed, is thus gratified. By this is not meant that dreams always deal with nakedly expressed sexual conceptions and feelings, but quite commonly that these elements are veiled or "symbolized" so that, the patient having related or written out his dream, the psychanalyst reads into them the fantasies of his own autosuggestions. To show the extent to which Freud has gone, he assumes that during the dream there is a "critic" or "censor" which concerns itself with the suppressed desire. The suppressed desire forms a compromise with this critic, is modified, symbolized, and the desire, so modified, is represented as fulfilled. In other words, according to this theory, just as a repressed sexual complex may give rise to a nervous or mental symptom by reaching the surface of consciousness in a transformed or converted shape, so may it reach the surface in the dream state in a converted form and thus bring about relief. For the introduction of the hypothetic "critic" or "censor" there is not the slightest justification; it is something created out of nothing.

The conditions under which a dream is elicited by the psychanalyst are similar to those employed in eliciting the history of sexual traumas. The patient is required to make an oral statement of the dream or to give an account in writing. This is to be as full as possible. Nothing is to be omitted. In addition, he is to communicate every idea without exception that occurs to him in connection with the dream. It is often retold and rewritten many times—after visits and discussions with the psychanalyst. That the material so obtained has the same value as that obtained by the other method is quite evident, and that the psychanalyst always secures the material which he seeks, goes without question.

Freud declares that it is the "critic" which causes the patient to reject certain things from his communication, but if the patient can withhold the "critic" in regard to the ideas which present themselves in thinking over the substance of a dream, a psychic material is furnished which leads to the solution or unravelling of the dream.

Every dream, according to Freud, has a **manifest** or **apparent content**, *i.e.*, that which appears on the surface of the recital; and a **latent content**, *i.e.*, the material derived from the dream when the patient gives himself up to the unrestrained association of ideas (*sic*) which ensues when he dwells upon the dream. Dreams also reveal a condensation; when we compare the number of ideas contained in a dream, as written down from memory, with the number of ideas revealed in the latent dream content, it becomes apparent that a very great condensation has taken place. According to Freud, we do not find a single factor of the dream content from which threads of association do not lead into three or more different channels; there is no situation which is not pieced together out of three or four impressions and experiences. During the process of eliciting the latent dream content, the mind passes from the thoughts and conceptions with which it is primarily concerned, to others which have no claim to emphasis or importance, and it is this process which has to do with the concealment of the meaning of the dream. This is termed by Freud "**dream displacement**." In it lies the explanation of the fact that we are compelled to break off in communicating the contents of a dream, because thoughts present themselves which cannot be spoken of to others without injury of important considerations, personal and private. It is the repression of these thoughts, the existence of which is thus revealed, that Freud believes gives rise to hysteric symptoms, phobias, obsessions and delusions. He also believes that a whole train of phenomena of the everyday life of normal individuals—forgetfulness, unconscious mistakes in speech, mistakes in simple acts and other errors—are due to similar causes.

It would be out of place in this volume to enter into a detailed discussion of dreams. Suffice it to say, however, that, in all probability, dream conceptions arise just before the sleeper awakens, *i.e.*, just before he is in the act of entering into consciousness; or, during such intervals or periods of the sleep in which the sleep becomes very light so that the level of consciousness is approached, or, it may be, nearly reached. Most frequently, it would appear that dream conceptions are part and parcel of the act of awakening. These conceptions form the material from which the dream is subsequently constructed. This construction occurs only after waking consciousness has been established. There is in every act of awakening an intermediate twilight state of mind, usually very brief, but sometimes prolonged, during which inroads, vague and indistinct, are made on the sensorium from without, and the conceptions thus arising, are, when the patient fully awakens, arranged automatically into some semblance of order and sequence both as to time and space. The arrangement of the dream pictures is automatic, begins at once in the act of awakening, and is, later, often elaborated and dramatized. It is probable that when the awakening occurs quickly, *i.e.*, when the transition to consciousness is sudden and complete, that the dream remains fragmentary. To take such a dream, especially in a case of hysteria, and submit its conceptions to a process, the essential features of which are indistinguishable from those of an autohypnosis, may lead to almost any vagary. That the ideas resulting from this method are determined by the personal peculiarities of the individual, by his training, his education and his habits of thought; by his desires, his instincts and his sex, goes,

I think, without saying; but that one has the right to ascribe to these ideas any value other than this, can be, to say the least, seriously questioned; to go so far as to say that because in one individual dreams usually have, or always have, a sexual content, therefore, we are to conclude that all dreams in all individuals have a sexual content, is, to say the least, not quite logical. To ascribe to ideas which are manifestly secondary abstractions— ideas evolved subsequently to the dream—a causal character, an etiologic value to explain preëxisting symptoms, is again not quite logical. To say that the dream analysis of Freud unearths a repressed dream-complex, the unearthing of which gives relief to the patient, is merely to say that the patient, dwelling on his dream and induced to speak without hindrance, merely tells the unpleasant, perhaps, secret and personal fact or facts of his history, which he would have told and constantly does tell, without reference to any dream. The danger, however, arises, just as it does in Freud's method of "free association," that the patient will fabricate, involuntarily or perhaps voluntarily, as did Löwenfeld's patient, and recite events that never occurred. Perhaps they are purely fictitious happenings to fill in inconsistencies and lacunæ, and yet, arising spontaneously in the patient's mind, may be accepted by the patient as true and find a place among the memories of his actual experiences. Such a patient is, I believe, damaged, just as is a patient who takes away with him after a hypnosis, a persistent suggestion as to fictitious past occurrences.

In addition to the theory of repressed memories of sexual traumas in childhood and of the repressed desires revealed in dreams, the psychanalysts employ a third method of unearthing repressed sexual complexes, namely, that of the **association test**. It may be briefly described as follows: A series of words is read to a patient, and he is instructed that as soon as he hears each word, he is to utter at once the first word or thought that comes into his mind. The examiner records with a stop watch the time elapsing between the reading of the word and the reply. If, now, it be found that the time elapsing—**the reaction time**—is suddenly increased as though there were a brief period of hesitation, it is probable that a complex has been aroused. The word read by the investigator is the stimulus-word; the word uttered in reply the reaction word; and a word which betrays an increase in time reaction may prove to be a complex indicator. An ordinary reaction may require between one and two seconds, say from one and two-tenth to one and eight-tenth seconds; if the reaction time is suddenly lengthened to three, four, or five seconds, there is reason to suspect the existence of a repressed complex. The list of words should be reasonably long, and should contain, in addition to miscellaneous words expressive of various objects and actions, also a carefully selected number, based upon the possibilities which a previous general study of the case has suggested to the examiner; these words should be interspersed at irregular intervals. In addition to the increased time required, the reaction word may also be significant if the association be unusually obscure or apparently non-existent. Again, it is also significant if, after a reaction word with increased time has been noted, delay, though less in degree, is observed in the next word or two following. It would seem as though the patient had been slightly disturbed and the disturbance transmitted to the immediately succeeding tests. It is quite unnecessary to add that the results obtained by this method are commonly quite trivial and, further, are subject to the vagaries of interpretation of the psychanalyst.

The Freudian psychology of the unconscious mind is, in several aspects, extremely peculiar. For instance, just as Freud does not hesitate to create out of the whole cloth a wide-awake "critic" guarding the dream, he equally, without hesitation, ascribes new qualities and peculiarities to the emotions. He makes the latter separate things, mobile somethings, capable of being detached, displaced, and producing effects which have no relation to the origin of the emotion. Again, he assumes that, as in the case of the "critic" or "censor" of the dream, there is in the unconscious mind in the waking state, a something which manifests itself as an effort at self-protection, so that thoughts with unpleasant emotional content are shoved into the subconscious, but the e only to give rise to other troubles. That this theory is not in accord with universal experience can, I think, be safely maintained. It is quite impossible, thus, to forget a real worry, as a crime, a financial disaster, death of a child, etc.; indeed, the greater the worry, the more insistently is it present to the mind.

Further, it should be emphasized that the Freudian psychology is peculiar in the fact that all of these detachable and movable emotions and suppressed memories have to do exclusively with sexual matters. No matter how obtained or how expressed, the phenomena observed are always interpreted by the "libido," the sexual desire. This is the invariable motif of the psychanalyst; sometimes it is recorded in terms of the grossest and most disgusting perversions, at other times it is sublimated and diluted, but it is always the same, always the libido. Lastly, the repressed ideas coming to the surface in dreams, in psychanalysis, in the association tests, do not signify what they appear to signify, but are masked and disguised; in other words, are symbols. The art of the psychanalyst lies in the interpretation of these symbols.

That with such hypotheses and under such circumstances, the psychanalyst can find in a given patient almost anything that he is looking for, goes without saying. Indeed, the interpretation depends on the imagination, the autosuggestion of the analyst, the figments and the fancies of his own brain. At times, the symbols indicate what they most readily suggest; at times and apparently without reason, the opposite. There can be no doubt that the psychanalyst always finds that for which he is seeking. There is not a single object in the universe in which a sexual significance cannot be discerned, whether it be a hat, a cup, a snake, a horse, a tooth-pick; even the physician's stethoscope is believed to be a phallic symbol. As a matter of course, the conclusion to be formed from the investigation of a given case already exists preformed in the psychanalyst's mind; namely, that there are present in the patient repressed sexual memories. The analyst regards this preformed conclusion as an axiomatic truth. The objection to this whole matter lies not so much in the unpleasant and repulsive character of its details, as in the hopelessly illogical character of its doctrines and the unscientific character of its methods.

To what extremes and how peculiar the beliefs in regard to psychanalysis have grown, is revealed by a cursory review of some of its later doctrines. It began with the theory of sexual traumas in childhood, but now it has been extended to include the period of intrauterine life. The psychic life of this period, according to Freud's Hungarian disciple Ferenczi, is one of "unconditioned omnipotence."* This term, whatever it may mean, Ferenczi applies to the child *in utero* because, without any effort on its part, it is supplied with nutriment and caloric!

Further, while being born, that is, during the act of passing through the pelvis of its mother, the child suffers from fear, and this fear is the prototype of the attacks of fear which come on at later periods in the life of the individual, for these attacks act by evoking the memory of this "birth fear." Again, the child is not asexual. It finds itself in a state of autoeroticism from which arise all of the determinations of its future soul-life. Still more, the child is a polymorphic pervert and universal criminal (Stekel). The first sexual tidal wave is reached at three or four years of age, and the dominating factor is incestuous love, the "Œdipus complex." In later life, the tendencies of the individual are likewise determined by his eroticism; thus the "sublimation of erotic and criminal tendencies" gives rise to the surgeon. Economy, love of order and obstinacy indicate anal eroticism. Luxurious water-closets, that is, hygienic water-closets, such as are universal in America, also indicate anal eroticism. The love of domesticated animals, the liking for sport, are likewise the outcome of the libido. The dream and the neuroses, alike, embrace not only the life of the child, but also that of the savage and primitive man. The epileptic attack is a retrogression into the infantile period of wish-fulfilment by means of incoördinate movements; it is an overpowering of the moral consciousness by the criminal unconsciousness; it replaces the sinful sexual act (Stekel). Melancholia and mania, we are told, are the product of the repressions and displacements of the converted sexual desire, the transformed libido. Delusions of jealousy have their origin in the projection by the husband of his repressed polygamous impulses on his wife. A cause of chronic paranoia is unmasked as an irritation of the anal

* Hoche: "Ueber den Werth der Psychoanalyse," Arch. f. Psychiat.," 1913, li, No. 3.

erogenous zone. The symptoms of dementia præcox are conditioned by thoughts, which, because of their unpleasant character, are repressed; the delusive ideas of the patient are merely symbols of thoughts. The patient suffers from "reminiscences of humanity" while "his history embraces all mythology." The real underlying, the fundamental, the central phantasy of dementia præcox is, of course, the incest—the Œdipus—complex. What a narrow escape paresis has made in this list of affections! Yet the prediction can be safely ventured that it, too, in spite of the spirochete, will be brought within the psychanalytic pale. Psychanalysis further explains migraine, every form of headache that is not organic, asthma, angioneurotic edema, hysteric sneezing, mucous colitis and what not. In what words shall we characterize such fantastic nonsense, such vacuous harebrained absurdities, such meaningless jargon! And such utterances are dealt with by the psychanalytic sect as though they were each and every one scientifically demonstrated facts, self-evident, axiomatic truths.

The psychanalysts have assumed a most exalted and expansive tone. They deal with the very "depths" of psychology, with the "weight of absolute fact." The publications of this or that member of the sect are spoken of as "revelations." Psychanalysis has "revealed the unsconscious soul-life in its entire extent" (Imago). The dream interpretation is the solution of a riddle which has defied solution for thousands of years. Sexual morality is now erected "in a new form;" "there is now beginning a healthier, more honest conception of life;" "for we know," say the psychanalysts, "that the future is ours." The hope is also expressed that the opponents of psychanalysts will be educated to assume a "respectable tone;" they are charged with harboring "unscientific prejudice" and "prejudiced science." They are also told that they are "ignorant prattlers." Psychanalysis has now expanded so as to embrace all departments of human knowledge. The journal, Imago, deals with the reformation of manners, of religion, of the science of religion, with right living, esthetics, literature, art, mythology, pedagogy, criminology and moral theology. The psychanalyst is now the great reformer who is putting everything to rights. He speaks with a smile of indulgence and condescension of the cavillers who fail to accept his doctrines; addresses himself to the "initiated" (Wissenden), speaks of the "Master" or of the "brethren"* of his cult.

At times it is proclaimed that the proof of the correctness of the psychanalytic interpretation lies in the cures effected. Breuer's original case of hysteria was the much-vaunted example of successful treatment. It is a matter, however, of everyday experience that the fact of recovery from hysteria is no evidence as to the specific value of any method of treatment, inasmuch as in hysteria recoveries occur under the most diverse conditions, so long as the suggestion is made that the patient will recover. In the instance of psychanalysis both physician and patient start with the presumption, that is, with the suggestion that the cause will be revealed, that the cause is revealed and that, with this unearthing of the cause, the symptoms will disappear. The discovery of repressed sexual complexes is exactly what we would be led to expect under these circumstances; as in hypnosis, the believing physician and the believing patient react on each other; both are under the influence of the same suggestion. The patient knows just what is expected of her and the physician finds just what he is expecting to find. In other words, psychanalysis, in spite of the special technique which its disciples say they pursue, is nothing more than suggestion in a new pseudo-scientific guise. That it achieves a measure of success in such affections as hysteria—so amenable to all forms of suggestion—is not astonishing. It is exactly what should have been expected.

Inasmuch as we are told that the successful treatment of a case requires from six months to three years, it is not suprising that success now and then follows the persistent use of the treatment in affections that are self-limited in duration or that pursue a wave-like course. A case of melancholia so treated naturally comes to an end after a number of months and is then regarded as cured by psychanalysis. It is probable, also, that such cases are often improperly diagnosticated and are then reported as cases caused by this or that painful complex, cured by psychanalysis. When

---

* Loc. cit.

the symptoms recur, which is almost inevitably the case, the patient usually has recourse to another physician and thus the failure becomes known, as in cases within my own experience. Stekel admits failures in periodic affections, in hypochondria and in homosexuals; but psychanalysis, rich in resources, explains failures by asserting that the patient did not want to recover and resisted his physician.

It is a matter of proper inquiry whether or not psychanalysis is harmful. Hoche some three years ago addressed a circular inquiry to a large number of clinicians, psychiatrists, neurologists and practising physicians, selecting colleagues who were experienced and whom he knew, personally or scientifically, sufficiently well to place dependence on their judgment. The results of this inquiry, secured independently and from the most varied sources, were remarkably uniform. It came to light in the first place, that psychanalysis is being applied in cases which one would think the psychanalysts themselves would regard as unsuitable—epilepsy, paresis, hebephrenia, catatonia, melancholia; such cases are doubtless submitted to the treatment as a result of gross diagnostic errors.

Numerous communications, received by Hoche, report an intense and often persistent feeling of indignation on the part of the patients because of the reckless and shameless questioning to which they have been subjected; a feeling which often leads to an abrupt cessation of the treatment. This feeling is evident not only in those who are ill and morbidly sensitive, but also, it need hardly be added, in persons of an entirely normal, moral and esthetic make-up. What must we think of the wounding of the feelings of a sensitive and innocent nature when to a loving son or daughter is suggested an incestuous love for the mother? What injury can be greater than to give to one of the most beautiful relations in human life the most shocking and the vilest of interpretations? Harm, also, is done by fixing sexual associations in the patient's mind. Often this leads the patient baldly to associate every object that he sees with either the male or female genitals. Hoche's reports show, too, that engagements and wedded life have alike been shattered, destroyed by psychanalysis. Most serious of all, perhaps, is the poisoning of the minds of youthful patients. In more than one instance, cases came to light in which illicit sexual living resulted from the procedure; at times indirectly, and at other times, monstrous as this seems, as a direct result of advice given. Besides this, Hoche found in his reports other serious outcomes, such as venereal diseases and illegitimate pregnancies.

The attachment of the patient to the physician, so prone to occur in hysteric patients and hypnotic subjects, if the physician be at all lax in his attitude, is peculiarly fostered by psychanalysis. There are the daily, or almost daily, long-continued conversations on sexual matters, extending over many months of time—sometimes as long as three years—conversations of the most intimate character, in which the patient, who is usually a woman, openly acknowledges her suppressed sexual desires and rehearses at length the memories connected with them. Human beings, men and women, are so constituted that intimate conversations on sexual matters cannot take place without being accompanied automatically by certain associated feelings and emotions, and, when we reflect that the very object of the treatment is to lay bare the repressed desires of the patient and to bring about relief by an emotional discharge—the so-called "abreaction"—we cannot but feel that the relation between physician and patient is, as a writer in Science has expressed it, a quasisexual one, no matter how guarded it may be. No wonder that the patient often acquires an attitude of absolute dependence on the physician, of being utterly unable to get along without him. Again, because of the long-continued mental concentration on their inner selves, on their sexual experiences, the patients become incapable of giving their attention to other matters, incapable of following a daily occupation, incapable of attending to any consecutive duties. They lose their self-confidence; they can do nothing without asking the doctor; they must give him an account of every thought, every incident, no matter how trivial. That such persons frequently become useless to themselves and their families is not surprising. States of excitement also are occasionally induced in hysteric persons and, also, in patients suffering from other affections. Another effect is to create in the patient a fear which may acquire the force of an obsession, that in the recital to the physician, or in making the record of the dream, she has forgotten something important; perhaps the most important thing in the entire matter. Depression, too, especially is fostered in those who already entertain delusions of self-accusation with a sexual content. The constant questioning of the patient on sexual matters, the constant delving for new sexual material, confirms the patient in her morbid self-accusation. Several cases have, according to Hoche, terminated, during such periods of depression, in suicide.

Finally, to sum up the therapeutic results claimed for psychanalysis, we find that the cures have the same unreality as those achieved under hypnotism. The treatment requires daily séances of long duration extending over six months to three years or longer. Indeed, it would appear that the treatment, once started, is never quite completed.

The psychology of insanity, the psychologic interpretation of the symptoms, is one thing, psychanalysis is another. The psychology of insanity is a legitimate field of inquiry; though from the very nature of the subject its results must be largely speculative. Psychanalysis, on the other hand, is a cult, a creed, the disciples of which constitute a sect. To be admitted to its brotherhood, it is merely necessary that the novice should be converted to the faith, not that he should be convinced by scientific proof; for none such is possible. If the convert claims that he has found psychanalysis followed by cures, he places himself side by side with those who claim cures by means of hypnotism, divine healing, Christian Science and like procedures.

Psychanalysis is an outcome of the general mystic tendency of the modern world. Occultism and symbolism in art, music, literature and the drama—cubism, futurism, modernism, the problem play—are all expressions of this tendency. On what basis are we to explain such phenomena? Factors which influence the social condition, the mode of living, of great masses of people, all have to do with this psychopathic tendency. Among them, we may enumerate the strain of modern living, the strain of the adaptation required by rapid rise in social level with its unaccustomed demands and new dissipations, the strain of the struggle of those who have not yet achieved their goal, and to this we should add the lateness of marriage and the difficulties of living a normal, a physiologic, a complete life. Under these circumstances the less stable and weaker minds lose their moorings. That which is old and has perhaps been acquired slowly, with difficulty and at great cost, is forgotten. Truth is rejected for no other reason than that it is old. New things are accepted for no other reason than that they are new. There is an abandonment of all previous standards. The mind is unhinged and takes refuge in mysticism. The real gives place to the unreal, the beautiful to the unbeautiful, the wholesome facts of life to the morbid untruths of disease; actual experiences are belied by pathologic illusions; the evidences of the senses are replaced by the phantasms of exhaustion. To the jaded and blasé psychopathic patient, to the chronic hysteric, psychasthenic, hypochondriac or what not, to the patient who has tried all sorts of procedures, psychanalysis presents something new, something interesting, something pruriently exciting.

METALLOTHERAPY

Metallotherapy is a mode of treatment in which various metals are applied to parts of the body affected by disease. Like many other methods, it is very old. Aristotle, Galen, Paul of Ægina, Ætius, Paracelsus, and others considered that it possessed special virtues in the treatment of the most diverse affections. They, however, attributed the curative powers to the magical inscriptions which the metals bore. It was not until the eighteenth century, when animal magnetism was the order of the day that the subject was seriously studied. In 1754, Lenoble, instead of using metals, made artificial magnets, with which he treated numerous affections. In 1774, as we have already learned (see p. 287), Hell, of Vienna, recovered from rheumatism, in consequence, as he believed, of the application of magnets. He also reported the case of a woman cured of cardialgia, while Bauer, of Vienna, was healed of a stubborn ophthalmia, and Osterwald, a director of the Academy of Sciences of Munich, became well of paralysis through the same means. Mesmer began a very extensive use of magnets, but soon abandoned them, finding that he could achieve the results he desired as readily without them, as with them. Various other physicians, Unzer, Bolten, Heinsius, Weber, Manduyt, Andry, and Thouret, published cases treated by metallotherapy, while Wichmann anticipated some of the results of Burq. It was the latter who, in 1849, made an elaborate study of metallotherapy and erected it into a well-defined method. In his thesis, published in 1851, he described his first experiences in regard to the influence of metals upon anesthesia, namely, the production of tingling sensations, heat, perspiration, redness, and the reappearance of sensation. Burq was vigorously opposed; but notwithstanding, succeeded, after a struggle of thirty years, in attracting to his method the serious attention of scientific men, and finally the Société de Biologie appointed Charcot, Luys, and Dumontpallier to investigate it; later Landolt, Gellé, and Regnard were added to this commission. Burq maintained that the application of metals to a limited part of the surface of the body was capable of causing the disappearance of the paralysis of sensation and motion produced by hysteria. He further asserted that the same metal is not suitable for every individual; that a special metal is required in each given case. He also believed that the internal use of metals produced the same therapeutic effect as the application of the metal to the skin. He went so far as to assert that the application of the metallic discs not only causes general sensation to return, together with dilatation of the capillaries and rise of temperature in the paralyzed limb, but also that it cures blindness, deafness, loss of smell, and loss of taste. For instance, in a case in which one-half of the tongue was not sensitive to colocynth, the tongue became perfectly normal after the application of plates of iron. Patients in whom gold produced similar results, remained entirely insensible to iron, copper, and zinc; while in cases in which the latter metals were effective, gold was without result. The same facts obtained when the metals were used internally.

The commission reported in 1877, first, concerning the phenomena resulting from the application of metals to the surface of the body of patients suffering from disturbances of sensation. On applying a disc of metal, generally of small dimensions—a piece of money, for example—on a hysteric patient, attacked by permanent (*sic*) hemianesthesia, a return of sensibility was effected at the end of ten or twenty minutes in a zone several centimeters above and below the site of application. This return was preceded by tingling, pricking, and a kind of "trouble in the perception of sensations," as a result of which a cold body like ice appeared hot. There were observed, at the same time, a local elevation of temperature in the part, appreciable by a thermometer, and, in the case of the upper extremities, an increase of strength that could be demonstrated by the dynamometer.

The extension of the sensitive area was more or less progressive around the metal; subsequently it involved the entire limb, and finally the whole anesthetic side. At the same time, there was effected a dilatation of the capillaries; when a pin puncture was made before the application of the metal, the puncture would not bleed, while if a puncture were made after the application, the puncture not only bled, but the escape of blood was considerable.

The experiments with the internal administration of the metals seemed no less convincing than the preceding. A patient, sensitive to gold, took each day a dose containing two centigrams of gold-and-sodium chlorid. Eight days later there was a complete return of sensibility, general and special, restoration of the muscular strength, a considerable improvement in the general condition, and a reappearance of the menses after two years' cessation! Another patient, equally sensitive to gold, experienced like good effects from the internal administration of gold chlorid. A third patient was placed on pills of copper dioxid and water of Saint-Christau, for which there were soon substituted pills of copper albuminate, containing each two centigrams. The number of these pills was gradually increased to five. There was first a very marked improvement, but the treatment having been suspended by reason of the appearance of "gastro-intestinal *attacks*" (!), the patient very quickly lost that which she had gained. When the intestinal disturbance had passed away, the water of Saint-Christau was resumed, and at the end of ten days the patient had made a satisfactory recovery. Two hystero-epileptics, sensitive to gold, were likewise submitted to an appropriate internal medication; sensation and motion became normal and the hysteric attacks disappeared.

The committee also noted a new fact, which had escaped Burq, namely, the so-called **phenomenon of transfer**, *i.e.*, that while the sensibility and muscular force reappeared on the paralyzed side, the normal side lost in general and special sensations, in temperature and strength. The committee further believed that hemianesthesia from organic lesion also could be cured. Thus, anesthesia of ten years' duration and due to cerebral lesion was said to have yielded to gold. In two cases with hemichorea and hemianesthesia, due to old lesions, and in which the anesthesia was permanent and never varied, the application of the metal was as successful as in hysteria. A hemianesthesia of even thirty years disappeared, though the return of sensibility was delayed for three hours. Charcot endeavored to explain these phenomena as the result of an electric current developed by the contact of the metal and the skin. Rabuteau explained them by a chemical action which he believed to take place between the metal and the moisture of the skin. It was also noticed that after the sensation returned from the internal use of the metal, the anesthesia could be made to reappear by a fresh application of the metal externally. Charcot gave to this symptom the name of **metallic anesthesia**. Burq maintained, however, that in such case the patient had not yet been entirely cured, and that treatment should have been continued. Charcot, and after him Debove, after a long experience with metals, electricity, and magnets, arrived at the conclusion that the last-named agents were more powerful and yielded more constant and more successful results. Subsequently, magnets only were used. Westphal visited Charcot in 1878 and afterward studied the question in Berlin; Westphal reported that in many cases of hysteria he obtained the same results as the French investigators, but that it took him longer. He also obtained, however, exactly the same results with mustard plasters, and even with other substances which were not metallic. Marigliano and Sepelli achieved results like those of the French, as did also Thompson, Wilks, Ost, Mader, and others. Bennett, in 1878, obtained identical results by the application of wooden buttons in a case of hemianesthesia and hemialgesia of one year's duration.   On the other hand, internal metallotherapy met with failure in his hands.   Bennett was inclined to the theory that the results were due to the influence upon the patient's mind, rather than to the application of the metals; he called attention to the fact that hysteric patients, being under the influence of emotion and attention, were apt to undergo rapid or sudden changes of symptoms.   At the Forty-seventh Congress of the British Medical Association, Beard called attention to the numerous sources of error in the reported experiments with metallotherapy, and also reported that he had treated a number of organic as well as functional affections by "mental therapeutics," as he called it, and that he had obtained far better results than by other methods.   Doubts concerning the value of metallotherapy then began to spread.   Douglas Aigre, in his thesis, "A Clinical Study of Metalloscopy and Metallotherapy in Anesthesia" (Paris, 1879), after a thorough consideration of the subject, came to the conclusion that the investigators had not paid sufficient attention to the hysteric factors present, and, therefore, constantly committed errors: he maintained that the success which was attributed to metallotherapy was due to the expectant attention of the patients. Following this severe criticism, various investigators in France, Germany, and Italy made experiments in both men and animals, in which they endeavored to exclude the factor of expectant attention, and the results were asserted to be very satisfactory.   Absolute success was reported, i.e., full recovery with no relapse, in hysteria—hystero-epilepsy with all the attendant phenomena, such as hemianesthesia, hyperesthesia, paraplegia, monoplegia, blindness, contracture—and also in chorea, diabetes, hemianesthesia from lead-poisoning and from alcoholism, and herpes zoster; also in hemianesthesia of organic origin.   In this connection it is interesting to note that in a case of hysteria, Thermes obtained similar results with a piece of ice.   Jourdanis, a pupil of Dujardin Beaumetz, investigated the subject of **xylotherapy,** i.e., the application of wood instead of metals.   He obtained results similar to those of metallotherapy.

These subjects are not at the present day awarded serious consideration.   After all, the assertions of the metallotherapists were merely those of Hell in another form—the assertions originally adopted by Mesmer and, subsequently, expanded by him into the theory and practice of healing by the magnetic fluid. The transition from metallotherapy to magnetotherapy, and the final transition from magnetotherapy to hypnotism, is both interesting and natural. It seems remarkable that it did not occur to any of the French investigators even to test the truth of their observations by control experiments. How easily it was done by Bennett with his wooden buttons and by Westphal with his mustard plasters! The history of metallotherapy is only another instance of the fact that physicians do not differ from the common man in their love of the mysterious. Like the common man, they time and again become the victims of self-deception and autosuggestion. The spell of mysticism beshrouds thought; accurate thinking and even accurate seeing become impossible; and, as in hypnotism, operator and subject react unconsciously upon each other in an endless chain of suggestion and autosuggestion.

In connection with metallotherapy, it is interesting to speak of a special form of this mode of treatment devised by one Elisha Perkins, an American physician, who was born in Norwich, Connecticut, on January 16, 1741, and who practised in Plainfield. About 1796, he invented a method of treatment with metallic tractors, so called because they were supposed to draw disease away. These consisted of two needles, one resembling brass and the other resembling steel; they were made of a composition of metals. They were three inches long and were pointed at the ends. The needles were united, and in using them, the pointed ends were passed over the affected parts, until some reaction occurred. They were chiefly used in local inflammations, pains in the head, face, teeth, rheumatism, and like diseases. The points were applied to the affected part and then drawn over it in a downward direction for about twenty minutes. Perkins obtained considerable support for his method of treatment in the United States, and it was also quite favorably received abroad. In Copenhagen physicians endorsed his method, while in London, a Perkinsian Institute was established for the treatment of the poor. The list of persons asserted to have been cured by the tractors amounted at one time to an almost fabulous number.   A few years, however, after Perkins's death, the wonder-working needles disappeared and were heard of no more.   Haygarth, of Bath, obtained identical results with wooden cylinders made to imitate the tractors, and the practice could not survive the consequent ridicule. Doubtless, both in metallotherapy and in Perkins's tractors, as in Charcot's magnets, the dominant factor at work was suggestion. How powerfully suggestion acts in hysteria, even in the waking state, we have already seen.   In addition, the monotonous impression produced upon the skin by the application of a metallic surface or the steady strokings of the Perkins's tractors, suggests the monotonous impression of the hypnotic experiment.

MIND CURE, FAITH CURE, EDDYISM

Mind Cure and Faith Cure

We come now to consider briefly the methods of treatment which have as their essential and common characteristic the induction of a **negative hallucination** (see p. 304).   We have already seen how, in hypnosis the pain of a neuralgia can be suggested away; that is, excluded from the field of consciousness.   A negative hallucination having been established in the patient's mind, pain no longer exists.   Similarly, in mind cure and in faith cure, the essential feature of the treatment is the suggestion to the patient, or by the patient to himself, of the absence of the various symptoms which he presents.   Combined with the negative hallucination of the absence of disease, or the non-existence of disease, there is also the positive belief of the patient in his wellbeing.   The suggestions are made or supposed to be made in the waking state.   In many of the reported cases, however, there is reason to believe that there was established some degree of hypnosis.   Indeed, the very monotony of the repetition of the suggestion, the fixation of the mind of the subject upon one idea, and the constant repetition of the idea to him, or by himself in some set phrase, embrace the common factors of the induction of hypnosis.   That powerful results, however, can be induced by suggestion in the waking state, we have already seen.   Bernheim repeatedly declared that hypnosis is not at all necessary to achieve startling effects by suggestion.

Numerous cases of striking results achieved by mind and faith cure and suggestions in the waking state, are upon record. Thus, Eastman has reported recovery from deafness, from aphonia, from traumatic paralysis, and from insomnia, through mind cure. A. H. Burr has reported a case of paralysis following injury, disappearing under faith cure; while Hudson, Desplat, Gorodichze, Anaeleto, Jacobs, Stadelman, Goudard, Cocke, Gallet, van Renterghem, and others have reported striking instances of cure as the result of suggestion in the waking state. The cases cited are similar to those which have been reported as cured by hypnotism; and, after the full discussion given to the latter subject, need no further elucidation. The cases placed on record by Hudson, however, of surgical operations performed painlessly in the waking state, are exceedingly interesting and instructive; though their authenticity is open to attack. The first is that of a boy in whom a hypnotist endeavored to induce anesthesia, previous to the amputation of a crushed leg. The hypnotist failed to induce sleep, but, notwithstanding, strongly suggested anesthesia. Amputation was performed without an anesthetic and the boy declared that he did not feel any pain. The second case is that of a country fiddler, in whom also a leg had to be amputated. He refused to take an anesthetic and insisted upon having his fiddle brought to him, saying that he had always fiddled his pains away and that he could do it now. He played while the operation was performed and declared that he felt no pain. In the third case, a patient who suffered from a disease of the knee-cap for which amputation was advised likewise refused an anesthetic. He declared that he wished to be an eye-witness of the operation, which was performed, and, it was said, instead of being painful, was actually pleasurable to him. Hudson also cites the case of an hysteric patient of the elder Hammond, whom Hammond could make insensible to pain by merely telling her positively that all feeling was abolished. He once opened a bone felon for her, carrying the knife to the periosteum, without the slightest sensation being experienced by the patient. In the fifth case, it was suggested to a woman by her husband, a physician, that she would not feel the slightest pain while a dentist operated upon a diseased tooth. She subsequently declared that she did not even know that the tooth had been operated upon. Cases such as those just cited are certainly remarkable—*if true*—as instances of successful surgery under waking suggestion, and they surely equal any thus far reported as having been performed under hypnosis.

Eddyism (Christian Science)

Eddyism, or so-called "Christian Science," is a complex system of mystic healing founded some fifty years ago by Mary Baker G. Eddy. She wrote a book, entitled "Science and Health, with a Key to the Scriptures." She speaks of her system as a discovery and as a divine revelation. She claimed as a child to have heard supernatural voices calling her by name. She opened a college for her teachings in Lynn, Mass., where she trained many thousands of pupils. She was regarded as the head of the sect or church which she organized and she had to be implicitly obeyed by her disciples.

The following citation can be considered as a statement—as nearly coherent as anything emanating from the same source—of the essentials of the Eddyist belief: "First, as adherents of truth, we take the Scriptures as our guide to eternal life. Second, we acknowledge the way of salvation demonstrated by Jesus to be the power of truth over all errors, sin, sickness, and death, and the resurrection of human life and understanding to seize the great possibilities and living energies of divine life."

In explaining her views upon disease and cure, Mrs. Eddy said first, that human beings in their higher qualities are not separate persons from God, but of one substance with Him; hence they are immortal. Second, there is an immortal mind which must be separated from a mortal mind, which last does all the mischief in the world. This last mind believes in disease and death. Third, matter has absolutely no existence in any form. All is mind or nothing. Human bodies do not exist, because God is ignorant of matter, disease, or death. Mrs. Eddy unfortunately contradicts herself not infrequently. Thus, she constantly assures her patients that there is nothing wrong with them, that they have no disease; and yet in reporting her cures to the world she speaks of having healed cancer, consumption, and other diseases. Further, she says that as the body and organs do not exist, it is of no use to examine them, and there is no disease; yet, notwithstanding, Eddyist practitioners affirm that they cure local diseases. Disease being a false belief in the mortal mind, Eddyists allow no medicine to be given to patients.

Patients are treated by one of two ways. First, by persuading the sufferer that he is well; second, by "silent influence," that is, the healer brings her mind to bear upon the patient; this influence may be exerted by her at any distance. If a death results in spite of the Eddyist treatment, the believers answer that the death is not a real death, but a delusion of the mortal mind. As to surgery, Eddyists have set dislocated bones without touching them. However, they advise calling in a surgeon!

It is interesting to note that Mrs. Eddy was from childhood on, fond of such subjects as metaphysics, moral science, philosophy, and logic, and that she was always very positive in her opinions.* She was at one time a practitioner of homeopathy, she was an ardent advocate of woman's rights, had remarkable energy and zeal, had the most implicit faith in herself and her mission, and communicated this faith to her disciples. Her followers are drawn largely from the well-to-do, those that can contribute moderate amounts to the wealth of the church. The ignorant and the uneducated classes furnish but a small proportion of the Christian Scientists; no special propaganda has been carried into the ranks of the poor. It is reported that Mrs. Eddy was herself quite poor before she "discovered" Christian Science, but that her material prosperity became very great. She had magnificent homes both in Boston and Concord, and is said to have given over $80,000 annually to charities!

The account of her discovery of Christian Science reads as follows: "In 1866 she was returning with her husband at Lynn,

*In this and following paragraphs, Dr. Harry T. Marshall's excellent paper, "A Study of Christian Science," "Johns Hopkins Hospital Bulletin," No. 111, June, 1900, p. 128, has been used freely.

Mass., from an errand of mercy, when she fell upon the ice and was carried helpless to her home. The skilled physicians declared that there was absolutely no hope for her, and pronounced the verdict that she had but three days to live. Finding no hope and no help on earth, she lifted her heart to God. On the third day, calling for her Bible, she asked the family to leave the room. Her Bible opened to the healing of the palsied man (Matt. ix, 2). The Truth which set him free, she saw; the Power which gave him strength she felt; the Life Divine which healed the sick of the palsy, restored her, and she rose from the bed of pain, healed and free. She walked into the midst of the family, they cried out in alarm, thinking that she had died and that they beheld her ghost! This miraculous restoration dates the birth of Christian Science." How she is regarded by her devotees, the following citation will show. Says the "Christian Science Journal:" "Surely the people of the coming centuries will vie with each other in doing homage to the Rev. Mary Baker G. Eddy, the greatest character since the advent of Jesus Christ, and her book, "Science and Health, with a Key to the Scriptures," will go down in history part of the sacred writings of the ages."

The method in detail which the Eddyist healer pursues is somewhat as follows: he or she sits beside the afflicted one and confidently, positively and repeatedly declares that the disease is non-existent. In addition, the healer, or both the patient and the healer, read from Mrs. Eddy's book. The following selections from the book illustrate the method of practice and the believer's point of view:

"Always begin your treatment by allaying the fear of the patient. Silently reassure the patient as to his exemption from disease and danger. Watch the result of this simple rule of Christian Science, and you will find that it alleviates the symptoms of every disease. If you succeed in wholly removing the fear, your patient is healed. The great fact that God wisely governs all, never punishing aught but sin, is your standpoint whence to advance and destroy the human fear of sickness. Plead the case in Science and for Truth, mentally and silently. You may vary the arguments to meet the peculiar or general symptoms of the case you treat;

but be thoroughly persuaded in your own mind, and you will finally be the winner.

"You may call the disease by name when you mentally deny it; but by naming it audibly, you are liable to impress it upon the thought. . . . To prevent disease or to cure it mentally, let Spirit destroy this dream of sense. . . . Argue with the patient (mentally, not audibly) that he has no disease, and conform the argument to the evidence. Mentally insist that health is the everlasting fact, and sickness the temporal falsity. . . . If the case is that of a young child or an infant, it needs to be met mainly through the parent's thought, silently or audibly, on the basis of Christian Science.

"If the case to be treated is consumption, take up the leading points included (according to belief) in this disease. Show that it is not inherited; that inflammation, tubercles, hemorrhage, and decomposition are beliefs, images of mortal thoughts, superimposed upon the body; that they are not the Truth of man; that they should be treated as error, and put out of thought. Then these ills will disappear. If the lungs are disappearing, this is but one of the beliefs of mortal mind. Mortal man will be less mortal, when he learns that lungs never sustained existence, and can never destroy God, Who is our life. When this is understood, mankind will be more Godlike. What if the lungs are ulcerated? God is more to a man than his lungs; and the less we acknowledge matter or its laws, the more immortality we possess.

"You say a boil is painful, but that is impossible, for matter without mind is not painful. The boil simply manifests your belief in pain, through inflammation and swelling; and you call this belief a boil.

"When the sick recover by the use of drugs, it is the law of a general belief, culminating in individual faith, which heals; and according to this faith will the effect be.

"Mortal mind confers the only power a drug can ever possess.

"A physical diagnosis of disease—since mortal mind must be its cause, if it exists—generally has a tendency to induce disease.

"The daily ablutions of an infant are no more natural or necessary than would be the process of taking a fish out of water every

day and covering it with dirt, in order to make it thrive more
vigorously thereafter in its native element.

"When there are fewer doctors and less thought is given to
sanitary subjects, there will be better constitutions and less
disease."

The discussion of so-called Christian Science as a religion is best
left to theologians. As a therapeutic method it concerns not only
medical practitioners, but every rational human being. Undeniably the treatment is one of **suggestion**, and, speaking more
specifically, of suggestion by the induction of the **negative hallucination.** The rise and spread of the cult, while remarkable, is,
however, far from being a phenomenon unparalleled in history.
Leaders of such movements not infrequently present striking instances of the force and power of persons who, developing mystic
ideas in early life, conceive, and finally firmly believe, that they
are endowed with a special mission for the reformation of the world,
and have thus been stimulated to exert themselves with remarkable
persistence and energy. They are often undeniably great in the
scope of their delusions and the force and persistence with which
they promulgate them—and what shall we say of their followers?
The latter are merely examples of the spread of a delusion, a true
folie communiqué. The leaders present instances of the mystic
form of paranoia. They are characterized by the existence of
hallucinations in their early years, by the gradual evolution and
systematization of delusions, and by the great mission which they
regard as the object of their lives. In due course they undergo
a veritable "transformation of the personality." It is this transformation which usually marks the beginning of the "mission."

Eddyism is more than a passing fad; it is a great and actual
danger. The denial of all disease, the neglect of all medical treatment, the defiance of all sanitary regulations, make the so-called
Christian Scientist dangerous not only to himself and his family,
but also to his neighbors. His tenets bring him into crass conflict
with the authorities and lead him to contemptuous defiance of the
law. Moreover, what can we think of the sanity of the creature

who allows his child to perish of diphtheria when the life-saving antitoxin is at hand, or who will suffer his child to become hopelessly blind rather than have its ophthalmia treated by a physician? Such insanity should be dealt with as crime; this is, indeed, the only remedy.

Other mystic methods could here be considered were such consideration of practical value. The literature of occult medicine, exclusive of works upon hypnotism, is quite considerable. All the methods, however, no matter under what name they are couched, "vital force," "psychic force," "mental medicine," "natural suggestion," "science of life," "power of mind," "power of will," "force of mind," "new thought," worcesterism, and what not, are based upon the induction of the **negative hallucination**. This we have already sufficiently discussed. With the especial negative hallucination as to the disease, there is associated the induction of the general positive hallucination of well-being. The subjective accompaniments of morbid processes alone are recognized by mystic medicine. The organic basis to which the pain or other unpleasant symptom owes its existence is ignored. It is, so to speak, hallucinated away. The advocates of mystic healing fail to realize the hopelessness of their situation. The seat of the higher psychic activities, the cortex, can only be cognizant of changes taking place within itself. Normally, these changes are correlated with the changes which take place in the body or in the environment. To interpret *artificially* induced changes—hallucinations and delusions—as correctly representing transformations in the organism or in the external world, is an absurdity which falls to the ground of its own weight.

Mystic medicine is as old as the race. Some forms have gone, others have come, still others will appear in the future; but no matter how the dress is changed, the method is always the same. The incantations of the "medicine man" differ in no essential from the incantations of the eddyist or the doweyite. Each deals with disease as the result of sin and crime, as evidence of the anger or the ill-will of the demons or of the gods, who must be appeased by prayer, charms, and magic rites; or who must be opposed by some occult knowledge or mystic power possessed by the healer. Civilization merely adds a complex outward raiment, but this raiment conceals the same old puerile superstition and magic that characterized the medical practice of our savage ancestors.

GENERAL INDEX

A

Abderhalden on blood ferments, 183

Abdomen, distention of, 112, 130

Abdominal reflex, 105

Abortion prevented by hypnosis, 312

Aboulia, 82, 235

Abreaction, 335, 337, 352

Accident compensation, 95, 99, 101, 112, 135

Accidents, trivial, ado about, 139

Accused person, sanity of, 332

Aches, occupation, 14

Achilles-jerk, 105

Acidosis, 249

Acne, bromid, 67

Activity and rest, alternations of, 5
  minimum of, 26

Adalin, use of, 66, 195

Adiposity, 69, 79, 253

Agoraphobia, 19, 143, 234

Aigre, Douglas, 358

Alcohol a cause of insanity, 176
  of neuritis, 165
  as a poison, 243
  as a sedative, 194
  drugs antagonistic to, 254
  in beef preparations, 52
  in delirium, 205
  in neurasthenia, 35
  withdrawal of, 248, 251, 254

Alcoholism, 243
  chronic, 244, 250, 253
    neuropathic factors in, 250, 256
    nursing in, 252, 256
    stimulation in, 254
    symptoms of, 250
  due to coca preparations, 267
  hypertonic intravenous injection in, 257
  physical signs of, 244

Alcoholism, relapses in, 256
  renal disease in, 248
  sleep in, 249
  treatment of, by hypnotism, 256
    by isolation, 252
    by medicines, 248, 254

Alloxuric bodies, 31, 33

Alteratives in insanity, 196
  in neuritis, 164

Ammonium acetate in alcoholism, 248

Amnesia with somnambulism, 336

Amputations, painless, 361
  under hypnosis, 311

Amusement as aid to suggestion, 282
  for paranoiacs, 233

Anal eroticism, 348

Analgesics for headache, 63
  in neuritis, 165, 166

Ancestors, nervous, 144

Anesthesia, geometric, 97
  hypnotic, 298, 300, 333
  hysterical, 90, 92, 301
  in a limb, 90
  islet-like, 96
  metallic, of Charcot, 357
  metallotherapy in, 355
  of genitals, 312, 326
  on examination, 93
  organic, as seat of injury, 92
  segmental, 96, 301
  surgical, hypnotic, 311

"Anesthesia, universal," 97

Animal magnetism, 287, 290, 354

Animals, catalepsy in, 299

Ankle clonus in hysteria, 105
  in neurasthenia, 11

Anorexia in neurasthenia, 59
  nervosa, 110, 127

Anthrophobia, 19

Antibodies, formation of, 183, 184, 190, 191, 193, 194, 261

Printed in the United States
by Baker & Taylor Publisher Services